Family Issues in Pediatric Psychology

Family Issues in Pediatric Psychology

Edited by

Michael C. Roberts
The University of Kansas

Jan L. Wallander
University of Alabama at Birmingham

Routledge
Taylor & Francis Group
LONDON AND NEW YORK

First published 1992 by Lawrence Erlbaum Associates, Inc., Publishers

2 Park Square, Milton Park, Abingdon, Oxon OX14 4RN
711 Third Avenue, New York, NY 10017, USA

Routledge is an imprint of the Taylor & Francis Group, an informa business

First issued in hardback 2017

Transferred to Digital Printing 2009 by Routledge

Chapters 2, 3, 4, 5, 8, 10, 12, 13, 15 from *Journal of Pediatric Psychology, 14*(2). Chapters 6, 7, 9, 14 from *Journal of Pediatric Psychology, 14*(3). All chapters reprinted with permission of the publisher.

ISBN 978-0-8058-0854-4 (pbk)
ISBN 978-1-138-45184-1 (hbk)

Library of Congress Cataloging-in-Publication Data

Family issues in pediatric psychology / edited by Michael C. Roberts and Jan L. Wallander.
p. cm.
Articles reprinted from the Journal of pediatric psychology.
Includes bibliographical references and index.
ISBN 0-8058-0854-X
1. Sick children—Psychology. 2. Sick children—Family relationships. 3. Teenagers—Diseases—Psychological aspects. I. Roberts, Michael C. II. Wallander, Jan Lance. III. Journal of pediatric psychology.
[DNLM: 1. Adolescent Psychology. 2. Child Psychology. 3. Family--psychology. 4. Family Therapy. WS 105.5.F2 F1985]
RJ47.5.F36 1992
155.4—dc20
DNLM/DLC
for Library of Congress 91-34578
CIP

Publisher's Note
The publisher has gone to great lengths to ensure the quality of this reprint but points out that some imperfections in the original may be apparent.

Contents

Preface

In 1989, pediatric psychology as an organized field recognized its 21st birthday and "coming of age" through the Society of Pediatric Psychology (Section V of the Division of Clinical Psychology, American Psychological Association). In its relatively brief period of existence, the field has evolved and expanded as a science and in clinical practice. One notable aspect of pediatric psychology's development has been the recognition of broader elements encompassing the field over time and correspondingly, inclusion of these elements in scientific study and practical interventions. Such elements have included, for example, integration of illness and health issues, consideration of both physical and mental health development, focus on prevention as well as remediation, and new attention to family roles in health and illness. This latter aspect became the theme of a special issue of the *Journal of Pediatric Psychology* to reflect the increased attention to family issues and to catalyst the field to even more work. The 14 special theme articles from two journal issues are published herein with an overview chapter as a single source for access to work at the "cutting edge" of pediatric psychology. They are relevant to a variety of fields and interests because family issues and pediatric medicine from psychosocial viewpoints inherently interact with numerous disciplines and approaches.

We want to recognize the authors who contributed their work for publication in the journal and here as well as the numerous editorial board members and ad hoc consultants who provided extensive reviews in selecting these articles. We also appreciate the enormous contributions of Lawrence Erlbaum Associations in publishing this volume and acknowledge the cooperation of Plenum Publishing Corporation, the journal's publisher.

The publication of this book is sponsored by the Society of Pediatric Psychology through its publication of the *Journal of Pediatric Psychology*. As with other of the society publications, such sponsorship recognizes the scholarly significance of the material presented in the volume and the care taken in development of the chapters on scientific and professional issues. The articles were peer reviewed and published in the *Journal of Pediatric Psychology*. The volume has not been considered by the American Psychological Association Council of Representatives, however, and therefore, does not represent official policy of the organization as a whole.

Michael C. Roberts
Jan L. Wallander

1

Family Issues in Pediatric Psychology: An Overview

Michael C. Roberts
The University of Kansas

Jan L. Wallander
University of Alabama at Birmingham

The field of pediatric psychology is a continually developing one of research and practice. This dynamic quality provides excitement, challenge, and employment for professionals in the field. Since its formal roots in Wright's classic (1967) overview and before, pediatric psychology has been characterized by attention to a wide variety of interacting components and processes. These elements have been delineated in the most recent expansion of the editorial statement for coverage of the *Journal of Pediatric Psychology* (JPP), the publication outlet of the Society of Pediatric Psychology:

> *Journal of Pediatric Psychology* publishes articles relating to theory, research, and professional practice in pediatric psychology. Pediatric psychology is an interdisciplinary field addressing the full range of physical and mental development, health, and illness issues affecting children, adolescents, and families. The journal publishes papers on a wide variety of topics exploring the relationship between psychological and physical well-being of children and adolescents including: understanding, assessment, and intervention with developmental disorders; evaluation and treatment of behavioral and emotional problems and concomitants of disease and illness; the role of psychology in pediatric medicine; the promotion of health and development; and the prevention of illness and injury among children and youth. Articles are welcome from authors in psychology and related disciplines serving children and families. (Roberts, La Greca, & Harper, 1988, p. 2)

This statement reflects an orientation, evident since the field's inception, to a diversity of problems and approaches to study and with which to intervene.

Over the years, attention in children's health care has seemingly shifted from an exclusive parental focus to almost an exclusive child focus. More recently, a new shift in focus recognizes the greater complexity of psychosocial phenomena involving children in the context of their families and support systems, with actors and procedures in the health-care system. This "ecological model" is daily demonstrated in clinical settings for pediatric psychology and has prompted a considerable amount of research.

A special topic issue of the *Journal of Pediatric Psychology* was developed on "Family Issues in Pediatric Psychology" to illustrate the advancement of research and practice with regard to family roles. The response to the call for papers was overwhelming. After a careful review process, 14 were selected for publication, 9 in the June 1989 issue (Volume 14, Number 2) and 5 more in the September 1989 issue (Volume 14, Number 3). These 14 articles are presented in this volume as a demonstration of what pediatric psychology is doing with the hope that they may provide catalysts for application and investigation of family roles. Other articles oriented to family issues will continue to appear in the journal subsequent to the special topical issue. As Roberts and Maieron (1989), noted in the issue's editorial, "the range of health conditions for family involvement *is* the range of pediatric psychology for research and practice. Thus, the articles generated for the special issue on families are but a sampling of this specialty's concern" (p. 155). This chapter provides an overview to the selected chapters by providing a context for family roles, aspects of intervention, policies with families in pediatric health care, and important theoretical and research paradigms.

DEFINITIONS OF FAMILY

Philippe Aries (1962) suggested that the concept of the family as a unit "bound by love rather than authority" only emerged about 1700. Although this is seemingly late as a developmental stage of civilization, the family as a social organization has continued to evolve (Olson & Habenstein, 1983). The concept of the family has, in recent years, become a politicized issue of what constitutes a family. A number of forces have produced a "rise of many alternative family styles and the decline of the traditional family structure of father as breadwinner, mother as full-time homemaker, and two-plus children" (Flomenhaft, 1982, p. 5).

These changes in society have become epitomized in antagonistic stances of conservative versus liberal politics regarding what has seemingly become a "bumper sticker" debate and politicians' claims on both sides of being "for the family." Further political debate has centered on how public policies should officially recognize family relationships. On one end of the continuum are those who argue for a narrow definition of only legally defined relationships of husband, wife, and biological or adopted children. At the other end are those who express a broader definition, based less on "blood" or legal ties, but more inclusive of supportive relationships.

Although pediatric psychology may utilize a formal family unit for study in clinical activity, professionals have had to recognize that the nuclear, intact family is not the norm. There are now more families where only one parent is present in the home; more mothers are working outside the home; more pregnancies for adolescents and pregnancies for older women; and more families are living below the poverty line (Johnson, 1990). These changes in the family within an evolving society have created changes in family relationships. Indeed, family relationships reflect the diversity of the humans making up the relationships. Thus, in pediatric psychology, the practitioner or researcher may look beyond parents and siblings to grandparents or aunts and uncles (or interested and involved "others" whether legally defined or based on functional roles) for assessment information and intervention.

A family may be seen as "two or more individuals who define themselves as family and who, over time assume those obligations to one another that are generally considered an essential component of family systems" (National Association of Social Workers, 1981, p. 43). Consistent with this, Turk and Kerns (1985b) presented that:

> . . . families are groups composed of members who have mutual obligations to provide a broad range of emotional and material support (Dean, Lin, & Ensel, 1981). ...No attempt is made to suggest that families necessarily consist of blood relatives nor is it assumed that families live together; rather the operative phrase is 'mutual obligations.' Furthermore, families within our perspective have (a) structure, (b) functions and assigned roles, (c) modes of interacting, (d) resources, (e) a life cycle, (f) a history, and (g) a set of individual members with unique histories. (pp. 2–3)

These definitions are pragmatic and realistic (a particularly notable characteristic of pediatric psychology; Roberts, 1986). Although each practitioner and researcher in the field does not necessarily assess a family's characteristics in each of these seven aspects, this broader definition makes clear that what constitutes a family defies prescriptive and proscriptive definitions. Thus in this orientation, families for pediatric psychology are a context–one that interacts with, fluctuates, and remains constant with other contexts such as the school and/or health-care setting. Given the definitional perplexities, each research project and each clinical intervention in pediatric psychology must necessarily define family for its uses (Baranowski & Nader, 1985). Family research or intervention does not mean all members of a family as a total unit are involved every time. Indeed, individuals or subunits (siblings, parents, all combinations, and interactions) may be considered within this rubric.

A major organization advocating for an increased role of families in pediatric health care, the Association for the Care of Children's Health (ACCH) stated that *family* "refers to each child's immediate and extended families, biological or not. The composition of one child's family may vary significantly from that of another; a child may have more than one family; and a child's family may change over time" (1988 working draft, Glossary p. 2). This articulation captures what most in the pediatric psychology field would endorse.

Shorr, as chairperson of the Select Panel for the Promotion of Child Health, described the importance of considering the family in health issues: "not only is the family the primary unit for the delivery of health services to infants and children, but the family environment is probably the greatest influence on a child's health" (in Harris, 1981, p. v). The Select Panel's report continued:

> a child is dependent upon his or her mother and the other family members not only for the physical necessities of life–food, shelter, clothing, and protection from harm–but also for the emotional support and intellectual stimulation needed for healthy growth and development...Our growing awareness of the psychological and social components of health has enhanced our awareness of the family's importance...the family is not only the principal influence upon a child's development, it is also the intermediary between the child and the outside world including the health care system. It is parents who decide when to seek health care for a child, where to seek it, and from whom. It is parents who provide the lion's share of all care to a sick or injured child. Health providers can support, encourage, and enhance the competence of parents in their role as caregivers, or they can directly or indirectly undermine and denigrate it. (Harris, 1981, pp. 52–53)

Earlier in the history of health care, the child was seen as a single unit with parents banished from medical wards (Johnson, 1990; Shore & Goldston, 1978). Later, parents, typically the mother, became included in this unit of involvement. And, still later, fathers and siblings were added (and much later, others such as grandparents) as it became better understood that interactions within the health-care system (such as with chronic or terminal illnesses) affect all in a family in reciprocal fashion (e.g., see Akamatsu, Stephens, Hobfoll, & Crowther, in press; Flomenhaft, 1982; Peterson, Mori, & Carter, 1985). This progression was paralleled in the development of pediatric psychology in which children's problems were viewed in a primary focus and when other family members (usually parents) were utilized as vehicles for professionals' prescribed interventions. Thus, for example, early discussions of pediatric psychology practice emphasized advising parents in child rearing (Salk, 1969; Wright, 1967).

Pediatric psychology in research and practice recognizes the family, in whatever constellation of actors, as an important context. The chapters in this volume delineate the family processes, resources, and support influencing psychological adjustment of the child and family, on family processes involved in development of physical disorders, on interventions on families and their constituent individuals such as siblings, and theoretical perspective for conceptualizing family roles.

INTERVENTIONS AND POLICIES WITH FAMILIES

One particular area of concern over the history of children's health care has been the hospital policy requiring separation of an ill child from his or her parents for hospitalization. For example, Johnson (1990) recently stated that 40–50 years ago, "families were expected to leave their child at the hospital and to pick them up either at discharge or death, with infrequent visiting between times" (p. 232). She cited that in a 1954 survey of hospitals serving children in New York City only 32% permitted daily visiting by parents. Research has clearly documented that separation of child and parents through hospitalization poses psychological and medical risks for the child (and for the parents, although this is less documented). Additional research supported positive effects of parents' presence and rooming in (Craig & McKay, 1958; Fagin, 1964; Shore & Goldston, 1978). Despite this research, there were instituted (and some remain) medical and hospital policies limiting parent–child contact. Other perspectives viewed a child's illness as a medical condition to be medically treated and not involving psychosocial aspects. This perspective certainly does not consider how the family might be affected or how the family might influence the illness (Flomenhaft, 1982).

To a large degree, these restrictive attitudes have been changed, but not totally eliminated because vestiges show up in various practices, policies, and attitudes of medical professionals. A survey for ACCH was conducted by Roberts, Maieron, and Collier (1988) of 286 hospitals serving children in the United States and Canada. This comprehensive survey found greater attention to families and psychosocial issues, although not in all aspects. For example, 98% of the hospitals now have unrestricted visiting hours for parents and 94% allow parent rooming in. About half the hospitals provide sleeping accommodations (whereas in 1966, less than 1% of general hospitals provided these facilities; Shore & Goldston, 1978). In 1988, only 46% of the hospitals allowed sibling visiting of a sick child and most hospitals still restrict parental presence during health-care experiences. Still, over 90% attempt to familiarize children and families with the hospital setting and procedures. Finally, 73% of the hospitals overall have written policies and/or philosophy delineating roles for families. Obviously, however, the degree to which actual personnel and procedures follow through is uneven (Roberts et al., 1988).

ACCH has provided several models of how families might be recognized through what is described as "Family Centered Care – A philosophy and approach that: 1) recognize and support the pivotal role of families in their child's health care; 2) promote the family's typical patterns of living; 3) support families in their natural roles by building upon their natural strengths; and 4) promote partnership between parents and professionals in planning and coordinating the child's health care" (1988 working draft, Glossary p. 2). These concepts were detailed in a monograph on *Family Centered Care for Children with Special Health Care Needs* (Shelton, Jeppson, & Johnson, 1987). The articulation of these elements was made specifically for children with special health needs. In 1990, a more general statement of the elements of family-centered care was articulated that recognized diversity of race, cultural and ethnic background, and economic conditions (Johnson, 1990):

- Recognizing that the family is the constant in a child's life, while the service systems and personnel within those systems fluctuate.
- Facilitating parent/professional collaboration at all levels of health care.
- Honoring the racial, ethnic, cultural, and socioeconomic diversity of families.
- Recognizing family strengths and individuality and respecting different methods of coping.
- Sharing with parents, on a continuing basis and in a supportive manner, complete and unbiased information.
- Encouraging and facilitating family-to-family support and networking.
- Understanding and incorporating the developmental needs of infants, children, and adolescents and their families into health-care systems.
- Implementing comprehensive policies and programs that provide emotional and financial support to meet the needs of families.
- Designing accessible health care systems that are flexible, culturally competent, and responsive to family-identified needs. (p. 237)

ACCH has extended these specific elements more generally in a manual of guidelines and strategies for hospitals and health-care professionals to use in implementing sound policies and practices. Developed by ACCH in conjunction with several organizations, including the Society of Pediatric Psychology, this document outlines psychosocially sound, developmentally appropriate, family-centered care of children in hospitals and health-care settings. The guidelines will cover how this care might be implemented through administrative issues, personnel, selection and training, facility design, patient care, and other aspects. All of these hospital and health-care policies and practices are important psychologically to the extent to which they implement a family orientation. Johnson (1990) articulated the goal "to ensure that every health care encounter in a hospital builds the competence and confidence of families and offers them a full range of choices for participating in their children's care" (p. 239). Family-centered care was found to be projected as one of the "top 10" issues for the future in psychosocial realms (Tucker & Roberts, 1990). This Delphic survey of experts suggested that the issues of concern are "empowering the family system (a) to secure services from the system and (b) to meet its own psychosocial needs" (p. 205).

The central role of families in children's health care is epitomized by the Surgeon General's report, *Healthy People,* which indicated that:

> The role as exemplar and guide is particularly critical for the parent who is shaping the health practices of another generation. Parents can enhance the opportunities for their children's health by fostering healthy personal habits, by ensuring availability and use of appropriate childhood health services, by participating in sound and enjoyable recreational activities, and by encouraging the development of effective health curricula in the school systems. (Califano, 1979, pp. 142–143)

Many professional organizations are also increasing professional's recognition of families. Certainly groups of family systems therapists have long advocated that families should be at the center of study and therapeutic interventions. Psychology, as an academic discipline and health-care profession, has become part of the movement for understanding and fostering families, especially with regard to physical and mental health. For example, the Division of Child, Youth, and Family Services (APA Division 37) and its quarterly publication provide a forum for

> the application of psychological knowledge to advocacy, service delivery, and public policies affecting children, youth, and families. The Division advances research, education, training, and practices through a multidisciplinary perspective. (APA, 1990, p. 12)

A newer division on Family Psychology (APA Division 43) was formed with an orientation to integrating:

> The understanding of individuals, couples, families, and other wider context. [This Division] ...seeks to promote human welfare through development, dissemination, and application of knowledge about the dynamics, structure, and functioning of families. (APA, 1990, p. 14)

Kaslow (1991) delineated the expansion of family psychology beyond family therapy while retaining the family as the basic unit of interest while helping the individual within the family. Other divisions of American psychology consider families less centrally, but as one context for human behavior such as the Division of Community Psychology. Although the Division of Health Psychology has somewhat neglected children and families relative to other foci, the voices and writings of pediatric and child health psychologists were present in the Report of the Work Group on Child Health Psychology at the 1988 Conference on Health and Behavior (Drotar et al., 1989). This report listed as one of four issues of priority for child health research the topic of "Family Influences on Child and Adolescent Health." This ad hoc group recommended attention be given to "(a) family mediators of health behavior and outcome, (b) impact of changes in family structure on health, (c) impact of child illness and handicap on the family, and (d) impact of family maltreatment" (Drotar et al., 1989, p. 783).

Of course, the Society of Pediatric Psychology, as a section (V) of the Division of Clinical Psychology of APA, provides considerable impetus regarding families in the field. As noted in the introduction, the masthead of the *Journal of Pediatric Psychology* describes the field as "addressing the full range of physical and mental developments, health, and illness issues affecting children, adolescents, and families (Roberts et al., 1988, p. 2).

We should note that the focus in most of pediatric psychology on families is less viewing the family as an interactional unit, but more as subsets of the unit as they might affect or be affected by a child. This child-centered view of families is appropriate given the *pediatric* aspects of the field's coverage. The child-centered focus is evident in the articles presented here, given the pediatric orientation of the journal, the sponsoring society, the authors, and readership. This orientation is worthy in itself.

There are a number of books, symposia, and articles now rising on family-related issues, often with a broader view of a "family health psychology" (e.g., Akamatsu et al., in press; Turk & Kerns, 1985a). Despite this, Kerns and Turk (1985) noted that the family has been historically neglected in behavioral medicine research. They analyzed articles published in the *Journal of Behavioral Medicine* and *Health Psychology* to determine low proportions of articles on family topics. Fanurik and Roberts (1986) similarly reported that the *Journal of Pediatric Psychology* over the same time had published a low proportion of articles relevant to the family. As a result, the special issue of the *Journal of Pediatric Psychology* on family issues in pediatric psychology was developed for enhancing the visibility of research on family variables. We should note that the impact of the journal issue has been a continuing level of submission as researchers have recognized the importance of family variables in pediatric psychology work as well as the receptive publication outlet of JPP. Routh (1991) viewed "the family as a frontier in child health psychology." Although he suggests the "research base is thin" (p. 326), the zeitgeist, as reflected by the research published herein, is to provide empirical support for family considerations.

Before, turning to the specific chapters presented in this volume, we want to outline some of the theoretical and research issues involved in family work in the field and discuss how these are addressed by these articles.

THEORETICAL PARADIGMS

A rich tradition exists in the field of family studies for elaborate, often complex, theories being proposed to explain phenomena of interest. In fact, one can argue that this is an area of inquiry where there may have been too much emphasis placed on theory compared to empirical investigation. For example, Routh (1991) found that in the 800-page *Handbook of Family Therapy,* only 5% of the cited journal articles were empirical research. However, in general, the theoretical work available on families does not seem to have influenced directly much of the pediatric psychology research. Part of the reason for this may be that the conceptual efforts pertaining to families are typically presented in sources outside the realm of pediatric psychology. There is a separate literature basically on family studies and some in family medicine, which may escape the attention of many pediatric psychology researchers (e.g., Doherty & Baird, 1983; Doherty & Campbell, 1988; Ramsey, 1989). This is unfortunate, we feel, because for the consideration of family issues in pediatric psychology to advance, the developments in family studies more generally must be recognized and, if possible, integrated. There is, in other words, too wide a gap between the study of family issues in pediatric psychology and family studies in general, especially when it comes to the use of theory.

Use of Theory

The value of theory for any area of inquiry is manyfold. We think that particularly salient advantages of conducting research, from a theoretical base is that it provides an explicit context for laying out ahead of time the research direction one desires to pursue, the specific questions to be addressed, and the assumptions that will influence one's decisions at a number of choice points in the conduct of one's research. Thus, one's choices regarding, for example, sampling, measurement, and analytical strategies should be easier to make, have a rationale, and be understandable to others. A theoretical base will similarly facilitate drawing appropriate and internally valid interpretations of the results, which also should be better understood by others.

Pediatric psychology is still very much in a descriptive and exploratory phase (Peterson & Harbeck, 1988; Roberts, 1986). The absence of overriding theory is apparent in this selection of research on family issues in pediatric psychology, issues for which there are theories available to help us understand observed phenomena. There are a few examples in this volume, however, of more or less theory-driven research. For example, Walker, Ortiz-Valdes, and Newbrough (chapter 11, this volume) test an explicit theoretical model of maternal effects on the adjustment in children with several different disorders. Kazak and Meadows (chapter 2, this volume) present a general theoretical context for their work on family, parental, and child adaptation when the child has cancer. Similarly, Murch and Cohen (chapter 3, this volume) base their hypotheses regarding the moderating role of family environment in the stress-adjustment relationship in children with spina bifida on the general stress theories available. Finally, Wallander and colleagues in two separate contributions (chapters 8 and 9, this volume) state two general conceptual models that both delineate hypothesized causal variables and operative paths of influence, one for understanding adaptation in children who have a chronic physical disorder and the other the adaptation of their mothers.

Family Systems versus Individualistic Family Perspectives

Although one may not always see it as a theoretical statement, all research in this volume is based, at least implicitly, on a particular view of family. Most researchers investigating family issues will agree with the general definition of *family* noted earlier: Family is a group composed of members who have mutual obligations to provide a broad range of emotional and material support (Dean, Lin, & Ensel, 1981; Turk & Kerns, 1985b). Moreover, most researchers will acknowledge that the family is a *system,* a unit with its own characteristics that cannot be totally understood by studying solely its individual members.

The notion of family system is almost legion (if not religion) among family researchers. Yet, very little research into family issues in pediatric psychology is conducted explicitly from the family systems perspective. Indeed, we cannot classify any of the studies reported in this volume as family systems research. Rather, most investigators who study family in pediatric psychology focus on individual family members or a dyad within the family (e.g., mother–child). This is the case in this volume.

A family systems research strategy can be worthwhile. However, if research does not reflect the family systems perspective, then alternative theoretical perspective can be utilized. A researcher may choose to investigate some set of family issues from another theoretical perspective. That is, as evident from the current collection of reports, it may be beneficial to study individual family members' behaviors, as well as individual family members' perspectives on the family. All but one of the studies reported in this volume indeed have adopted an individualistic perspective on family, obtaining the report from one family member on family variables of interest. The exception is the calculation of a family score on the Family Adaptability and Cohesion Evaluation Scale by Chaney and Peterson (chapter 7, this volume), thus obtaining a family perspective.

The advantages of using such an individualistic perspective include important information on individual behavior vis-á-vis family is gained. Moreover, in utilizing this approach, researchers need not deal with the complex and difficult to understand theoretical notions inherent in family systems theory, nor the corresponding complex methodological and analytical strategies necessitated in studying these notions. Nonetheless, the most prominant theoretical models are now reviewed.

The Family Systems Theory

Although there are many family systems theories, a commonality is the explicit recognition that members of the family are related to one another in a network of interactions. As Turk and Kerns (1985b) have pointed out, what is important is the relationship or interaction between family members. Emphasis therefore is placed on the modes of communication and the position of different family members in the family system, rather than on specific content of the communication. The individuals can then be understood as members of a larger social context–the family. Their behavior are thought to be formed through interaction with their family environment. Linear causation is largely disregarded in preference for invoking circular causes, in which many interacting variables are taken into consideration.

The dynamics of the whole family consequently are emphasized in family systems theory, whereas observation of the component parts and their attributes are given less attention. A major property of a system is the need to maintain a steady state. Changes in any family member thus would necessitate that other family members adapt to the change. This notion is paramount in Minuchin's (1974) work, whose specific family systems theory could thus far have been most influential in pediatric psychology, inasmuch as he investigated children with chronic physical disorders. He and his colleagues proposed, for example, that physical illness in a child might serve as a stabilizing function in the family.

As noted, none of the current investigators have made use of an explicitly stated family systems theory in conducting the research reported herein. However, several investigators incorporate family systems notions in discussing their results, after the fact rather than as a guiding framework. Family systems theory is rich in its possibilities. More work in pediatric psychology would benefit from this perspective.

Family Stress Theory

Family stress theory is another theoretical perspective that is represented to some extent in the current selection of pediatric psychology research. Indeed, many problems studied in pediatric psychology can be viewed in terms of stress (e.g., the child with a chronic illness or one undergoing an aversive medical procedure). Inasmuch as family aspects influence these situations and are influenced by them, several family stress theories have been developed. For example, McCubbin and Patterson (1983) have proposed the Family Adjustment and Adaptation Response (FAAR) model. Actually incorporating a family systems perspective, it proposes that the family attempts to maintain balanced functioning or homeostasis by meeting its *demands* (what it happening to them), and using its *capabilities* (what they have available for dealing with these demands). The *meanings* the family ascribes to the demands and their capabilities are critical factors in achieving balanced functioning.

The outcome is conceptualized in terms of *family adjustment* and *family adaptation*, which represent two phases in the FAAR model. The adjustment phase denotes a relatively stable phase. The patterns of family interaction are predictable and stable at that point. A *crisis*, or state of disequilibrium, emerges in the family system when demands exceed capabilities and this imbalance persists. During adaptation, the family attempts to restore homeostasis by increasing capabilities, reducing demands, or changing the meanings of the demands.

Proposed and utilized primarily in family sociology, none of the investigations in this volume employed this specific extension of the family systems perspective. However, many of the problems tackled by the current investigators might have been studied using the FAAR model. It has distinct advantages, such as being explicit, transactional, and developmental. Also, McCubbin and associates have developed a set of questionnaires for measuring the constructs in their model, which may be applicable to pediatric psychology research.

Stress and Coping Theory

Although developed independently, the disease/disability-stress-coping (DSC) model proposed by Wallander and Varni and colleagues shares some of the notions contained in the FAAR model (cf. Wallander & Varni, in press). As can be gleaned in two contributions by Wallander et al., the DSC is a stress-coping model, like the FAAR model, but it utilizes primarily an individualistic perspective. That is, it is proposed to explain chronically ill or handicapped children's adjustment or the adjustment of parents of such children. As such, it incorporates, among many purported causal variables, some family characteristics, such as family resources and family dynamics. There are several non-family variables included in this model as well.

As can be seen in the figures accompanying the two contributions of Wallander et al. in this volume, the model hypothesizes that disease or disability parameters, functional implications, and psychosocial stressors are risk factors for children's or parents' adaptation, and that personal style, socioecological, and stress-processing variables serve as resistance factors in the relationships between these risk factors and adaptation. The DSC model is complex, with one consequence being it is difficult to evaluate in its entirety. However, this model may be used as a heuristic as much as an explanatory model, and used to guide and organize different research efforts. As it is relatively new, researchers aside from Wallander and Varni have not yet tested this model. However, Singer and Irvin (1989) have proposed a stress model that incorporates in a simpler model some of the elements of the DSC model.

Role Theories

Role theories conceptualize individuals within the family context. In contrast to explicit system theories, each family member's behavior is considered along with the interactional workings of the family (e.g., Nye & Berardo, 1973; Quick & Jacob, 1973). Various health-related behaviors, such as the impact of illness on functioning in the family, are purported to be related to the role that members play in the family (e.g., breadwinner, scapegoat, caretaker). Various schemes for categorizing are available (e.g., Baric, 1970). The outcome expected in the family from an illness or an interaction with the medical system then is in large part dependent on the role the family member in question has within the family.

For example, if a young child acquires a chronic illness requiring hospitalization, the family caretaker, which typically is the mother, may then have to shift her attention solely to the ill child, leaving her larger role within the family unfilled. The functioning in that family may be understood in light of this. Notions such as the flexibility versus rigidity of assumed roles may also be invoked to better understand outcomes (Pratt, 1976). Also relevant to pediatric psychology issues may be the gender roles adopted by the parents. There has been discussion at various points in the literature about the degree to which raising a disabled or chronically ill child requires the adoption of more or less traditional gender roles by parents, and which arrangement may be more beneficial for the welfare of the family, the target child, and the individual parents.

Attachment Theory

Because close emotional attachment is thought to be imperative for good adjustment throughout life (e.g., Bowlby, 1980), attachment theory has been invoked to understand development in children with chronic physical conditions and developmental disabilities (Blacher, 1984). In particular it has been applied in study of high-risk infants. Mother–infant attachment is an adaptive process serving both the infant and the species. The infant receives physical protection and comfort, whereas the adult fulfills a need to love, protect, and interact. Presumably, the dyadic bonding that occurs early on serves as a role throughout life. Severing such an attachment would lead to crisis in adjustment, although bonding with other individuals is possible. There is a well-known standardized model available for studying early attachment, which employs the "Stranger Procedure" (Ainsworth & Wittig, 1969). Blacher (1984) has, from this starting point of attachment theory, proposed a more general ecological model of bi-directional levels of influence on a handicapped child, which may be generalizable to other conditions. This model hypothesizes child characteristics, emotional climate in the family, social network supports, and cultural influences as different levels of influence on these children's attachment and therefore socioemotional development.

Health Promotion and Problem Prevention Models

The discussion thus far has focused on family issues within pediatric psychology related to illness and handicapping conditions. An important aspect of the field has been a concern for the prevention of health-related problems and the promotion of healthy states and behavior (Roberts, 1986). Health psychology paradigms have not yet fully embraced family roles, although exceptions are beginning to appear, such as involving families in treatment and prevention of obesity (Epstein, McCurley, Wing, & Valoski, 1990), in preparation for surgery and hospitalization (Zastowney, Kirschenbaum, & Meng, 1986), and in prevention of injuries (Roberts, Fanurik, & Wilson, 1988). However, most prevention efforts have been primarily geared toward changing individuals' behavior and outcomes (Roberts, Fanurik, & Layfield, 1987).

A family orientation to prevention is reflected in Patterson et al. (chapter 13, this volume) in which aggregation of changes within families were assessed resulting from a cardiovascular health promotion program. Roberts and McElreath (in press) summarized these types of family-focused interventions and noted that an all-encompassing model for promotion and prevention has not yet been developed. They suggested that a transactional perspective of family health decision making and behavior might be useful, such as outlined by Fiese and Sameroff (chapter 15, this volume). Roberts and McElreath (in press) proposed that:

> families are *one* appropriate target and vehicle for prevention, but are not necessarily *the* only or necessarily the *most* appropriate. A clearer understanding of the role and functioning of family systems is needed in prevention for mental and physical health.

METHODOLOGICAL ISSUES

Research on family issues in pediatric psychology carries with it a number of methodological issues, most of which also apply to research in pediatric psychology more generally. Only a selection of these issues can be discussed here.

Correlational versus Experimental Designs

Either correlational or experimental designs may be preferable for family-oriented research, depending on the questions being addressed and the context in which the research is being conducted (natural setting or laboratory). Although an oversimplication, these two research approaches trade off investigator control and basis for making causative arguments for greater generalizability of the results and applicability of the research into real-life situations. Often by virtue of their employment settings, pediatric psychologists appear to utilize the latter more than the former. For example, all but one of the reports contained herein are based on nonexperimental research. It is strictly true that causation cannot be proven with a correlational design, but may be with an experimental design. However, there are considerable arguments for the use of correlational data as a basis for drawing causal *inferences*. Many actions related to health promotion and disease prevention have been taken based on such causal inferences (e.g., policies regarding tobacco smoking). Conducting correlational research from a theoretical basis and setting up designs where the most salient alternative explanations can be addressed enhance those prospects.

Because many problems germane to family issues in pediatric psychology cannot be studied practically using experimental manipulations, there are, fortunately, sophisticated correlational designs available. These would be applicable particularly to theory-driven, multivariate, large-sample size, prospective research where complex relationships can be analyzed, such as through the use of structural equations analysis. Although none of the research presented herein meets all of these aspects, some of the work in this volume does test relationships in one sample (e.g.,

Wallander, Varni, Babani, Banis, & Wilcox, chapter 8; Murch & Cohen, chapter 1). Other work in this volume examines differences in two different but existing groups, such as children with and without a physical disease (Kazak & Meadows, chapter 2; Dyson, chapter 10; Walker & Green, chapter 4). Comparing two naturally occurring groups is, of course, a correlational design, even when ANOVA-type statistics are being used. The investigator does not control individuals' assignment to groups in these cases, which is the crucial feature of an experiment.

Experimental research in pediatric psychology may be mostly found when comparing treatments or preparations. In this volume on family issues research, this approach is represented by Satin et al.'s (chapter 12) test of effects of family intervention on patients' health and adjustment as well as on the family's adjustment when a child has diabetes. Although it is perhaps understandable that correlational research may predominate in investigations of family issues in pediatric psychology, experimental research should not be excluded from the research armamentarium of pediatric psychology. Both correlational and experimental strategies are needed, because different questions can be addressed; such different questions do need to be addressed for the field to advance.

Selection of Variables

The issue of variable selection is related to the exploratory versus theory-driven research aspects discussed earlier under the rubric "Use of Theory." The researchers' conceptual base clearly influences selection of variables to use in research. In exploratory research, there may be included a host of seemingly important variables, whereas in more theory-driven work, the investigator carefully decides which variables to investigate based on some conceptual rationale. This rationale often might be in the form of previous research findings which the researcher can organize into some conceptual schema or even a formal theory. However, both exploratory and theory-driven research have a place in a developing field such as pediatric psychology. However, as the field moves from the intuitive to the empirical (Roberts, 1986) and eventually to the theoretical, the articles in the *Journal of Pediatric Psychology* will necessarily reflect this scientific trend–and to the benefit of the applications base. Because most of the research on family issues found in this volume do not seem to spring from an explicit conceptual base, they would be better characterized as exploratory. Some, however, do provide a more distinct theoretical tie-in.

Measurement

The actual measurement of the variables of interest is a crucial component of any research, inasmuch as this amounts to operationally defining those constructs or notions about which researchers have questions. A variety of issues enter into the consideration of measurement of variables. A significant one is which measurement method is being used. We commonly think about self-report, independent report, and physiological recording as the primary sources of data, although each can be further subdivided. Each contains advantages and disadvantages. No one measurement type is better in all cases. The choice should be guided first by the nature of the variable and the questions which are being asked about that variable, but it would be unrealistic not to also consider practical matters. Research in pediatric psychology is not typically conducted in a vacuum, but more often in clinical settings with real patients and their family members and health-care providers.

Reliance on self-report measures in much psychological research must be noted. For example, all but three of the investigations in this volume relied exclusively on self-report. Of course, some variables, such as perceptions of the environment or internal states, may best be measured through self-report. Supplementing these measures with others may be appropriate to provide more information. The most common self-report procedure is the traditional psychometric method, using a scale consisting of a number of questions. Originally advocated under the rubric of behavioral assessment, many variables typically measured through such questionnaires can also, or rather, be measured using self-monitoring. In this case the individual tracks behaviors (which can be covert or overt) concurrently or with a very short time lag (e.g., at the end of the day). Patterson et al.'s (chapter 13) measurement of physical activity in this volume exemplifies the use of self-monitoring.

Examples of independent reporting as an alternative strategy, include parents or teachers reporting on target child's behavior, health-care providers providing ratings of disease status of health behaviors, or specially trained "professional" observers or judges using formal schemes to translate target individual's behavior into quantitative data. The latter can often be seen, for example, in research on familial influences on child's anxiety and distress related to medical procedures (Jay, 1988).

Finally, physiological recording is exemplified in the research of Satin et al. (chapter 12, this volume), where a biochemical assay was used as one outcome measure for children with diabetes (glycosylated hemoglobin A1), and that Patterson et al. (chapter 13, this volume), where blood pressure and body mass were measured as outcomes in participants in a heart health promotion program. Certain areas of inquiry lend themselves better to this type of measurement, but status regarding most pediatric disorders can be indexed, at least in part, by a physiological measure. Often enough, these can be obtained in the normal course of events of a health-care provider contact (e.g., blood pressure, biochemical lab tests) that would not require extra cost or effort on the part of the investigator. Although physiological measures can be seductive in their apparent objectivity and clarity, most such measures have their own problems and subjective influences. They are not the panacea for measurement concerns. Nonetheless, the creative use of physiological measures can bolster our research.

In general, we would do well to obtain multiple measures of most of our variables because no one perspective is likely to hold "the truth." Most variables furthermore are multidimensional in nature. For example, adjustment in various pediatric populations is often of interest to researchers. Aside from the importance of measuring adjustment using multiple methods, adjustment can be reflected in different realms. At a gross level, a distinction may be made among social connectedness, overt behavior, and internal states. Internal states, in turn, may be constituted by traditional considerations for depressive and anxious states, but also perceptions of oneself now and what one's life in the future may hold, to only identify a couple of possibilities. Interpretation of multiple measures may be problematic (cf. Peterson, 1984). Although it would be desirable to consider multiple dimensions of various variables, researchers inevitably run into the problem of the time and effort this would take and other significant practical concerns. Here again, a strong conceptual basis may help make such decisions.

Comparison Groups

Control groups can be extremely helpful for addressing many questions and for comparing interventions or conditions for individuals clustered in groups. However, control groups may not be as necessary for answering other questions. For example, some research questions concern themselves with describing something or investigating relationships among variables *within* a certain target group. Examples of this latter type of research included in this volume are Murch and Cohen (chapter 3), Hatcher et al. (chapter 14), Mason et al. (chapter 6), and Wallander, Varni, Babani, DeHaan, Wilcox, and Banis (chapter 9).

Control groups were used in other investigations reported in this volume where status of the target group vis-á-vis some other group was of interest. Examples include Kazak and Meadows' (chapter 2) comparison of families with a child who was 10–15 years past a diagnosis of cancer to families who were their neighbors or friends, and Drotar and Eckerle's (chapter 5) comparison of the family environment of babies with non-organic failure to thrive and healthy babies. Different types of control groups may be employed for these purposes. Often the question is whether the target groups are different from the general population or some variant thereof (e.g., healthy patients at the same medical setting). Other times a distinction from some alternative patient group is important. Walker and Greene (chapter 4) compared adolescents with recurrent abdominal pain, separated into those with and without identifiable organic etiology, to healthy controls in terms of somatic, mental, and family status.

For some purposes, it makes sense to use a normative comparison group, rather than a control group specifically assembled for the current research. Many of the instruments in use today have moderately to very extensive normative data readily available. An example is the commonly used Child Behavior Checklist (Achenbach & Edelbrock, 1983), for which data are available on 1,300 children–a sample well stratified and representative of the U.S. population around 1980 in addition to 2,300 children referred to mental health clinics. Advantages of using normative comparison groups are their size, enhancing power and possibility of detecting differences, and often better representation of children in general than is feasible to obtain by an individual investigator. However, the comparability between the target group and the norm group on all important variables cannot be ensured. Therefore, the use of these normative comparison groups necessitates care.

Another use of control group is present in treatment-outcome research, where random assignment is typically made to active target treatment and either or all of other active comparison treatment, placebo treatment, or waiting-list control conditions. Satin et al. (chapter 12, this volume), investigated adjustment and health as a function of two active treatments, one being enhanced, and a waiting-list control in youngsters with diabetes and their families.

Sample Definition and Target Group

In the research presented here, the research samples are constituted by volunteers, as can be expected. Most of the research on family issues in pediatric psychology is of the type where potential subjects are asked to give of their time for the benefit of the research and possibly other individuals with the same condition at some elusive point in the future. Volunteer samples, furthermore, are typically drawn from specific settings, such as one medical clinic, which serves only a certain portion of all individuals with the target condition. However, there may be explicit medical or implicit demographic and economic selection criteria operating in defining that group. The role of such factors in pediatric psychology research is not evaluated often enough. Research would improve, furthermore, by using multiple recruitment strategies and/or research settings, such as through cross-institutional collaboration. Related to these issues is the inclusion of members of ethnic minority and low SES groups in pediatric psychology research. A concerted effort should be made at targeting some of the research specifically on these underserved, and understudied, segments of our society.

The research contained in this volume typically targets either a specific disorder or health goal (e.g., spine bifida, heart health promotion) or it includes several disorders. Some of the latter type of research adopts a noncategorical approach to studying psychosocial issues in pediatric conditions, either explicitly such as in Wallander, Varni, Babani, Banis, and Wilcox (chapter 8, this volume) or implicitly such as in Walker et al. (chapter 11, this volume). The noncategorical approach is based on the notion that different pediatric conditions hold many more similarities than differences, particularly when considering the psychosocial processes that are involved and outcomes in which we typically are interested. Adopting this approach does not negate that there are different biological processes present in different pediatric conditions, nor that different specific treatments are often employed for them. Indeed the role of these in, for example, psychosocial outcomes, can and ought to be addressed. Much previous research, however, show that, for many purposes, distinct disorders can be combined when studying psychosocial processes and outcomes, such as is the case in much of the research represented in this volume. Several advantages are thus gained. Larger sample sizes can be obtained, enhancing statistical treatment and inferences and the generalizability of the results. More widespread impact may also be achieved if the results can be made directly applicable to several distinct conditions. Quicker advances can be made toward the goal of developing some general psychological theories applicable to phenomena of interest in pediatric psychology.

Developmental Perspective

Pediatric psychology obviously concerns itself with developing beings, children who grow and change. So too do their families, both related to the children's development and independently. However, a distinct developmental perspective is absent in most of the research in pediatric psychology and as presented in this volume. Such a lack of explicit attention to developmental issues is exemplified in the use of wide age ranges without much study of age differences in the variables of interest, little study of changes over time, and few references to basic developmental theory and literature. Pediatric psychology, and the study of family issues in it, must place itself more generally in the body of developmental psychology and use its theories and methods (Roberts, Maddux, & Wright, 1984). We cannot hope to learn much about children and their families without respecting the notion of development.

SUMMARY

Much remains for pediatric psychology to integrate families fully into conceptualizations for research and practice. The chapters presented here represent a fundamental stage of development in the process of understanding and intervening through considerations of families, as composites of individuals and as interactive units. The chapters were peer reviewed through the *Journal of Pediatric Psychology*. As independent submissions, they offer a variety of approaches and topics revolving around family issues. We have organized the chapters into sections on Individual Disorders, Noncategorical Disorders, Intervention Issues and Programs, and A Theoretical Perspective. They might also have been organized along lines of methodology, theory, or conceptualization of families. The pediatric psychology field, however, is still progressing toward increased sophistication on these aspects. There is a strong focus on Individual Disorders and family issues represented by more articles on such pediatric problems as failure to thrive, recurrent abdominal pain, spina bifida, arthritis, AIDS, and cancer. The articles in the Noncategorical Disorders section combine different disorders for comparisons where psychosocial issues are considered similar or share commonalities. Thus, the articles study in combination conditions of spina bifida, cerebral palsy, arthritis, diabetes, mental retardation, and cystic fibrosis along with aspects of siblings, maternal and family functioning. The section on Intervention Issues and Programs demonstrate a few approaches to aspects of therapeutic strategies such as diabetes care in adolescents, a heart health promotion program, and parental anxiety about their children's health care. Finally, the Theoretical Perspective section presents an article outlining application of the transactional perspective to pediatric psychology research and practice.

REFERENCES

Achenbach, T.M., & Edelbrock, C. (1983). *Manual for the Child Behavior Checklist and Revised Child Behavior Profile*. Burlington: University of Vermont.

Ainsworth, M.D., & Wittig, B.A. (1969). Attachment and exploratory behavioral of one-year-olds in a strange situation. In B.M. Foss (Ed.), *Determinants of infant behavior Vol. 4* (pp. 11–136). London: Methuen.

Akamatsu, T.J., Stephens, M.A.P., Hobfoll, S.E., & Crowther, J.H. (Eds.). (in press). *Family health psychology*. New York: Hemisphere.

American Psychological Association. (1990). *Apportionment ballot: Division/state association: Purpose/activities brochure*. Washington, DC: Author.

Association for the Care of Children's Health. (1988). *ACCH psychosocial guidelines for pediatric care in hospitals* (working draft). Washington, DC: Author.

Aries, P. (1962). *Centuries of childhood: A social history of family life* (R. Baldick, Trans.). New York: Alfred A. Knopf.

Baranowski, T., & Nader, P.R. (1985). Family involvement in health behavior change

programs. In D.C. Turk & R.D. Kerns (Eds.), *Health, illness, and families: A life-span perspective* (pp. 81–107). New York: Wiley.
Baric, L. (1970). Conjugal roles as indicators of family influence on health directed action. *International Journal of Health Education, 13*, 58–65.
Blacher, J. (1984). A dynamic perspective on the impact of severely handicapped child on the family. In J. Blacher (Ed.), *Severely handicapped young children and their families: Research in review* (pp. 3–50). New York: Academic.
Bowlby, J. (1980). *Attachment and loss: Vol. 3. Loss, sadness, and depression.* New York: Basic Books.
Califano, J. (1979). *Healthy people.* Washington, DC: U.S. Government Printing Office.
Craig, J., & McKay, E. (1958). Working of mother and baby unit. *British Medical Journal, 1*, 275–277.
Dean, A., Lin, N., & Ensel, W.M. (1981). The epidemiological significance of social support systems in depression. In R.G. Simmons (Ed.), *Research in community mental halth: Vol. 2. A research annual* (pp. 77–109). Greenwich, CT: JAI.
Doherty, W.J., & Baird, M.A. (1983). *Family therapy and family medicine.* New York: Guilford Press.
Doherty, W.J., & Campbell, T.L. (1988). *Families and health.* Newbury Park, CA: Sage.
Drotar, D., Johnson, S.B., Iannotti, R., Krasnegor, N., Matthews, K.A., Melamed, B.G., Millstein, S., Peterson, R.A., Popiel, D., & Routh, D.K. (1989). Child health psychology. *Health Psychology, 8*, 781–784.
Epstein, L.H., McCurley, J., Wing, R.R., & Valoski, A. (1990). Five-year follow-up of family-based behavioral treatments for childhood obesity. *Journal of Consulting and Clinical Psychology, 58*, 661–664.
Fagin, C. (1964). The case for rooming-in when young children are hospitalized. *Nursing Science, 2*, 324–333.
Fanurik, D., & Roberts, M.C. (1986). Review of Turk, D.C., & Kerns, R.D. (Eds.), *Health, illness, and families: A life-span perspective.* New York: Wiley, 1985. In *Journal of Pediatric Psychology, 11*, 307–209.
Flomenhaft, K. (1982). The family and medical illness. In A.E. Christ & K. Flomenhaft (Eds.), *Psychosocial family interventions in chronic pediatric illness* (pp. 5–12). New York: Plenum.
Harris, P.R. (1981). *Better health for our children: A national strategy.* Washington, DC: U.S. Government Printing Office.
Jay, S.M. (1988). Invasive medical procedures: Psychological intervention and assessment. In D.K. Routh (Ed.), *Handbook of pediatric psychology* (pp. 401–425). New York: Guilford Press.
Johnson, B.H. (1990). The changing role of families in health care. *Children's Health Care, 19*, 234–241.
Kaslow, F.W. (1991). The art and science of family psychology: Retrospective and perspective. *American Psychologist, 46*, 621–626.
Kerns, R.D., & Turk, D.C. (1985). Behavioral medicine and the family: Historical perspectives and future directions. In D.C. Turk & R.D. Kerns (Eds.), *Health, illness, and families: A life-span perspective* (pp. 338–353). New York: Wiley.
McCubbin, H.I., & Patterson, J.M. (1983). The family stress process: The Double ABCX Model of adjustment and adaptation. In H. McCubbin, M. Sussman, & J. Patterson (Eds.), *Advances and developments in family stress theory and research* (pp. 1–34). New York: Haworth.
Minuchin, S. (1974). *Families and family therapy.* Cambridge, MA: Harvard University Press.
National Association of Social Workers. (1981). *Family policy.* Silver Spring, MD: Author.
Nye, F.I., & Berardo, F.M. (1973). *The family, its structure and interactions.* Columbus, OH: Ross Laboratories.
Olson, R., & Habenstein, R. (1983). Families and children in history. In C.E. Walker & M.C. Roberts (Eds.), *Handbook of clinical child psychology* (pp. 3–25). New York: Wiley.
Peterson, L. (1984). A brief methodological comment on possible inaccuracies induced by

multimodal measurement analysis and reporting. *Journal of Behavioral Medicine, 7,* 307–313.
Peterson, L., & Harbeck, C. (1988). *The pediatric psychologist.* Champaign, IL: Research Press.
Peterson, L., Mori, L., & Carter, P. (1985). The role of the family in children's responses to stressful medical procedures. *Journal of Clinical Child Psychology, 14,* 98–104.
Pratt, L. (1976). *Family structure and effective health behavior. The energized family.* Boston, MA: Houghton-Mifflin.
Quick, E., & Jacob, T. (1973). Marital disturbance in relation to role theory and relationship theory. *Journal of Abnormal Psychology, 82,* 399–412.
Ramsey, L.R., Jr. (Ed.). (1989). *Family systems in medicine.* New York: Guilford Press.
Roberts, M.C. (1986). *Pediatric psychology: Psychological interventions and strategies for pediatric problems.* New York: Plenum.
Roberts, M.C., Fanurik, D., & Layfield, D. (1987). Behavioral approaches to prevention of childhood injuries. *Journal of Social Issues, 43,* 105–118.
Roberts, M.C., Fanurik, D., & Wilson, D. (1988). A community program to reward children's use of seat belts. *American Journal of Community Psychology, 16,* 395–407.
Roberts, M.C., La Greca, A.M., & Harper, D.C. (1988). *Journal of Pediatric Psychology:* Another stage of development. *Journal of Pediatric Psychology, 13,* 1–5.
Roberts, M.C., Maddux, J.E., & Wright, L. (1984). The developmental perspective in behavioral health. In J.D. Matarazzo, N.E. Miller, S.M. Weiss, J.A. Herd, & S.M. Weiss (Eds.), *Behavioral health: A handbook of health enhancement and disease prevention* (pp. 56–68). New York: Wiley.
Roberts, M.C., & Maieron, M.J. (1989). Editorial: Family issues in pediatric psychology. *Journal of Pediatric Psychology, 14,* 153–155.
Roberts, M.C., Maieron, M.J., & Collier, J. (1988). *Directory of hospital psychosocial policies and programs (1988 Edition).* Washington, DC: Association for the Care of Children's Health.
Roberts, M.C., & McElreath, L. (in press). The role of families in the prevention of physical and mental health problems. In T.J. Akamatsu, M.A.P. Stephens, S.E. Hobfoll, & J.H. Crowther (Eds.), *Family health psychology.* New York: Hemisphere.
Routh, D.K. (1991). The family as a frontier in child health psychology. In J.H. Johnson & S.B. Johnson (Eds.), *Advances in child health psychology.* (pp. 323–330). Gainesville, FL: University of Florida Press.
Salk, L. (1969, September). The purposes and functions of the psychologist in a pediatric setting. In *Issues concerning the expansion of psychology within pediatric settings.* Symposium presented at the 77th Annual Convention of the American Psychological Association, Washington, DC.
Shelton, T., Jeppson, E., & Johnson, B. (1987). *Family-centered care for children with special health care.* Washington, DC: Association of the Care of Children's Health.
Shore, M.F., & Goldston, S.E. (1978). Mental health aspects of pediatric care: Historical review and current status. In P. Magrab (Ed.), *Psychological management of pediatric problems: Vol. 1: Early life conditions and chronic diseases* (pp. 15–31). Baltimore: University Park Press.
Singer, G.H.S., & Irvin, L.K. (1989). Family caregiving, stress, and support. In G.H.S. Singer & L.K. Irvin (Eds.), *Support for caregiving families: Enabling positive adaptation to disability* (pp. 3–25). Baltimore: Brooks.
Tucker, H.S., & Roberts, M.C. (1990). Future issues in children's health care: Addressing psychosocial concerns. *Children's Health Care, 19,* 199–208.
Turk, D.C., & Kerns, R.D. (Eds.). (1985a). *Health, illness, and families: A life-span perspective.* New York: Wiley.
Turk, D.C., & Kerns, R.D. (1985b). The family in health and illness. In D.C. Turk & R.D. Kerns (Eds.), *Health, illness, and families: A life-span perspective* (pp. 1–22). New York: Wiley.
Wallander, J.L., & Varni, J.W. (in press). Adjustment in children with chronic physical disorders: Programmatic research on a disability-stress-coping model. In A.M. La

Greca, L. Siegal, J.L. Wallander, & C.E. Walker (Eds.), *Stress and coping with pediatric conditions*. New York: Guilford Press.
Wright, L. (1967). The pediatric psychologist: A role model. *American Psychologist, 22,* 323–325.
Zastowney, T.R., Kirschenbaum, D.S., & Meng, A.L. (1986). Coping skills training for children: Effects of distress before, during, and after hospitalization for surgery. *Health Psychology, 5,* 231-247.

I

INDIVIDUAL DISORDERS

2

Families of Young Adolescents Who Have Survived Cancer: Social-Emotional Adjustment, Adaptability, and Social Support[1]

Anne E. Kazak and Anna T. Meadows
University of Pennsylvania

Young adolescent (10–15 year old) survivors of childhood cancer and their families (n = 35) completed self-report measures of perceived self-competence, social support, child behavior, parental distress, and family adaptability and cohesion, at two data points, 6 months apart. Relative to instrument norms and a comparison group (n = 13), survivors and their families scored within normative levels. The overall lack of group differences is discussed in terms of the implications of tests of the null hypothesis for families with chronically ill children. Changes over time for the survivors suggest a decline in available social support. Parents of survivors who received educational assistance reported less family adaptability and more distress than parents of survivors not receiving these services.

Although childhood cancer is recognized as one of the most distressing experiences a family may encounter, the psychological implications of *surviving* a life-threatening illness in childhood are not well understood at present. Research on children in treatment has emphasized the importance of the quality of marital relationships, social support, and the changes that occur

[1]Support for this study was provided by the Joan B. Kroc Foundation. We thank Tamara Klerr for her assistance in data collection and coding and Maxine Field, Virginia Peckham, and Jerilyn Radcliffe for their feedback on earlier drafts of the paper.

over time as the family adjusts to treatment regimes, remissions, and eventual cure or death (Blotcky, Raczynski, Gurwitch, & Smith, 1985; Kupst et al., 1982, 1984; Kupst & Schulman, 1988). In the case of a life-threatening disease in which cure has been achieved, the challenge to family and pediatric researchers is to understand these children and families as they would other, presumed normal, groups, and at the same time appreciate the specific ways in which they may differ from others.

Statistical projections indicate that in 1990 one in 1,000 20-year-olds will have survived cancer (Meadows, Krejmas, & Belasco, 1980). Furthermore, the population of younger survivors will increase. Acute lymphocytic leukemia (ALL), the most common type of childhood cancer, with an overall cure rate of about 65%, is diagnosed at a median age of 3–4 years (Sather, 1986; Silverberg & Lubera, 1987). With an average length of treatment of 2–3 years, survivors of this once fatal illness are still young children. Although the child's memory of the illness and treatment experience may be sketchy, parents and older siblings retain direct memories of the experience. Consistent with work on early childhood trauma it would be expected that the children themselves will be affected psychologically, although the nature of the impact may be subtle. It is also likely that certain aspects of the experience could leave a positive effect while other impacts might be negative, or neutral.

There are definite long-term effects of cancer and its treatment. Among them are the cognitive impairments sometimes associated with radiation and chemotherapy (Meadows et al., 1981). Depending upon the nature of the treatment, and when it occurred, effects on learning ability and school performance may be marked or subtle (Peckham, Meadows, Bartel, & Marrero, 1988). Additional consequences of treatment, such as growth abnormalities, potential sterility, or amputations may have psychological ramifications, particularly for adolescents (Meadows & Silber, 1985).

Based upon general measures of psychological adjustment, childhood cancer survivors have been found to be functioning at normative levels in young adulthood (Teta et al., 1986). However, in a study of 118 survivors, Koocher and O'Malley (1981) reported that 47% experienced adjustment problems, based upon a clinical rating scale. They suggest that factors such as type and course of illness, developmental period in which the child was ill, time since recovery, and a generally optimistic outlook may help to differentiate between more and less successful coping among survivors. Only a few studies have examined the psychological adjustment of cancer survivors during adolescence, a time typically associated with difficult processes of growth and independence, leading into adulthood. Wallace, Reiter, and Pendergrass (1987) found that over half of their sample of parents of adolescent survivors express concerns about their offspring's emotional and social adjustment. Wasserman, Thompson, Wilimas, and Fairclough (1987) reported that although school achievement among survivors is high, memories of difficult school and peer relationships persist. Studying survivors age 7 to 21 years ($n = 50$), Fritz, Williams, and Amylon (1988) provided data supporting age-appropriate adjustment and heterogeneous coping styles.

In a study of 138 8- to 16-year-old survivors, Greenberg, Kazak, and Meadows (1989) reported normative levels of self-concept among survivors. Those former patients with more severe medical late effects of the disease and treatment (e.g., organ damage that limits activity, blindness, severe learning problems) had significantly worse adjustment than those with few or no late effects. Consistent with other research on children with cancer who are currently in treatment (Worchel et al., 1988), the childhood cancer survivors reported depressive symptoms that were well above norms for clinical and nonclinical groups (that is, denying the types of depressive symptoms that one would expect even in a nonclinical sample) (Greenberg et al., 1989). Other important areas for childhood cancer survivors have not been the topic of empirical investigation. These include potential overprotection of the once ill child and the ways in which families may continue to organize themselves around the illness even when it occurred many years before. Also neglected in the research has been a close look at the social and peer relationships of children who once had cancer. Since cancer treatment entails school absences and may evoke fear and uncertainty from peers, social interactions with peers may be affected in the long-term.

From these reports, one is left with the optimistic news that most childhood cancer survivors look generally well adjusted, although some experience more difficulties in adjustment than others. Although this does not seem different from the general population, the research in this area has not been very satisfying in terms of looking at family variables that may mediate and affect the course of psychological adjustment after cancer. Nor has the research been conceptualized within relevant theoretical frameworks.

Among the criticisms that may be directed towards previous research are four that are addressed in the present study:

1. Cross-sectional designs are commonly used when longitudinal (prospective) data are critical in order to understand complex processes that occur over time. The present study presents data from two time periods (the beginning and middle of an academic year).

2. There is a general lack of consideration given to the developmental point at which children and families are studied. Studies that sample a broad age range (as nearly all research in this area does) miss important developmental implications. In the present paper we report data on young adolescents (10–15 years old). This age group was chosen because of its neglect in past research in this field and because of the importance of individual and family variables during this developmental period in predicting later adjust-

ment (Cohen, Adler, Beck, & Irwin, 1986; Compas, 1987). In addition, these young adolescents were all diagnosed as young children, and thus experienced the disease at the same developmental stage.

3. There has been a tendency to measure multiple family traits and processes without a clear theoretical understanding of their interrelationships and clinical importance, and often with instruments with unimpressive psychometric histories. In the present study, emphasis is placed upon the adaptability of the family. Although much of the literature on childhood chronic illness and families has focused upon cohesion, there is evidence that it is the families' ability to change and adjust to the demands of the illness that may be more predictive of positive outcome (Kazak, 1989; Kazak, Reber, & Snitzer, 1988).

4. Cancer is not one disease but rather encompasses many different diseases. The type of disease and treatment are important variables to consider in research in this field. In the present study, we have limited the sample to three specific related types of cancer.

In recent studies of families with chronically ill or handicapped children, the extent to which many of these families appear to be coping well, or at normative levels, has been emphasized (Kazak & Marvin, 1984; Kazak et al., 1988). Rather than expecting to find deficits in the families of childhood cancer survivors, it was expected that these families would differ from matched comparison families and norms in the following ways:

1. Ten- to 15-year-old survivors of childhood cancer will have poorer perceptions of their academic ability and their social interactions than children who have not had cancer. They will not differ with respect to other aspects of self-concept and behavior. This hypothesis is tested by examining group differences and discrepancies from norms for scores on the Self-Perception Profile for Adolescents (Harter, 1986) and on the Social Support Rating Scale (Cauce, Felner, & Primavera, 1982). In addition, group and normative differences from mothers and fathers on the Social Competence factor of the Child Behavior Checklist (Achenbach & Edelbrock, 1978) are examined.

2. With respect to family variables, it is expected that adaptability will be an area in which the potential overprotectiveness and rigidity of families of childhood cancer survivors will be seen. This hypothesis is tested by examination of group and normative differences on the Family Adaptability and Cohesion Evaluation Scales-Second Version (Olson, Portner, & Bell, 1982).

3. A third hypothesis concerns the role of cognitive difficulties in childhood cancer survivors. It is expected that those children who have been identified as having a learning disability or difficulties in academic achievement will show poorer self-concept with respect to academic achievement, have

poorer peer relationships, and come from families in which there is lower adaptability.

4. Differences in scores between the beginning and end of a school year are examined for each group. Relative consistency is expected, although it is hypothesized that the survivor group will undergo more changes. This is presumed to be related to their higher risk status, as stated in the first three hypotheses.

METHOD

Subjects

Tumor registry records at The Children's Hospital of Philadelphia were used to identify survivors of three types of childhood cancer (acute lymphocytic leukemia, acute myelomonocytic leukemia, non-Hodgkin's lymphoma), presently 10–15 years old and off treatment and free of disease for at least 5 years. They became ill between 1974–1981, with 85% diagnosed since 1977. There were only minor variations in the therapy these children received. All completed 2–3 years of intravenous chemotherapy and intrathecal chemotherapy. A letter describing the study was sent to 65 eligible families, with follow-up phone calls to describe the study in detail. Of the 47 families who were contacted successfully, 35 (74.5%) completed initial data collection, 3 (6.4%) refused, and 9 (19.1%) who agreed to participate did not return data. 71.4% of these ($n = 25$) completed a second data collection point 6 months later. Letters and phone calls were used to encourage participation in the follow-up part of the study.

Chi-square analyses were performed in order to test for differences between those survivors who participated and those who did not, with respect to data available from the tumor registry (age, age at diagnosis, sex, radiation therapy, medical late effects of treatment, educational placement). There were no significant differences between the groups on these variables.

A comparison group was recruited by asking families to identify friends/neighbors who have children of the same age. Nineteen families were identified with 13 (68%) completing initial data collection. Of these families, 9 (69.2%) provided data 6 months later. Although this recruitment strategy generated fewer families than anticipated, it did provide a small group of families that were well matched with the cancer survivor families. Since all the instruments utilized in this study were well-validated, norms provided additional comparative data.

In order to compare families that completed both data points and those who completed only the first one, *t* test and chi-square analyses were used to test for possible biases. In the survivor group there were no differences between the families with respect to age, sex, age at diagnosis, treatment, and family demographic variables. *T* tests conducted on the dependent variables also showed no differences between those who continued in the study and those who did not. Similarly, no differences were found for the comparison group with respect to these variables. There is, therefore, no reason to suspect a systematic bias in the sample that provided data at both times.

The subjects in this study were categorized by the educational consultant to the Oncology Late Effects Clinic into two groups. The first group (45.7%, $n = 16$) were those who had some learning difficulties at present (i.e., low achievement, memory problems, used school resource rooms, had tutoring). Only one child had a full-time special education placement. The remaining subjects (54.3%, $n = 19$) had no reported learning or school difficulties. None of the comparison group children received special educational services.

Procedure

Families were mailed self-report questionnaires, with self-addressed stamped return envelopes for the first week of school in September 1987 and at a point later in the academic year (March 1988). This interval was chosen in order to assess functioning at the beginning of the school year and to be able to compare that with adjustment approximately 6 months later when students would be expected to have adjusted to their classroom and to have completed the majority of the curricula. Basic demographic data were collected, including grade in school, special education placement, and whether the child was a new student in the school. Data on diagnosis, treatment, physical effects of treatment, and pubertal status were obtained from oncology records.

Measures

At each data collection point, the 10- to 15-year-old participants completed the following instruments:

Family Adaptability and Cohesion Evaluation Scales-Version II (FACESII). This is a self-report scale based upon the Circumplex Model of Marital and Family Systems (Olson et al., 1982). The model is based upon the importance of cohesiveness and adaptability in family functioning. Four levels of cohesion (disengaged, separated, connected, enmeshed) and four levels of adaptability (rigid, structured, flexible, chaotic) are posited, with midrange values expected to be most adaptive. Alpha reliabilities range from

.78 to .87 (Barnes & Olson, 1985). Separate norms are provided for adolescents and adults. The scales are useful in differentiating functional and dysfunctional families (Garbarino, Sebes, & Schellenbach, 1984; Rodick, Henggeler, & Hanson, 1986) and are a valuable tool for identifying parent–child dyads that may develop destructive interaction patterns during adolescence (Garbarino et al., 1984).

The Self-Perception Profile for Adolescents (Harter, 1986). This is a self-report scale assessing perceptions of competence and self-worth with nine subscales: scholastic competence; social acceptance; athletic competence; physical appearance; job competence; romantic appeal; conduct/morality; close friendship; and global self-worth. The scale is an extension of earlier work on younger children (Harter, 1982; Harter & Pike, 1984) and has alpha reliabilities ranging from .85 to .95.

The Social Support Rating Scale. The SSRS (Cauce, 1986; Cauce et al., 1982) was modified slightly to include 17 sources of social support on three factors (family, friends, school/other adults). Adolescents indicated the extent to which persons provided emotional support and caring, help, and guidance, and the extent to which each person may have upset them on a 5-point Likert-type scale. They also indicate the extent to which they are satisfied with the emotional support and help, and the extent to which they are the sort of person who seeks help, on a 7-point Likert-type scale. Each subscale consists of items loading above 0.5 and each has an eigenvalue greater than or equal to 1.0. The scale factors have internal consistency coefficients (Cronbach's alpha) exceeding .75. Normative data are provided only for total scores. Since the scale was modified, comparisons with the normative data would not be valid. The SSRS is one of the few social support scales for children and adolescents and is unique in examining separate sources of support. Subscales have been shown to correlate significantly with ratings of self-competence (Cauce, Hannan, & Sargeant, 1987).

At each data collection point, mothers and fathers completed the following instruments:

The Langner Symptom Checklist. The LSC (Langner, 1962) is a 22-item scale assessing symptoms of anxiety and depression. The LSC has been established as a good measure of general mental health and is used widely in assessing adjustment and demoralization (Billings & Moos, 1984; Dohrenwend, Shrout, Egri, & Mendelson, 1980) and in studies of families with chronically ill and disabled children (Kazak, 1987; Kazak et al., 1988).

The Child Behavior Checklist. The CBCL (Achenbach & Edelbrock, 1978) is a widely used 113-item self-report questionnaire to assess childhood and adolescent psychopathology. Four scales have been identified through factor analysis: internalizing, externalizing, behavior problems, social competence. Median test–retest reliability is .89, with evidence that the scale differentiates disturbed and nondisturbed children (Achenbach & Edelbrock, 1983).

FACESII. (See description above.)

RESULTS[3]

Sample Description

The mean age of the 35 childhood cancer survivors was 12.2 years with a mean age at diagnosis of 3.7 years. All but 3 had been diagnosed with ALL. The majority of subjects received cranial irradiation as part of their treatment, with 46% (n = 16) having received 1,800 rad and 37% (n = 13) 2,400 rad. The remaining 17% (n = 6) did not receive radiation to their heads. With the exception of one patient who suffered a testicular relapse 2 years off therapy, subjects remained free of reoccurrence throughout treatment and since discontinuing treatment at least 5 years ago. In combination with the sampling criteria, these data show the homogeneity of our subjects with respect to disease and treatment.

The overwhelming majority of participants were white, including two with Asian mothers and one with an Asian father. Mean parental age was in the late 30s and early 40s, with 44% completing high school, 36% college educated, and 20% with graduate education. Median income was $35,000. There were no differences between the childhood cancer survivors and the comparison group with respect to these variables. The only significant difference between the groups was with respect to sex of the target child, $\chi^2(1) = 3.75, p < .05$, with only one girl in the comparison group. Simple t tests on sex differences indicated no relationship between sex and scores on the dependent variables. Although the predominance of boys in the comparison group could affect the outcome, we chose to include all subjects in the analyses. (See Table I.)

Scores on Dependent Variables and Group Differences

Child Variables. In general, scores on standardized instruments for the survivors of childhood cancer were within normative limits and did not differ significantly between the survivor and comparison groups. At Time 1, the

[3]Despite the increasing number of childhood cancer survivors, sample sizes are limited when the inclusion criteria are strict, as in the present study. Due to the multiple comparisons made, we urge readers to interpret the results cautiously.

Table I. Demographic Data

Variable	Cancer survivors (n = 35)	Comparison group (n = 13)
Child age (years)	M = 12.2	M = 12.3
Child sex[a]		
Female	13	1
Male	21	11
Mother's age (years)	M = 39.7	M = 37.6
Father's age (years)	M = 40.8	M = 38.8
Mother's education		
Completed high school	16	6
Some college	7	4
College degree	5	1
Graduate school	7	1
Father's education		
Completed high school	15	2
Some college	5	5
College degree	9	3
Graduate school	6	2
Marital status		
First marriage	26	9
Separated	1	0
Divorced	4	2
Widow	1	0
Remarried	2	1
Income		
Less than $10,000	1	
$10,000–$14,999	4	1
$15,000–$19,000	2	1
$20,000–$24,999	2	1
$25,000–$34,999	8	3
$35,000–$50,000	15	3
More than $50,000	3	3

[a]Difference between the number of male and female subjects in the two groups is significant, $p < .05$.

survivors perceived their families as significantly less adaptable than the comparison group, $t(46) = 2.00$, $p < .05$. According to normative values on FACESII, the cancer survivors rated their families as "structured," whereas the comparison group rated theirs as falling within the "flexible" range. (See Table II.) Similar patterns in terms of group differences were seen at Time 2. Cancer survivors and the comparison group differed with respect to feelings of competence on school-related issues, $t(35) = 2.03$, $p < .05$, with the survivors reporting lower levels of competence. In addition, the survivors reported less help and guidance from friends than the comparison group, $t(31) = 2.28$, $p < .05$.

Table II. Means and Standard Deviations—Child Measures

	Cancer survivors		Comparison group		Norms	
	M	*SD*	*M*	*SD*	*M*	*SD*
Time 1	n = 35		n = 13			
FACES Cohesion[b]	59.1	11.8	64.5	8.2	56.3	9.2
FACES Adaptability[a]	44.5	8.5	49.0	6.3	45.4	7.9
Social support						
Family						
Emotional support	4.21	4.5	4.32	0.5		
Help and guidance	4.07	0.6	4.22	0.5		
Upset	3.37	0.9	3.15	1.2		
Mean total	11.65		11.69			
Friends						
Emotional support	3.75	0.7	3.80	0.8		
Help and guidance	3.60	0.8	3.57	0.8		
Upset	2.71	1.4	2.57	1.3		
Mean total	10.06		9.94			
School and other adults						
Emotional support	3.66	0.9	3.80	0.8		
Help and guidance	3.62	1.1	3.66	0.7		
Upset	2.70	1.2	2.53	0.9		
Mean total	9.98		9.99			
Satisfaction with emotional support	5.72	1.3	6.16	1.0		
Satisfaction with help and guidance	5.82	1.2	6.33	1.2		
Time 2	n = 25		n = 9			
FACES Cohesion	58.7	7.8	63.3	5.0	56.3	9.2
FACES Adaptability	43.1	7.2	47.9	3.8	45.4	7.9
Social support						
Family						
Emotional support	3.86	0.6	4.14	0.7		
Help and guidance	3.94	0.6	4.10	0.7		
Upset	3.02	1.0	2.64	1.2		
Mean total	10.82		10.88			
Friends						
Emotional support	3.38	0.8	3.87	0.7		
Help and guidance[a]	3.34	0.7	3.90	0.6		
Upset	2.52	0.7	2.71	1.1		
Mean total	9.24		10.48			
School and other adults						
Emotional support	3.08	1.2	3.34	0.7		
Help and guidance	3.28	1.0	3.37	0.8		
Upset	2.31	0.8	2.12	0.7		
Mean total	8.67		8.83			
Satisfaction with emotional support	5.69	1.3	6.12	1.1		
Satisfaction with help and guidance	5.60	1.4	6.12	1.0		

[a] $p < .05$.
[b] $p < .10$.

Parental Variables. There were no significant differences between the two groups on the parental variables at Time 1, with all scores consistent with normative values. At Time 2, mothers of the childhood cancer survivors rated their families as significantly less adaptable than the comparison group mothers, $t(32) = 2.32$, $p < .05$. (See Table III.)

Change Scores (Time 1 – Time 2)

There were more statistically significant changes over time in the cancer survivor group than in the comparison group. At Time 2, mothers of cancer survivors rated their families as significantly more cohesive than at Time 1, $t(23) = 2.52$, $p < .05$, and less adaptable, $t(23) = 2.24$, $p < .05$. Fathers of childhood cancer survivors rated their children as having significantly lower levels of behavior problems, $t(16) = 2.63$, $p < .05$, at Time 2 than at Time 1. The survivors themselves had a significant decline in one area of their perceived competence, that related to their athletic abilities, $t(23) = 2.27$, $p < .05$. There were significant changes for all the social support variables related to emotional support and caring and help and guidance. At Time 2 the survivors perceived that they received significantly less emotional support and caring from their families, $t(22) = 4.64$, $p < .0001$, friends, $t(22) = 4.05$, $p < .0005$, and teachers and other nonfamily adults, $t(22) = 4.71$, $p < .0001$, than they had previously. Similarly, they reported receiving less help and guidance from friends, $t(22) = 3.03$, $p < .001$, and teachers and other nonfamily adults, $t(22) = 2.47$, $p < .05$. There were no differences over time in the amount of upset they reported in their social network.

For the comparison group, two significant changes are seen in social support: These adolescents reported significantly less emotional support and caring, $t(8) = 3.71$, $p < .001$, and less help and guidance from school and other nonfamily adults, $t(8) = 3.26$, $p < .05$, in March than in September.

Effects of Learning/Achievement Problems

Survivors who were receiving help for learning difficulties were not significantly different from those with no identified learning problems on the Harter scales or FACESII, with the exception that those children receiving help rated themselves as having significantly less romantic appeal at Time 2 than did their peers, $t(18) = 2.46$, $p < .05$. Survivors receiving educational assistance reported receiving significantly more help and guidance from their friends, $t(22) = 2.38$, $p < .05$, and school and other nonfamily adults, $t(22) = 2.15$, $p < .05$, at Time 2 than did the other survivors.

At Time 1, $t(32) = 2.43$, $p < .05$, and Time 2, $t(23) = 2.37$, $p < .05$, mothers of survivors receiving assistance in learning difficulties reported

Table III. Means and Standard Deviations—Parental Measures

	Cancer survivors		Comparison group		Norms	
	M	*SD*	*M*	*SD*	*M*	*SD*
Time 1/Mothers	*n* = 35		*n* = 19			
FACES Cohesion	65.3	7.7	63.6	10.8	64.9	8.4
FACES Adaptability	49.2	5.3	48.0	6.5	49.9	6.6
Langner	2.20	2.3	3.20	1.6	2.60	2.7
Child Behavior Checklist						
Internalizing	53.1	8.5	54.8	7.8	50.0	10.0
Externalizing	51.3	6.2	51.7	4.8	50.0	10.0
Behavior problems	49.5	10.8	52.4	7.0	50.0	10.0
Social competence	46.6	11.7	48.5	10.1	50.0	10.0
Time 1/Fathers	*n* = 35		*n* = 19			
FACES Cohesion	61.3	11.6	60.9	11.1	64.9	8.4
FACES Adaptability	48.3	7.1	49.0	8.7	49.9	6.6
Langner	1.97	2.6	2.20	.24	2.60	2.7
Child Behavior Checklist						
Internalizing	53.3	9.2	59.4	9.4	50.0	10.0
Externalizing	50.8	5.9	54.4	7.7	50.0	10.0
Behavior problems	50.3	8.44	56.0	8.2	50.0	10.0
Social competence	47.4	10.7	47.1	9.9	50.0	10.0
Time 2/Mothers	*n* = 25		*n* = 9			
FACES Cohesion	61.4	7.7	64.2	8.7	64.9	8.4
FACES Adaptability[a]	46.8	4.8	50.4	6.6	49.9	6.6
Langner	2.1	2.1	2.8	2.3	2.60	2.7
Child Behavior Checklist						
Internalizing	51.7	8.4	56.2	7.8	50.0	10.0
Externalizing	49.7	8.0	50.6	6.9	50.0	10.0
Behavior problems	47.8	9.5	51.8	7.7	50.0	10.0
Social competence	45.8	10.7	47.8	11.8	50.0	10.0
Time 2/Fathers	*n* = 25		*n* = 9			
FACES Cohesion	61.8	8.6	56.2	8.3	64.9	8.4
FACES Adaptability	47.9	7.3	42.0	9.6	49.9	6.6
Langner	1.8	2.9	1.9	2.8	2.60	2.7
Child Behavior Checklist						
Internalizing	50.2	6.6	53.6	6.8	50.0	10.0
Externalizing	47.1	5.9	48.6	4.8	50.0	10.0
Behavior problems	45.7	9.1	49.2	6.3	50.0	10.0
Social competence	45.4	8.5	44.0	6.2	50.0	10.0

[a] $p < .05$.

their families to be significantly less cohesive than mothers of survivors without learning problems. At Time 1 but not at Time 2 there were significant differences for maternal reports of adaptability, $t(32) = 2.50$, $p < .05$, and maternal distress ratings, $t(32) = 2.38$, $p < .05$. Mothers of the children receiving educational assistance perceived their families as significantly less adaptable and themselves as having significantly more symptoms of anxiety and depression than mothers of the other survivors. They also rated their children as having lower levels of social competence on the CBCL at Time 1, $t(32) = 3.19$, $p < .01$, and Time 2, $t(23) = 2.19$, $p < .05$. Fathers of the survivors receiving educational help rated their families as less cohesive, $t(27) = 1.94$, $p < .05$, and less adaptable, $t(27) = 2.22$, $p < .05$, than the other fathers at Time 1. They also concurred with the maternal data in reporting lower levels of social competence at Time 1, $t(26) = 2.36$, $p < .05$.

Predicting Perceived Social Acceptance and Scholastic Competence

After inspection of Pearson product-moment correlations, stepwise multiple regressions were performed, predicting perceived social acceptance and scholastic competence on the Harter scales for the cancer survivors from selected background, support, and family variables. A four-variable model accounted for 57% ($R^2 = .57$) of the variance in perceived social acceptance. The significant predictors were satisfaction with emotional support (partial $R^2 = .35$), age at diagnosis (partial $R^2 = .11$), changing schools (partial $R^2 = .07$), and the child's perceived family adaptability (partial $R^2 = .05$). A three-variable predictor model accounted for 29% of the variance ($R^2 = .29$) in perceived scholastic competence. Significant predictors were age at diagnosis (partial $R^2 = .11$), mother's perceived family adaptability (partial $R^2 = .13$), and child's age (partial $R^2 = .06$).

DISCUSSION

This study provides data on a population previously neglected in pediatric psychology and family research—early adolescent survivors of childhood cancer and their parents. In general, the results support previous research on childhood cancer survivors in verifying that most score near normative levels in terms of psychological and social functioning (Greenberg et al., 1989; Wallace et al., 1987; Wasserman et al., 1987).

The overall lack of differences between the survivor and comparison groups merits further consideration. On the one hand, limited sample size, attrition, reliance on self-report measures, and a potentially elevated experimental error rate could all affect the analysis and interpretation of the data. An alternative view is to suggest that research on families with chronically ill children may have reached a point at which we can consider accepting the null hypothesis (Greenwald, 1975). Historically, research on families with chronically ill children has been based upon the notion that these families were expected to be different (and often deficient) from other families. As Greenwald (1975) noted, scientific theory can advance by rejecting theories as well as supporting them, particularly when, as in the present study, the design (i.e., unbiased sample, carefully matched controls), measures (reliable, valid), and analysis (liberal) favor finding significant differences. This notion has been advanced in other social and clinical psychological research (cf. Delamater et al., 1988; Schroeder, Dovidio, Sibicky, Matthews, & Allen, 1988). What is most striking for the field of family research in chronic childhood illness are recent empirical and review papers that describe relatively minor group differences between families with ill children and others (cf. Kazak & Marvin, 1984; Kazak et al., 1988; Lobato, Faust, & Spirito, 1988; Sabbeth & Levanthal, 1984). From these conclusions it may be possible to design investigations than will help us understand what differentiates more and less positive adaptation, and to develop measures that can assess relevant structural and functional characteristics of these families, rather than expecting group differences on relatively gross dimensions of family adaptation.

The points that follow are based upon within-group (survivor) findings. Survivors reported lower levels of perceived social support at the second data point than they did early in the school year, from family, friends, and teachers. One possibility is that subtle effects of having had cancer combined with possible parental overprotectiveness and time away from peers may be reflected in these perceptions of social support. Although not affecting their overall evaluation of their perceived self-competence, it suggests that over the course of the year the cancer survivors may feel more alienated from others.

It is interesting that while there were few differences in the child variables between survivors receiving special educational assistance and those who did not, parental differences were seen. The students receiving special assistance perceived that they received more help and support from friends and teachers than the other survivors. However, parents of the group receiving assistance tended to rate their families as less adaptable, themselves as more distressed, and their children as having lower social competence. This may reflect the fact that those children receiving special assistance are those with more severe late effects, and that the families experience more distress and more demands for reorganizing in order to cope effectively with the child's difficulties.

The variables selected in the present study were able to explain a large amount of the variance in perceived social acceptance. Consistent with other literature on social support, satisfaction with support was an important predictor of well-being. The association of being younger at diagnosis with higher perceived social acceptance may indicate a lessened impact on social relationships when diagnosis and treatment occurs during infancy and toddler years, as opposed to during the early years of formal education. The data suggest that school transitions that occur during this developmental period (e.g., leaving grade school for junior high or junior high for senior high) may affect feelings of social acceptance. Family adaptability was an important predictor for both regression models. With respect to perceived scholastic competence, the regression model explained a modest amount of the variance and suggests that the older children in the sample, who were also older at diagnosis feel better about their school performance than the younger survivors. There was no statistically significant association between age at diagnosis and receiving educational assistance. Therefore, this association may be due to simply being in school for a longer period of time.

As predicted, family adaptability proved to be an important variable in understanding family functioning. Adaptability scores differed significantly for parents of survivors receiving educational assistance and those who were not and were significant predictors of perceived social acceptance and scholastic competence. These conclusions support the notion that the family's flexibility and ability to change in response to demands may be among the most critical variables to explore in future research on families with ill children.

A few general points can be made regarding the clinical implications of the data. The importance of family adaptability and the changes over time in the survivor group suggest closer attention to how survivors and their families change over time and how these changes might be either adaptive or stressful. Psychologists can help families understand the benefits of flexibility and the ways in which adaptability may relate to developmental transitions of the child and family. Social support available to survivors and the potential strain of special education placement emerge as two areas meriting particular clinical attention.

Adjustment of these survivors, diagnosed as young children, appears good overall. The results highlight the importance of family adaptability and understanding the impact of the educational system and the potential learning problems of this group. The focus on one age group allows for a more in-depth understanding of this population than previous studies. The results support further investigation of child and family processes during early adolescence, with prospective research to understand predictors of later adjustment. Future research looking at the interaction of child, family, and school system variables, particularly during periods of transition, will enhance our understanding of this group of children, and of families in general.

REFERENCES

Achenbach, T., & Edelbrock, C. (1978). The classification of child psychopathology: A review and analysis of empirical efforts. *Psychological Bulletin, 85,* 1275-1301.

Achenbach, T., & Edelbrock, C. (1983). *Manual for the Child Behavior Checklist and Revised Child Behavior Profile.* Burlington: University of Vermont, Department of Psychiatry.

Barnes, H., & Olson, D. (1985). Parent-adolescent communication and the Circumplex Model. *Child Development, 56,* 438-447.

Billings, A., & Moos, R. (1984). Coping, stress, and social resources among adults with unipolar depression. *Journal of Personality and Social Psychology, 96,* 877-891.

Blotcky, A., Raczynski, J., Gurwitch, R., & Smith, K. (1985). Family influences on hopelessness among children early in the cancer experience. *Journal of Pediatric Psychology, 10,* 479-493.

Cauce, A. (1986). Social networks and social competence: Exploring the effects of early adolescent friendships. *American Journal of Community Psychology, 14,* 607-628.

Cauce, A., Felner, R., & Primavera, J. (1982). Social support in high-risk adolescents: Structural components and adaptive impact. *American Journal of Community Psychology, 10,* 417-428.

Cauce, A., Hannan, K., & Sargeant, M. (1987). *Negative events, social support, and locus of control in early adolescence: Contributions to well-being.* Paper presented at the annual meeting of the American Psychological Association, New York.

Cohen, M., Adler, N., Beck, A., & Irwin, C. (1986). Parental reactions to the onset of adolescence. *Journal of Adolescent Health Care, 7,* 101-106.

Compas, B. (1987). Coping with stress during childhood and adolescence. *Psychological Bulletin, 101,* 393-403.

Delamater, A., Bubb, J., Kurtz, S., Kuntze, J., Smith, J., White, N., & Santiago, J. (1988). Physiologic response to acute psychological stress in adolescents with type I diabetes. *Journal of Pediatric Psychology, 13,* 69-86.

Dohrenwend, B., Shrout, P., Egri, G., & Mendelson, F. (1980). Nonspecific psychological distress and other dimensions of psychopathology. *Archives of General Psychiatry, 37,* 1229-1238.

Fritz, G., Williams, J., & Amylon, M. (1988). After treatment ends: Psychosocial sequalae in pediatric cancer survivors. *American Journal of Orthopsychiatry, 58,* 552-561.

Garbarino, J., Sebes, J., & Schellenbach, C. (1984). Families at risk for destructive parent-child relations in adolescence. *Child Development,* 174-183.

Greenberg, H., Kazak, A., & Meadows, A. (1989). Psychological adjustment in 8- to 16-year-old cancer survivors and their parents. *Journal of Pediatrics, 114,* 488-493.

Greenwald, A. (1975). Consequences of prejudice against the null hypothesis. *Psychological Bulletin, 82,* 1-20.

Harter, S. (1982). The Perceived Competence Scale for Children. *Child Development, 53,* 87-97.

Harter, S. (1986). *Self-Perception Profile for Adolescents.* Denver, CO: University of Denver, Department of Psychology.

Harter, S., & Pike, R. (1984). The pictorial scale of perceived competence and social acceptance for young children. *Child Development, 55,* 1969-1982.

Kazak, A. (1987). Families with disabled children: Stress and social networks in three samples. *Journal of Abnormal Child Psychology, 15,* 137-146.

Kazak, A. (1989). Families of chronically ill children: A systems and social ecological model of adaptation and challenge. *Journal of Consulting and Clinical Psychology, 57,* 25-30.

Kazak, A., & Marvin, R. (1984). Differences, difficulties, and adaptation: Stress and social networks in families with a handicapped child. *Family Relations, 33,* 67-77.

Kazak, A., Reber, M., & Snitzer, L. (1988). Childhood chronic disease and family functioning: A study of phenylketonuria. *Pediatrics, 81,* 224-230.

Koocher, G., & O'Malley, J. (1981). *The Damocles Syndrome: Psychosocial consequences of surviving childhood cancer.* New York: McGraw-Hill.

Kupst, M., & Schulman, J. (1988). Longterm coping with pediatric leukemia: A six year follow-up study. *Journal of Pediatric Psychology, 13,* 7-22.

Kupst, M., Schulman, J., Maurer, H., Honig, G., Morgan, E., & Fochtman, D. (1982). Family coping with childhood leukemia: One year after diagnosis. *Journal of Pediatric Psychology, 7,* 157-174.

Kupst, M., Schulman, J., Maurer, H., Honig, G., Morgan, E., & Fochtman, D. (1984). Coping with pediatric leukemia: A two year follow-up. *Journal of Pediatric Psychology, 9,* 149-163.

Langner, T. (1962). A 22-item screening score of psychiatric symptoms indicating impairment. *Journal of Health and Human Behavior, 3,* 269-276.

Lobato, D., Faust, D., & Spirito, A. (1988). Examining the effects of chronic disease and disability on children's sibling relationships. *Journal of Pediatric Psychology, 13,* 389-408.

Meadows, A., Krejmas, N., & Belasco, J. (1980). Medical cost of cure: Sequalae in survivors of childhood cancer. In J. van Eys & M. Sullivan (Eds.), *Status of the curability of childhood cancers* (pp. 273-276). New York: Raven.

Meadows, A., Massari, D., Fergusson, J. Gordon, J., Littman, P., & Moss, K. (1981). Declines in IQ scores and cognitive dysfunctions in children with acute lymphocytic leukemia treated with cranial irradiation. *Lancet, 2,* 1015-1018.

Meadows, A., & Silber, J. (1985). Delayed consequences of therapy for childhood cancer. *Cancer, 58,* 529-533.

Olson, D., Portner, J., & Bell, R. (1982). Family Adaptability and Cohesion Evaluation Scales. In D. Olson et al. (Eds.), *Family Inventories: Inventories used in a national survey of families across the family life cycle.* St. Paul: University of Minnesota, Department of Family Social Science.

Peckham, V., Meadows, A., Bartel, N., & Marrero, O. (1988). Educational late effects in long-term survivors of childhood ALL. *Pediatrics, 81,* 127-133.

Rodick, J., Henggeler S., & Hanson, C. (1986). An evaluation of the Family Adaptability and Cohesion Evaluation Scales and the Circumplex Model. *Journal of Abnormal Child Psychology, 14,* 77-87.

Sabbeth, B., & Leventhal, J. (1984). Marital adjustment to chronic childhood illness. *Pediatrics, 73,* 762-768.

Sather, H. (1986). Age at diagnosis in childhood acute lymphoblastic leukemia. *Medical and Pediatric Oncology, 14,* 166-172.

Schroeder, D., Dovidio, J., Sibicky, M., Matthews, L., & Allen, J. (1988). Empathic concern and helping behavior: Egoism or altruism? *Journal of Experimental Social Psychology, 24,* 333-353.

Silverberg, E., & Lubera, J. (1987). Cancer statistics, 1987. *Ca—A Cancer Journal for Clinicians, 37,* 2-19.

Teta, M., Po, M., Kasl, S., Meigs, J., Myers, M., & Mulvihill, J. (1986). Psychosocial consequences of childhood and adolescent cancer survival. *Journal of Chronic Diseases, 39,* 751-759.

Wallace, M., Reiter, P., & Pendergrass, T. (1987). Parents of longterm survivors of childhood cancer: A preliminary survey to characterize concerns and needs. *Oncology Nursing Forum, 14,* 39-43.

Wasserman, A., Thompson, E., Wilimas, J., & Fairclough, D. (1987). The psychological status of survivors of childhood/adolescent Hodgkin's Disease. *American Journal of Diseases of Childhood, 141,* 626-631.

Worchel, F., Nolan, B., Willson, V., Purser, J., Copeland, D., & Pfefferbaum, B. (1988). Assessment of depression in children with cancer. *Journal of Pediatric Psychology, 13,* 101-112.

3

Relationships Among Life Stress, Perceived Family Environment, and the Psychological Distress of Spina Bifida Adolescents[1]

Renee L. Murch and Lawrence H. Cohen
University of Delaware

Fifty-three teen-agers with spina bifida participated in a mail survey and completed measures of recent life events, perceived family environment, and psychological distress. Low levels of perceived family conflict and control served as life stress buffers in the prediction of distress, whereas a high level of perceived independence served as a life stress exacerbator. These interaction effects differ from those obtained for a normal sample of adolescents in the lone previous study (Burt, Cohen, & Bjorck, 1988) that reported comparable analyses. The results suggest that the process by which family environments moderate stress adjustment differs for able-bodied vs. spina bifida adolescents.

Research on adults, adolescents, and children has shown that an accumulation of recently experienced negative life events is positively related to psy-

[1]This article is based on a master's thesis completed by Renee L. Murch under the direction of Lawrence H. Cohen in the Department of Psychology at the University of Delaware. We thank the adolescents who participated in this study and the staff of the A. I. duPont Institute, especially Wayne Adams and Rosalyn Gleeson. Anne Kazak read an earlier version of this article and provided invaluable feedback. We also acknowledge the helpful comments of the two anonymous reviewers.

chological distress, broadly defined (Johnson, 1986; Thoits, 1983). Adolescent studies have documented this relationship for nonclinical samples (e.g., L. Cohen, Burt, & Bjorck, 1987), samples from families identified as psychiatric risks (e.g., Hirsch, Moos, & Reischl, 1985), and for samples with a chronic medical illness (e.g., Bedell, Giordani, Amour, Tavormina, & Boll, 1977).

Not all adolescents, however, are vulnerable to life stress (e.g., Garmezy, 1983). Recent interest in a developmental model of coping (e.g., Compas, 1987; Garmezy & Rutter, 1983) underscores the need for research on the variables that moderate (buffer) a child's/adolescent's response to life stress. Stress-buffering refers to a variable's ability to protect an individual from the negative effects of a high level of life stress (S. Cohen & Wills, 1985). In the child/adolescent literature, the overwhelming majority of studies concerned with stress-buffering have tested the effects of social support (e.g., Barrera, 1981; Burke & Weir, 1978; Gad & Johnson, 1980; Greenberg, Siegel, & Leitch, 1983; Hotaling, Atwell, & Linsky, 1978; Kaplan, Robbins, & Martin, 1983; Sandler, 1980). Other studies have tested the stress-buffering roles of attachment to parents (Greenberg et al., 1983), internal locus of control (Siddique & D'Arcy, 1984), specific coping strategies (Wills, 1986), and positive life events (L. Cohen et al., 1987; Siegel & Brown, 1988).

Current notions of adolescent development hold that, regardless of psychiatric or medical status, family functioning is a powerful predictor of an adolescent's overall adjustment as well as his or her resistance to the deleterious effects of life stress (e.g., Rutter, 1983). Measurement of families' social climates has been advanced by the work of Moos and Moos (1981), who developed the widely used Family Environment Scales (FES) to assess perceptions of such family variables as cohesiveness and conflict. Several adolescent studies have used the FES and documented the psychological benefits of a positive family environment, independent of life stress. These *direct* effects have been found in nonclinical samples of adolescents (e.g., Bell & Bell, 1982; Billings & Moos, 1983; Burt, Cohen, & Bjorck, 1988; Daniels, Moos, Billings, & Miller, 1987; Farber, Felner, & Primavera, 1985; Felner, Aber, Primavera, & Cauce, 1985; Friedrich, Reams, & Jacobs, 1982; Slater & Haber, 1984) as well as in adolescent psychiatric samples (e.g., Asarnow, Carlson, & Guthrie, 1987), adolescents from families identified as psychiatric risks (e.g., Billings & Moos, 1983; Hirsch et al., 1985), and in samples of chronically ill adolescents (e.g., Hauser, Jacobson, Wertlieb, Brink, & Wentworth, 1985).

Despite the conceptualization of family climate as a potential life stress buffer (e.g., Moos & Moos, 1981; Rutter, 1983), to our knowledge only two studies to date (Boyce et al., 1977; Burt et al., 1988) have specifically examined the life stress-moderating role of a child's/adolescent's family environment, that is, the *statistical interaction* between life stress and family climate in the prediction of psychological or physical functioning. Obviously, some social support studies have indirectly assessed family relations, but as conceptualized by Moos, family climate encompasses a range of processes including relationship, personal growth, and system maintenance variables. Both the Boyce et al. and Burt et al. studies sampled nonclinical populations, with the former employing an exploratory index of family climate and the latter employing the FES.

Boyce et al. (1977) found that young children under high life stress had more severe respiratory illnesses when part of a family characterized by high rather than low adherence to routine. Burt et al. (1988) tested the cross-sectional and longitudinal life stress-moderating effects of FES variables for young adolescents. None of their significant interaction effects supported the hypothesized stress-buffering role of positive family climate. In fact, several effects suggested a stress-*exacerbating* role of positive family climate. Burt et al. speculated that when confronted with a high level of life stress, normal young adolescents who are accustomed to a positive family climate might be at a disadvantage relative to those accustomed to a more negative climate, because the latter are more familiar with disruptive life experiences. Another possibility raised by Burt et al. is that it is the healthy family that responds to an adolescent's disrupted life by increased conflict and decreased cohesiveness.

The generalizability of these findings to high risk samples of adolescents is unknown, however. To our knowledge, no published study to date has examined the stress-moderating effects of family environment on the psychological functioning of chronically ill children or adolescents, including those with spina bifida, the focus of the present study. Despite the recognized importance of family functioning to the handicapped child's adjustment to life stress (e.g., Gallagher, Beckman, & Cross, 1983; Kazak, 1989), there apparently is no empirical data base to guide theory and clinical intervention.

Research on variables that affect spina bifida adolescents' adjustment to life stress requires an appreciation of the physical and behavioral handicaps that characterize this disability. Spina bifida (myelomeningocele) is one of the most common congenital birth defects in the world, with incidence estimates ranging from 0.67 to 2.50 per thousand births, depending on geographical area (Myers & Millsap, 1985). In spina bifida, the spinal column fails to develop fully resulting in a protrusion of neural material in the midline of the newborn's back. The degree of motor and sensory impairment in spina bifida is quite variable, depending on the location of the spinal lesion, insertion and revisions of shunts, orthopedic deformities, and neurological involvement. Most children require some mechanical aids (e.g., wheelchairs, crutches, or braces) to ambulate, and the majority incur bladder and bowel control difficulties. Most research suggests that spina bifida children and adolescents, on average, are within the normal range of intelligence (e.g., Leonard & Freeman, 1981), although learning disabilities and perceptual problems are not uncommon. The extant empirical literature suggests that spina bifida children and adolescents experience significantly more emotional and behavioral problems than nondisabled controls (e.g., Connell & McConnel, 1981; Dorner, 1975, 1976; McAndrew, 1979; Tew & Laurence, 1985).

There are a number of studies that have addressed social-ecological variables as they relate to spina bifida children and adolescents. Most studies report that families of children with spina bifida experience greater degrees of stress than normal comparison families (e.g., Gallagher et al., 1983; Kazak, 1987; Kazak & Marvin, 1984), and that the former families are relatively isolated socially and have smaller, denser social networks (e.g., Kazak, 1987; Kazak & Wilcox, 1984). The extant data, however, suggest no differences in overall marital satisfaction between spina bifida families and controls (e.g., Kazak, 1987; Martin, 1975; Spaulding & Morgan, 1986).

In the present study, adolescents with spina bifida were administered measures of perceived family environment (FES), recent life stress, and psychological distress (anxiety, depression, and self-esteem). The primary purpose of the study was to employ regression analyses to test the direct and life stress-moderating effects of the adolescents' perceived family climate on the distress criteria. Specifically, it was hypothesized that positive family environment (high cohesion, organization, expressiveness, and independence, and low conflict and control) would be negatively related to anxiety and depression and positively related to self-esteem. It was also hypothesized that positive family climate would serve to buffer the deleterious effects of high recent life stress, that is, significant FES × negative events effects in the prediction of the distress criteria. Although Burt et al. (1988) did not find stress-buffering effects for normal adolescents' positive family climate, it was expected that such effects would be obtained for a high-risk sample of adolescents who seemingly require a protective family to cope with high life stress. Other purposes of the study included documenting the specific negative life events recently experienced by spina bifida teen-agers and testing the relationship between recent life stress and the distress criteria.

METHOD

Subjects

Ninety adolescents with a primary diagnosis of spina bifida (34 male and 56 female; 86 Caucasian and 4 black), ranging in age from 12 to 18, were recruited at a large children's hospital in a mid-Atlantic state. Of these, 53 (59%) agreed to participate and obtained their parents' consent. Twenty-one (40%) were male and 32 (60%) were female (M = 15.68 years; SD = 1.94); 50 were Caucasian and 3 were black.

Complete data on the location of the spinal lesion were available for 52 of the 53 respondents. Ten (19%) had thoracic lesions, 39 (75%) had lumbar lesions, and 3 (6%) had sacral lesions. Twenty-three (43%) required a wheelchair, 19 (36%) required braces, crutches, or a walker, and 11 (21%) required no mechanical aid for locomotion. Fifteen (28%) of the respondents had a shunt, and the remaining 38 (72%) did not. Forty-two (79%) attended a public school; of these, 11 used a resource room in those schools. The remaining adolescents attended a private or parochial school (9%) or a special type of school (12%).

Mothers of 20 randomly selected respondents were asked over the phone to report on the educational background of themselves and the respondents' fathers. The following scale was used: (1) *less than high school,* (2) *finished high school,* (3) *some college,* (4) *finished college,* and (5) *education beyond college.* The average of the scores for both parents was 2.88 (SD = 1.06).

Respondents Versus Nonrespondents

Two-tailed t tests were computed to compare those adolescents who participated in the study with those who did not. Respondents and nonrespondents were compared on the following variables obtained from the hospital's medical files: sex, age, locomotion status (wheelchair, braces/walker/crutches, no mechanical aid), level of myelomeningocele, neurogenic bowel, and shunt status. No significant differences were obtained (all ts < 1.85).

Measures[3]

Demographic and Medical Information

Most of the demographic and medical information was obtained from the hospital's medical files. This information included sex, age, the presence of bladder and bowel control problems, the presence and type of shunt, and the level of spinal impairment. Information about the type of school the subjects attended, their grade in school, and their main means of locomotion was obtained from a brief self-report questionnaire.

[3]The questionnaire battery included exploratory measures of social support and social network. These measures and data obtained from them are not described in this article.

Recent Life Events

The Adolescent Life Experiences Survey (ALES), a 46-item self-report questionnaire designed specifically for adolescents, was administered as the measure of recent life events. This questionnaire is a slightly longer version of the 39-item Junior High Life Experiences Survey (JHLES) developed by Swearingen and Cohen (1985b). Subjects checked which life events had occurred in the past 6 months and indicated each experienced event's impact (negative, neutral, or positive) at the time of occurrence. The ALES was scored by unit scores (a simple count) of the number of self-rated positive, neutral, and negative life events, respectively, experienced by each subject. The unit scoring method has been found more efficient and predictive than normative methods based on psychologist-judges' ratings of the desirability or the life change associated with each event (Swearingen & Cohen, 1985b). L. Cohen et al. (1987) have demonstrated the JHLES' test–retest reliability and validity (parental confirmation of reported events). The JHLES has already been used successfully in three large-scale longitudinal studies of adolescents (L. Cohen et al., 1987; Glyshaw, Cohen, & Towbes, 1989; Swearingen & Cohen, 1985a).

Previous studies of adolescent life stress adjustment have shown the value of testing for differential effects as a function of negative event *controllability* (L. Cohen et al., 1987; Swearingen & Cohen, 1985a). Swearingen and Cohen (1985b) surveyed child clinicians to determine which JHLES events are uncontrollable or controllable by young adolescents. (For example, the item "my mother or father lost a job" is classified as uncontrollable, whereas the item "I ran away from home" is classified as controllable.) For the seven new items (e.g., "I began a job") added to the JHLES for relevance to middle adolescents, controllability classification was based on categorization by eight advanced clinical psychology graduate students. Seventy-five percent (6/8) or greater agreement was required for a new event to be categorized as controllable or uncontrollable. Therefore, in addition to total number of experienced negative events, each subject also had scores for number of controllable negative events and number of uncontrollable negative events, respectively.

Perceived Family Environment

The short form of Moos and Moos's (1981) Family Environment Scale (FES) was used to assess perceived family environment. The FES short-form scales are very highly correlated (most *r*s = about .90) with their long-form counterparts (Moos & Moos, 1981).

The following subscales were used: Cohesion, Expressiveness, Conflict, Independence, Organization, Control, and Achievement, the last for exploratory purposes. Each subscale has four items, and each item was rated on a 4-point scale, (1) *very false,* (2) *somewhat false,* (3) *somewhat true,* and (4) *very true.* Each subscale was scored by computing the mean response for those four items. These FES short-form scales were used successfully in a previous large-scale longitudinal study of adolescents' life stress adjustment (Burt et al., 1988).

Psychological Distress

Three self-report measures were used to assess psychological distress, broadly defined. Subjects' trait anxiety was measured by the Trait Anxiety Inventory for Children (Spielberger, 1973). This 20-item measure assesses relatively stable levels of anxiety among children and adolescents. Depression was measured by the Child Depression Inventory (Kovacs, 1980/1981), a 27-item questionnaire designed to assess depressive symptoms that have occurred in the past 2-week period. (One item concerning suicide potential was deleted at the request of the hospital research review committee, resulting in 26 items.) Self-esteem was measured by the Coopersmith Self-Esteem Inventory, Form B (Coopersmith, 1982). This 25-item questionnaire is a shortened version of the original scale, comprised of the items that have the highest correlations with the original scale's total score. Previous research has found these three widely used measures are sensitive to adolescents' recent life stress (L. Cohen et al., 1987; Swearingen & Cohen, 1985a).

Procedure

Names and addresses of all adolescents treated for spina bifida at the hospital were obtained. Upon admission to the hospital, patients' guardians signed a waiver allowing access to the medical file for research purposes. All potential subjects were mailed (a) a cover letter to parents and a cover letter to the adolescent; (b) a parental consent form and an adolescent consent form; (c) an instruction letter; (d) questionnaires; and (e) a postage-paid return envelope. Questionnaires could be completed in any order.

RESULTS

Descriptive Data

Means and standard deviations for the measures are presented in Table I.[4] The most frequently experienced negative life events were having a close family member die (17% of the respondents), arguing more with parents (11%), having a sibling leave home (9%), and having a close friend die (9%). The most frequently experienced positive life events were making a new friend (64%), having an outstanding personal achievement (e.g., award) (42%), being accepted into an extracurricular activity (25%), and beginning a job (19%).[5]

Correlational Analysis

The correlations are presented in Table II. As a conservative strategy, only correlations that were significant at $p < .01$ or lower are highlighted in this table and reported in the text. As is evident from this table, negative life events were significantly related to anxiety, depression, and self-esteem in the expected directions. (The correlations for controllable and uncontrollable negative events were virtually identical.) Positive and neutral life events were unrelated to the distress criteria.

[4]Separate 2 (Sex) × 2 (Age: 12–15 vs. 16–18) multivariate analyses of variance (MANOVAs) were conducted on the following dependent variable sets: (a) the seven FES scores; (b) the life events scores (respective number of negative, positive, and neutral life events); and (c) the psychological distress measures (anxiety, depression, and self-esteem). The FES MANOVA revealed a near significant effect for sex, $F(7, 43) = 2.08$, $p < .07$, with significant ANOVA results for Independence and Control (Fs > 4.50, ps $< .05$). Males' scores on Independence ($M = 3.03$) and Control ($M = 2.91$) were higher than those obtained by females (Ms $= 2.74$ and 2.45, respectively). No other MANOVA revealed significant or near significant sex, age, or sex × age effects (all Fs < 1.95).

[5]Fishers Exact Probability analyses were performed on individual ALES items to determine which life events were differentially experienced and perceived as negative by the spina bifida teenagers in this study and by a comparison group of able-bodied adolescents (Glyshaw et al., 1989) who also completed the ALES. These analyses, which were conducted separately by respondent sex, revealed very few significant or near significant group differences in specific negative event occurrences. Specifically, able-bodied males reported arguing more with their parents (18%) and experiencing the breakup with a girlfriend (14%) as negative events more often than the spina bifida males (0% for both events; $p < .05$ and $p < .09$, respectively). On the other hand, spina bifida males were more likely to have a brother or sister leave the household (10 vs. 2%; $p < .10$). Females with spina bifida experienced divorce or separation of parents (6%) and the loss of a job (6%) more often than did the comparison females (1% for both events; $p < .06$ for both events). These differences in negative event occurrence should be interpreted with caution, because a total of 92 analyses were conducted (46 ALES items, each sex analyzed separately).

Table I. Means and Standard Deviations for Life Events, Perceived Family Environment, and Psychological Distress

Variable	*M*	*SD*
Total negative events	1.56	2.10
Controllable negative events	0.50	0.91
Uncontrollable negative events	0.94	1.30
Positive events	3.16	2.38
Neutral events	0.78	1.03
Perceived cohesion	3.14	0.57
Perceived expressiveness	2.42	0.63
Perceived conflict	2.24	0.69
Perceived independence	2.85	0.47
Perceived achievement	2.77	0.48
Perceived organization	2.95	0.54
Perceived control	2.63	0.72
Anxiety	34.81	6.66
Depression	8.87	7.37
Self-esteem	15.42	5.69

Scatterplots were generated relating the FES scores to depression, anxiety, and self-esteem. No curvilinear relationships were revealed in this visual inspection of the data. The correlations for the FES scales were in the expected directions. In general, negative family climate was positively related to distress, whereas positive family climate was negatively related to distress. Specifically, Conflict was positively related to depression and negatively related to self-esteem. Independence was positively related to self-esteem. Similarly, Cohesion and Expressiveness were positively related to self-esteem, while the former was also negatively related to depression. Control, Organization, and Achievement were not significantly related to any of the distress criteria at $p < .01$.

Regression Analyses

Multivariate regression analyses were conducted, with depression, anxiety, and self-esteem constituting the multivariate criterion set. A multivariate regression analysis is analogous to a canonical correlation. The distress measures were analyzed as a multivariate set because of their high intercorrelations (see Table II) and to guard against Type 1 error. As an additional control, significant effects on the individual distress criteria are not reported unless the multivariate analysis was significant or near significant.

For each analysis, the predictor variables were (a) number of negative life events; (b) an FES score; and (c) the a × b interaction effect. Each main effect was tested with the other predictor statistically controlled (i.e., the main

Table II. Correlations Among Life Events, Perceived Family Environment, and Psychological Distress

Variable	2	3	4	5	6	7	8	9	10	11	12	13
1. Negative events	$.48^b$	.03	−.13	−.16	.08	−.29	−.21	.03	−.13	$.53^b$	$.55^b$	$-.39^a$
2. Positive events		−.30	.14	−.06	−.14	−.15	−.11	.29	−.27	.14	−.11	.02
3. Neutral events			−.11	−.17	.06	.13	−.06	−.12	−.13	.05	.01	−.13
4. Cohesion				$.43^b$	$-.40^a$	.14	.06	$.43^b$	−.21	.05	$-.42^a$	$.38^a$
5. Expressiveness					$-.35^a$	$.43^b$	.15	.15	.09	−.14	−.20	$.38^a$
6. Conflict						−.24	.33	−.17	$.43^b$	.34	$.42^a$	$-.41^a$
7. Independence							.11	−.01	−.13	−.29	−.30	$.44^b$
8. Achievement								.16	.24	.00	−.16	.10
9. Organization									−.10	.09	−.12	.14
10. Control										.17	.32	−.18
11. Anxiety											$.61^b$	$-.65^b$
12. Depression												$-.74^b$
13. Self-esteem												

$^a p < .01$.
$^b p < .001$.

Table III. Multivariate Regression Analyses of Psychological Distress on Negative Life Events and Perceived Family Environment

	Main effects[a]		
FES predictor	Negative events	FES	Interaction
Expressiveness	8.92[e]	3.12[c]	0.83
Conflict	10.14[e]	5.66[d]	5.53[d]
Independence	9.15[e]	2.23[b]	2.68[b]
Control	16.71[e]	8.10[e]	5.15[d]
Cohesion	9.26[e]	6.84[e]	5.06[d]
Organization	9.34[e]	1.51	1.82
Achievement	8.98[e]	0.37	0.33

[a]FES = Family Environment Scale. Each main effect predictor was tested with the other predictor controlled. For all analyses, $F(3, 41)$.
[b]$p < .10$.
[c]$p < .05$.
[d]$p < .01$.
[e]$p < .001$.

effects of the FES scores were tested after statistical control of recent life stress). Sex and age were entered as a multivariate first-step predictor in every regression analysis. (All regression analyses were also conducted with level of spinal lesion (dichotomized by a median split) entered as the first predictor, immediately before sex and age. Statistical control of lesion level had no effect on the results obtained.) Significant interaction effects are graphed in accordance with J. Cohen and Cohen (1975); predictor-criterion regression lines are portrayed for various levels of the other predictor conceptualized as the moderator variable.

Table III presents the results of the multivariate regression analyses. Table IV presents the FES main and interaction effects on the individual distress criteria.

Main Effects of Negative Life Events

Negative life events were a significant main effect predictor in every regression analysis involving an FES score (see Table III). The univariate analyses revealed that, with the exception of a few suppression effects, recent life stress was positively related to depression and anxiety and negatively related to self-esteem (Fs > 6.29, ps $< .05$; $.09 < R^2 < .31$).[6]

[6]According to J. Cohen and Cohen (1975, pp. 89-90), one form of *net suppression* in a regression analysis is characterized by an inconsistency between the sign (direction) for a predictor's partial regression coefficient and the sign for that predictor's correlation with the criterion. It can occur when a predictor is tested after statistical control of other predictor variables (i.e., sex and age, and an FES variable) and it is not uncommon in multivariate life stress studies (e.g., L. Cohen et al., 1987).

Main Effects of Perceived Family Environment

As is evident from Table III, significant or near significant multivariate main effects for FES Expressiveness, Conflict, Control, Cohesion, and Independence were found in the regression analyses. All significant univariate effects were in the hypothesized directions. With the exception of the Expressiveness effects, the FES main effects were qualified by significant interaction effects involving negative life events.

FES Conflict and Control were positively related to anxiety and depression and negatively related to self-esteem. Expressiveness, Cohesion, and Independence were positively related to self-esteem. Expressiveness and anxiety were negatively related. Cohesion and depression were also negatively related (see Table IV).

Life Stress × Family Environment Effects

Significant or near significant multivariate interaction effects were found in the regression analyses involving Conflict, Control, Cohesion, and Indepen-

Table IV. FES Main and Interaction Effects From Regression Analyses of Anxiety, Depression, and Self-Esteem on Negative Life Events and Perceived Family Environment[a]

	Anxiety		Depression		Self-esteem	
FES predictor	F	R^2	F	R^2	F	R^2
Conflict	10.65[d]	.11	10.78[d]	.13	13.27[e]	.18
Conflict × negative events	1.18	.01	5.18[c]	.06	0.70	.01
Independence	1.59	.02	0.94	.01	6.91[c]	.09
Independence × negative events	7.20[d]	.08	3.68[b]	.05	4.69[c]	.07
Achievement	0.12	.00	0.47	.01	0.00	.00
Achievement × negative events	0.37	.00	0.71	.01	0.06	.00
Organization	0.21	.00	1.46	.02	1.18	.03
Organization × negative events	0.55	.01	1.51	.02	0.21	.00
Expressiveness	3.78[b]	.04	0.47	.01	6.67[d]	.10
Expressiveness × negative events	2.51	.03	0.86	.01	1.07	.02
Cohesion	0.11	.00	9.56[d]	.12	7.76[d]	.12
Cohesion × negative events	0.05	.00	2.66	.03	2.34	.03
Control	4.34[c]	.05	19.66[e]	.20	5.72[c]	.09
Control × negative events	0.03	.00	11.88[e]	.10	0.48	.01

[a]FES = Family Environment Scale. Each effect was tested with statistical control of negative life events.
[b]$p < .10$.
[c]$p < .05$.
[d]$p < .01$.
[e]$p < .001$.

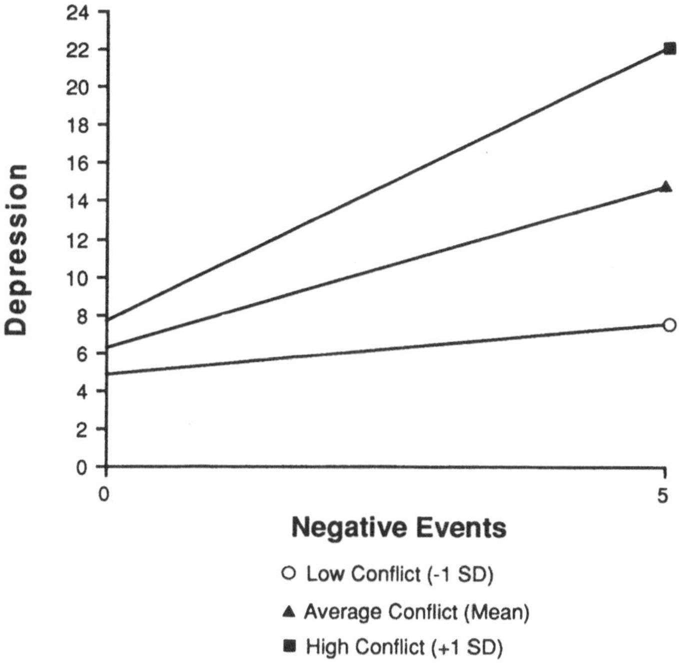

Fig. 1. Regression of depression on negative events for high, average, and low Conflict values.

dence (see Table III). None of the univariate predictions involving Cohesion were significant, however (ser Table IV).

For both Conflict and Control, the interaction effects were significant in the prediction of depression only (see Table IV). Figures 1 and 2 reveal the hypothesized stress-buffering effects of low FES Conflict and Control; the relationship between negative events and depression becomes decreasingly positive at lower levels of Conflict and Control.

The interaction involving FES Independence was significant in the prediction of anxiety and self-esteem, and approached significance in the prediction of depression (see Table IV). Figure 3 shows that at low levels of life stress, high Independence is slightly protective with respect to anxiety, but that at high levels of life stress, high Independence is slightly detrimental. The interaction for depression was virtually identical to that shown in Figure 3. Figure 4 shows that at low levels of life stress, high Independence is protective with respect to self-esteem, but that at high levels of life stress, self-esteem is vulnerable regardless of perceived Independence.

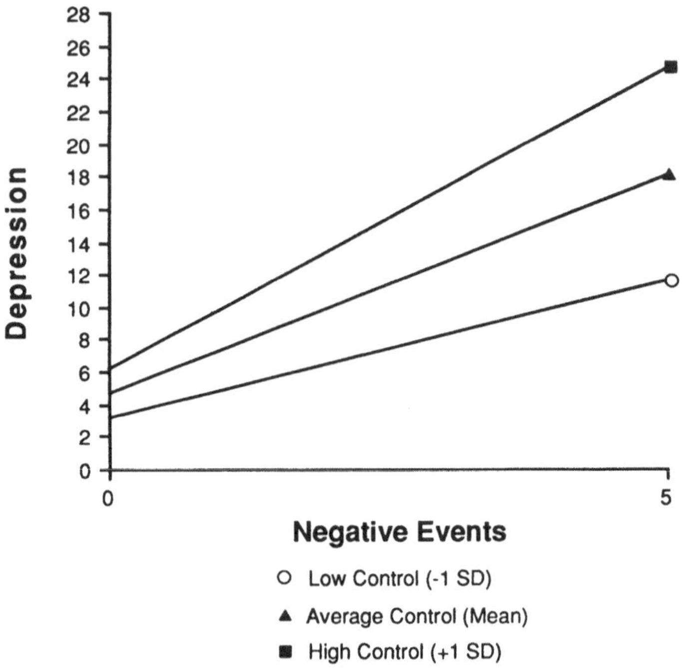

Fig. 2. Regression of depression on negative events for high, average, and low Control values.

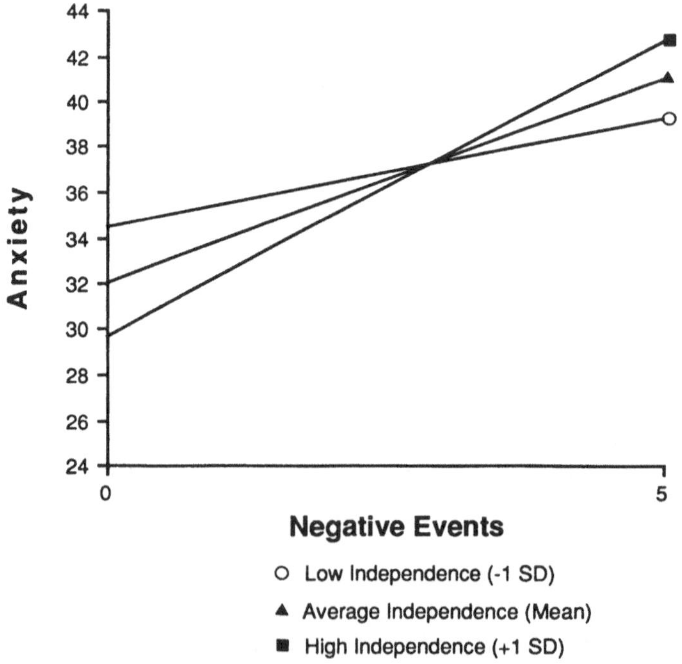

Fig. 3. Regression of anxiety on negative events for high, average, and low Independence values.

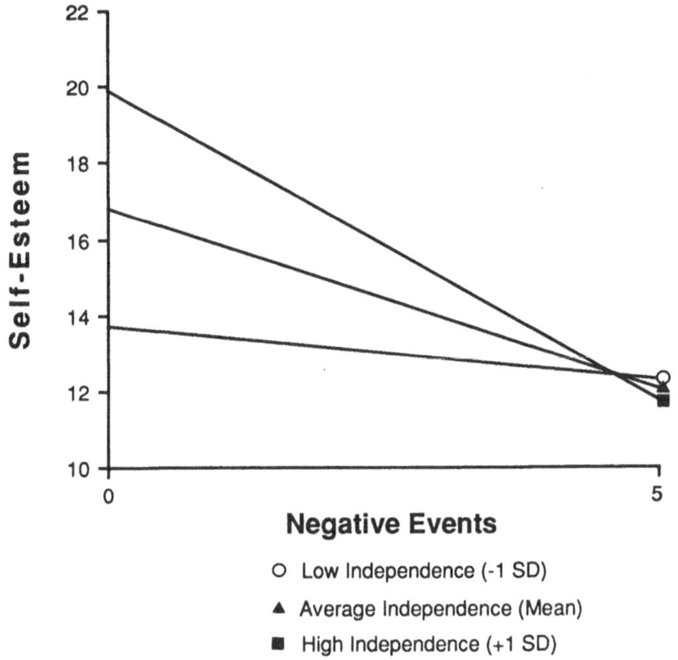

Fig. 4. Regression of self-esteem on negative events for high, average, and low Independence values.

Controllable Versus Uncontrollable Negative Events

For exploratory purposes, separate multivariate regression analyses were conducted, substituting controllable negative events, and then uncontrollable negative events, as a predictor variable in place of the *total* negative event score. These analyses revealed consistently significant main effects for both controllable and uncontrollable negative events on the distress criteria. The substitution of controllable or uncontrollable negative events as the life stress predictor had no impact on the FES main effects. As before, significant multivariate main effects were found for FES Expresiveness, Conflict, Control, Cohesion, and Independence, regardless of whether controllable or uncontrollable negative events were included in the prediction model.

On the other hand, the Negative Events × FES interaction effects did differ as a function of which life stress predictor was tested. The stress-buffering effects for low Conflict and Control, in the prediction of depression, were found only in the uncontrollable stress analyses; these interactions were nonsignificant in the controllable stress analyses. In addition, a new stress-buffering effect for high Cohesion, in the prediction of depression, was found in the uncontrollable stress analysis, whereas this interaction was nonsignificant in the controllable stress analysis. All of the significant

Independence interaction effects found in the original analyses were duplicated in the controllable stress analyses, but emerged nonsignificant in the uncontrollable stress analyses.

DISCUSSION

The adolescents' scores on the family environment, life events, and psychological distress measures were very similar to those obtained in previous studies of normal samples of adolescents (e.g., Burt et al., 1988; L. Cohen et al., 1987; Glyshaw et al., 1989; Swearingen & Cohen, 1985a). For example, in Burt et al.'s study of young adolescents, the mean number of negative events (also reported in the late spring) was 1.53 (SD = 2.13), whereas it was 1.56 (SD = 2.10) in the present study. Mean depression (also assessed by the CDI) was 8.54 (SD = 7.03) in the former study and 8.87 (SD = 7.37) in the present study. Mean FES Conflict and Control were 2.32 (SD = 0.69) and 2.63 (SD = 0.52), respectively, in the former study and 2.24 (SD = 0.69) and 2.63 (SD = 0.72) in the present study.

There are a number of other findings that parallel those obtained with previous samples of adolescents. Both correlational and regression analyses document that negative life events are positively related to anxiety and depression and negatively related to self-esteem, whereas positive and neutral life events are nonsignificant predictors, patterns previously obtained with a variety of child and adolescent samples (Johnson, 1986). As hypothesized, both correlational and regression analyses document that, in general, positive family climate is related to the adolescents' psychological adjustment, a pattern previously obtained with clinical and nonclinical samples of children and adolescents (e.g., Asarnow et al., 1987; Billings & Moos, 1983; Burt et al., 1988; Daniels et al., 1987; Hauser et al., 1985; Hirsch et al., 1985; Slater & Haber, 1984). Even scores on the global index of parents' education (M = 2.88) are quite comparable to those reported in a recent large-scale study of normal adolescents (M = 3.14; Glyshaw et al., 1989).

The present study obtained a near significant multivariate main effect for FES Independence. At the univariate level, this main effect is significant in the prediction of self-esteem, although it is qualified by a significant Life Stress × Independence interaction effect. Similar main effects for FES Independence have also been reported in previous studies of high-risk children and adolescents, such as Hauser et al.'s (1985) study of diabetic adolescents, Felner et al.'s (1985) study of minority adolescents, and Hirsch et al.'s (1985) study of children of depressed parents. Interestingly, analyses of "normal" children and adolescents have not revealed significant FES Independence main effects on measures of psychological adjustment (e.g., Burt et al., 1988; Hirsch et al., 1985). The differential role of perceived family independence in normal versus high risk or physically handicapped children and adolescents might be due in part to the differential ability of the individuals to achieve independence from their families. For example, many physically disabled adolescents must rely on family members to help with the activities of daily life (e.g., dressing and bathing)—tasks that able-bodied adolescents accomplish with ease. Therefore, achieving independence is a relatively greater accomplishment for the disabled (and high risk) adolescent, and as such, it (or the *perception* of same) seems to contribute more powerfully to self-esteem—at least at relatively low levels of recent life stress.

Only one other published study to date tested the life stress-moderating effects of adolescents' perceived family environment (Burt et al., 1988). In this longitudinal study of able-bodied young adolescents, no analysis revealed the hypothesized stress-buffering role of positive family climate. In fact, some analyses suggested the stress-*exacerbating* role of high FES Organization, Cohesion, and Expression, and low FES Control, on the criterion measures of depression, anxiety, and self-esteem. As mentioned earlier, they presented two possible explanations for these unexpected results. First, adolescents from positive family environments might be less familiar with disruptive life situations and therefore might be more adversely affected by them when they occur. Second, healthy families might respond to a high number of adolescent negative life events with increased control and decreased cohesion.

The interaction findings of the present study stand in sharp contrast to those obtained by Burt et al. (1988). The discrepant life stress × FES effects are even more compelling given that, in every other way, the descriptive and predictive findings involving the life events, FES, and distress measures are virtually identical to those reported in the Burt et al. study as well as in other related studies of adolescents.

Specifically, as hypothesized, low levels of FES Conflict and Control serve as life stress buffers in the prediction of depression. These stress-buffering effects were found only in the context of *uncontrollable* negative events, as was a stress-buffering effect for high FES Cohesion, also in the prediction of depression. One possible explanation for these findings is that families who are able to deal with the stress of raising a disabled adolescent and still maintain a positive family environment (low Conflict and Control, high Cohesion) are better equipped to cope appropriately with additional (uncontrollable) life stress. That is, dealing with the stress of the disability has, in effect, primed the family to respond constructively to other stressful situations. When faced with a high number of uncontrollable negative events, these families are able to *protect* the handicapped adolescent from feelings of depression.

Burt et al.'s speculations concerning the stress-moderating role of family environment are seemingly not applicable to these spina bifida teen-agers and perhaps other high-risk adolescents: (a) The teen-agers in our study are all too familiar with life disruption, independent of family climate, and therefore a negative family environment does not serve to "inoculate" them from high levels of life stress; and (b) whereas healthy families of able-bodied teen-agers might respond to high life stress with decreased cohesion and increased control, for handicapped teen-agers and perhaps other high-risk adolescents, whose resilience to life stress is brittle, it is the healthy family that responds in a protective rather than confrontive manner.

Unexpectedly, a high level of FES Independence serves as a life stress exacerbator in the prediction of depression and anxiety. These effects were found only in the context of *controllable* negative events.

In retrospect, this data pattern can be easily explained. One might assume that for these youngsters, achieving and maintaining a sense of independence is stressful in and of itself. During periods of low life stress, these adolescents might be able to maintain a relatively high level of family independence, but during stressful times, it might be necessary for them, in light of their physical limitations, to depend more on family members for support and assistance. At such times, the family that is perceived as placing a high value on independence might cause the spina bifida adolescent to feel that he or she is being pushed beyond his or her capabilities.

Additional studies are needed to clarify the findings that low FES Conflict and Control, and high Cohesion, serve as life stress buffers for uncontrollable stress only, whereas high FES Independence serves as a life stress exacerbator for controllable stress only. Burt et al.'s (1988) study of normal adolescents failed to find any meaningful FES pattern associated with event controllability. The present study's pattern is difficult to interpret in the absence of a more sensitive categorization of negative event type, because even those events *within* a controllability category are themselves extremely heterogeneous with respect to content and theme (Monroe & Peterman, 1988).

Unfortunately, Moos and Moos's (1981) classification of the FES scales into relationship (Cohesion, Expressiveness, Conflict), personal growth (Independence, Achievement), and system maintenance (Organization, Control) dimensions do not contribute much to the interpretation of the FES interaction effects. Specifically, stress-buffering effects were found for family environments perceived as positive on the first and the last dimensions. Burt et al.'s (1988) findings were similarly insensitive to these global environmental dimensions.

Methodological Limitations

Interpretation of the findings must be made in light of methodological considerations. The present sample was primarily middle-class, Caucasian, and intellectually competent. The family environment and criterion measures were based on the adolescents' self-reports, and future research should include more objective, behavior-based indices of family environment and psychological adjustment. The ALES does not adequately capture chronic, daily stress, stress that might be especially relevant to the lives of physically handicapped youth. The criterion measures allowed for comparison to studies conducted with able-bodied adolescents, but they are not appropriate for conclusions regarding "psychiatric status."

The present study employed a cross-sectional design, and therefore the data cannot address the causal relations among the variables. Previous longitudinal studies of able-bodied adolescents have cast doubt on the causal role of recent life stress and perceived family environment in the prediction of psychological functioning (Burt et al., 1988; L. Cohen et al., 1987; Swearingen & Cohen, 1985a), although there is no published study to date that bears on the etiological role of these variables for *at-risk* adolescents. Although our method of testing and interpreting stress-moderating (interaction) effects is normative in the life stress field (S. Cohen & Wills, 1985), it should be acknowledged that this method has not gone unchallenged (e.g., Kessler, 1983; Turner, 1983). The Burt et al. data do not provide an ideal comparison, in that they were collected several years ago and pertain to young adolescents only (although the present study's analyses statistically controlled for respondent age and sex). Finally, without other clinically identified comparison groups, it is unclear if the present findings are generalizable to other physically handicapped and at-risk teen-age samples.

Major Conclusions

The spina bifida teen-agers in this study were highly similar to able-bodied teen-agers sampled in previous studies on measures of recent life stress, perceived family environment, and anxiety, depression, and self-esteem. As expected, recent life stress was a positive predictor, and positive family climate a negative predictor, of the distress criteria. Low family conflict and control served as life stress buffers, a finding that is consistent with the theoretical literature but inconsistent with the findings of the one previous study of able-bodied adolescents that specifically tested these effects (Burt et al., 1988). In addition, the data pattern suggested that high family independence served as a life stress exacerbator for these handicapped adolescents. The results suggest that the family environments of able-bodied and spina bifida teen-agers are important moderators of their reactions to recent life stress, but in strikingly different ways.

REFERENCES

Asarnow, J., Carlson, G., & Guthrie, D. (1987). Coping strategies, self-perceptions, hopelessness, and perceived family environments in depressed and suicidal children. *Journal of Consulting and Clinical Psychology, 55,* 361-366.

Barrera, M. (1981). Social support in the adjustment of pregnant adolescents. In B. Gottlieb (Ed.), *Social networks and social support* (pp. 69-96). Beverly Hills: Sage.

Bedell, J., Giordani, B., Amour, J., Tavormina, J., & Boll, T. (1977). Life stress and the psychological and medical adjustment of chronically ill children. *Journal of Psychosomatic Research, 21,* 237-242.

Bell, L., & Bell, D. (1982). Family climate and the role of the female adolescent: Determinants of adolescent functioning. *Family Relations, 31,* 519-527.

Billings, A., & Moos, R. (1983). Comparisons of children of depressed and nondepressed parents: A social-environmental perspective. *Journal of Abnormal Child Psychology, 11,* 463-486.

Boyce, W., Jensen, E., Cassel, J., Collier, A., Smith, A., & Ramey, C. (1977). Influence of life events and family routines on childhood respiratory tract illness. *Pediatrics, 60,* 609-615.

Burke, R., & Weir, T. (1978). Benefits to adolescents of informal helping relationships with their parents and peers. *Psychological Reports, 42,* 1175-1184.

Burt, C., Cohen, L., & Bjorck, J. (1988). Perceived family environment as a moderator of young adolescents' life stress adjustment. *American Journal of Community Psychology, 16,* 101-122.

Cohen, J., & Cohen, P. (1975). *Applied multiple regression/correlation analysis for the behavioral sciences.* Hillsdale, NJ: Erlbaum.

Cohen, L., Burt, C., & Bjorck, J. (1987). Life stress and adjustment: Effects of life events experienced by young adolescents and their parents. *Developmental Psychology, 23,* 583-592.

Cohen, S., & Wills, T. (1985). Stress, social support, and the buffering hypothesis. *Psychological Bulletin, 98,* 310-357.

Compas, B. (1987). Coping with stress during childhood and adolescence. *Psychological Bulletin, 101,* 393-403.

Connell, H., & McConnel, T. (1981). Psychiatric sequelae in children treated operatively for hydrocephalus in infancy. *Developmental Medicine and Child Neurology, 23,* 505-517.

Coopersmith, S. (1982). *Self-esteem inventories.* Palo Alto: Consulting Psychologists Press.

Daniels, D., Moos, R., Billings, A., & Miller, J. (1987). Psychosocial risk and resistance factors among children with chronic illness, healthy siblings, and healthy controls. *Journal of Abnormal Child Psychology, 15,* 295-308.

Dorner, S. (1975). The relationship of physical handicap to stress in families with an adolescent with spina bifida. *Developmental Medicine and Child Neurology, 17,* 765-776.

Dorner, S. (1976). Adolescents with spina bifida: How they see their situation. *Archives of Disease in Childhood, 51,* 439-444.

Farber, S., Felner, R., & Primavera, J. (1985). Parental separation/divorce and adolescents: An examination of factors mediating adaptation. *American Journal of Community Psychology, 13,* 171-185.

Felner, R., Aber, M., Primavera, J., & Cauce, A. (1985). Adaptation and vulnerability in high-risk adolescents: An examination of environmental mediators. *American Journal of Community Psychology, 13,* 365-379.

Friedrich, W., Reams, R., & Jacobs, J. (1982). Depression and suicide ideation in early adolescents. *Journal of Youth and Adolescence, 11,* 403-407.

Gad, M., & Johnson, J. (1980). Correlates of adolescent life stress as related to race, SES, and levels of perceived social support. *Journal of Clinical Child Psychology, 9,* 13-16.

Gallagher, J., Beckman, P., & Cross, A. (1983). Families of handicapped children: Sources of stress and its amelioration. *Exceptional Children, 50,* 10-19.

Garmezy, N. (1983). Stressors of childhood. In N. Garmezy & M. Rutter (Eds.), *Stress, coping and development in children* (pp. 43-84). New York: McGraw-Hill.

Garmezy, N., & Rutter, M. (Eds.). (1983). *Stress, coping and development in children.* New York: McGraw-Hill.
Glyshaw, K., Cohen, L., & Towbes, L. (1989). *Coping strategies and psychological adjustment: Prospective analyses of early and middle adolescents.* Manuscript submitted for publication.
Greenberg, M., Siegel, J., & Leitch, C. (1983). The nature and importance of attachment relationships to parent and peers during adolescence. *Journal of Youth and Adolescence, 12,* 373-386.
Hauser, S., Jacobson, A., Wertlieb, D., Brink, S., & Wentworth, S. (1985). The contribution of family environment to perceived competence and illness adjustment in diabetic and acutely ill adolescents. *Family Relations, 34,* 99-108.
Hirsch, B., Moos, R., & Reischl, T. (1985). Psychosocial adjustment of adolescent children of a depressed, arthritic, or normal parent. *Journal of Abnormal Psychology, 94,* 154-164.
Hotaling, G., Atwell, S., & Linsky, A. (1978). Adolescent life changes and illness: A comparison of three models. *Journal of Youth and Adolescence, 7,* 393-403.
Johnson, J. (1986). *Life events as stressors in childhood and adolescence.* Beverly Hills: Sage.
Kaplan, H., Robbins, C., & Martin, S. (1983). Antecedents of psychological distress in young adults: Self-rejection, deprivation of social support, and life events. *Journal of Health and Social Behavior, 24,* 230-244.
Kazak, A. (1987). Families with disabled children: Stress and social networks in three samples. *Journal of Abnormal Child Psychology, 15,* 137-146.
Kazak, A. (1989). Families of chronically ill children: A systems and social ecological model of adaptation and challenge. *Journal of Consulting and Clinical Psychology, 57,* 25-30.
Kazak, A., & Marvin, R. (1984). Differences, difficulties and adaptation: Stress and social networks in families with a handicapped child. *Family Relations, 33,* 67-77.
Kazak, A., & Wilcox, B. (1984). The structure and function of social support networks in families with handicapped children. *American Journal of Community Psychology, 12,* 645-661.
Kessler, R. (1983). Methodological issues in the study of psychosocial stress. in H. Kaplan (Ed.), *Psychosocial stress: Trends in theory and research* (pp. 267-341). New York: Academic Press.
Kovacs, M. (1980/1981). Rating scales to assess depression in school-age children. *Acta-Paedopsychiatry, 46,* 305-315.
Leonard, C., & Freeman, J. (1981). Spina bifida: A new disease. *Pediatrics, 68,* 136-137.
Martin, P. (1975). Marital breakdown in families of patients with spina bifida cystica. *Developmental Medicine and Child Neurology, 17,* 757-764.
McAndrew, I. (1979). Adolescents and young people with spina bifida. *Developmental Medicine and Child Neurology, 21,* 619-629.
Monroe, S., & Peterman, A. (1988). Life stress and psychopathology. In L. Cohen (Ed.), *Life events and psychological functioning: Theoretical and methodological issues* (pp. 31-63). Newbury Park, CA: Sage.
Moos, R., & Moos, B. (1981). *Family Environment Scale manual.* Palo Alto, CA: Consulting Psychologists Press.
Myers, G., & Millsap, M. (1985). Spina bifida. In N. Hobbs & J. Perrin (Eds.), *Issues in the care of children with chronic illness* (pp. 214-235). San Francisco: Jossey-Bass.
Rutter, M. (1983). Stress, coping and development. In N. Garmezy & M. Rutter (Eds.), *Stress, coping and development in children* (pp. 1-41). New York: McGraw-Hill.
Sandler, I. (1980). Social support resources, stress, and maladjustment of poor children. *American Journal of Community Psychology, 8,* 41-52.
Siddique, C., & D'Arcy, C. (1984). Adolescence, stress, and psychological well-being. *Journal of Youth and Adolescence, 13,* 459-473.
Siegel, J., & Brown, J. (1988). A prospective study of stressful circumstances, illness symptoms, and depressed mood among adolescents. *Developmental Psychology, 24,* 715-721.
Slater, E., & Haber, J. (1984). Adolescent adjustment following divorce as a function of familial conflict. *Journal of Consulting and Clinical Psychology, 51,* 920-921.
Spaulding, B., & Morgan, S. (1986). Spina bifida children and their parents: A population prone to family dysfunction? *Journal of Pediatric Psychology, 11,* 359-374.

Spielberger, C. (1973). *State-Trait Anxiety Inventory for Children: Preliminary manual.* Palo Alto, CA: Consulting Psychologists Press.

Swearingen, E., & Cohen, L. (1985a). Life events and psychological distress: A prospective study of young adolescents. *Developmental Psychology, 21,* 1045-1054.

Swearingen, E., & Cohen, L. (1985b). Measurement of adolescents' life events: The Junior High Life Experiences Survey. *American Journal of Community Psychology, 13,* 69-85.

Tew, B., & Laurence, K. (1985). Possible personality problems among 10-year-old spina bifida children. *Child: Care, Health and Development, 11,* 375-390.

Thoits, P. 1983). Dimensions of life events that influence psychological distress: An evaluation and synthesis of the literature. In H. Kaplan (Ed.), *Psychosocial stress: Trends in theory and research* (pp. 33-103). New York: Academic Press.

Turner, R. J. (1983). Direct, indirect, and moderating effects of social support on psychological distress and associated conditions. In H. Kaplan (Ed.), *Psychosocial stress: Trends in theory and research* (pp. 105-155). New York: Academic Press.

Wills, T. (1986). Stress and coping in early adolescence: Relationships to substance use in urban school samples. *Health Psychology, 5,* 503-529.

4

Children with Recurrent Abdominal Pain and Their Parents: More Somatic Complaints, Anxiety, and Depression than Other Patient Families?[1]

Lynn S. Walker and John W. Greene
Vanderbilt University School of Medicine

*Patients presenting with abdominal pain were classified into two groups: the recurrent abdominal pain (RAP) group (*n *= 41), consisting of patients without identifiable organic etiology for abdominal pain, and the organic group (*n *= 28), consisting of patients with organic findings (primarily ulcer-related conditions). A control group of well patients (*n *= 41) also participated. RAP and organic patients had higher anxiety, depression, and somatic complaints than well patients, but did not differ from each other. Anxiety, depression, and somatization were greater in RAP mothers than well mothers. Father symptomatology did not differ for the groups. Results suggest that psychological distress does not discriminate between patients with and without identifiable organic etiology for abdominal pain. The high levels of anxiety and depression in RAP and organic patients suggest that they should be targeted in efforts to address "the new hidden morbidity" in pediatrics.*

Recurrent abdominal pain (RAP) is one of the most common symptoms of childhood, with an estimated prevalence of 10 to 15% in school-aged chil-

[1]This research was supported by a grant from the Vanderbilt University Research Council. The authors are grateful for the assistance of the Vanderbilt Division of Pediatric Gastroenterology which made this research possible. Thanks to Leonard Bickman and William Altemeier for comments on a draft of the manuscript.

dren (Apley 1975; Apley & Naish, 1958; Liebman, 1978). RAP is a diagnosis of exclusion; its key feature is the absence of identifiable organic findings to explain the child's repeated episodes of abdominal pain. When the medical evaluation produces negative findings, it is often assumed that the child's symptoms are the manifestation of an emotional disorder. The psychological adjustment of the parents is brought into question by implication when it is suggested that parental anxiety and overprotection reinforce the child's symptoms.

Recent investigations with RAP children provide some empirical evidence supporting the assumption of emotional disturbance in these children and their parents. Several investigations have demonstrated higher levels of anxiety in RAP children compared to healthy children in the community (Apley, 1975; Barr & Feuerstein, 1983; Hodges, Kline, Barbero, & Woodruff, 1985; Wasserman, Whitington, & Rivara, 1988). Furthermore, children with RAP typically have several additional nonspecific physical symptoms (Liebman, 1978, Stone & Barbero, 1970) that increase in number with age, suggesting that these children may reach the criteria for Somatization Disorder by adulthood (Ernst, Routh, & Harper, 1984).

With respect to the parents, mothers of children with RAP report higher levels of anxiety and depression than mothers of children without abdominal pain (Hodges, Kline, Barbero, & Flanery, 1985; Hodges, Kline, Barbero, & Woodruff, 1985; Zuckerman, Stevenson, & Bailey, 1987). The picture is less clear for fathers, who have not often been the object of study. Hodges and her colleagues compared the fathers of RAP children who were evaluated by a pediatric gastroenterology service to fathers of children in a community sample (Hodges, Kline, Barbero, & Flanery, 1985; Hodges, Kline, Barbero, & Woodruff, 1985). The RAP fathers reported more anxiety, but not more depression, than the comparison group. Finally, a study focusing on first-degree relatives of RAP children found that half of the children had one or more family members, primarily mothers and other female relatives, who met the criteria for Somatization Disorder (Routh & Ernst, 1984).

This research literature seems to suggest a high incidence of emotional disturbance, particularly anxiety and somatization, in RAP children and their parents. However, the literature is limited by reliance on community samples as control groups for clinic-referred RAP patients. In two studies that compared RAP patients to other pediatric patients, emotional and behavioral problems were not greater for RAP than for other patients (McGrath, Goodman, Firestone, Shipman, & Peters, 1983; Routh & Ernst, 1984).

There are several reasons that community control groups limit interpretation of results and should be supplemented with patient control groups in research on pediatric RAP patients. First, children in a community sample are not necessarily representative of users of the clinic who constitute the population from which the RAP sample is drawn. Consequently, a variety of factors other than child health status may account for differences in the emotional adjustment of the two groups. For example, differences in social class could account for differences in depression (cf. Hollingshead & Redlich, 1958). Second, nonpatient comparison groups cannot control for the possibility that group differences are due to patient versus nonpatient status at the time of research participation. Thus, the finding of greater anxiety in parents of RAP patients than a community group of parents (Hodges, Kline, Barbero, & Woodruff, 1985) could be due to a tendency for most parents, regardless of the child's condition, to be anxious at a clinic visit. Finally, and most important from the perspective of health service providers, use of a nonpatient comparison group does not allow one to address the question of whether psychological factors distinguish patients with recurrent abdominal pain from patients whose abdominal pain has an identifiable organic etiology that can be treated medically.

The goal of the present study was to determine whether patients with recurrent abdominal pain and their parents could be distinguished from other patient families on the basis of their patterns of somatic complaints, anxiety, and depression. Patients with abdominal pain referred to the pediatric outpatient clinics of a university medical center were evaluated and classified into two groups: those with and those without identifiable organic etiology for their pain. These patient groups were compared to each other and to a third group of well children who had previously attended the clinic for routine examinations or minor illnesses.

METHOD

Sample

Subjects for the study were recruited from patients at the pediatric outpatient clinics of a university medical center. Mothers, fathers, and the patients' schoolteachers were also invited to participate. Consecutive new patients, ages 8 to 17, who presented for evaluation of abdominal pain of at least 1-month duration were eligible for the study. Patients with a handicap or mental retardation were excluded. Patients were classified into two groups on the basis of results of their medical evaluation: (a) the recurrent abdominal pain (RAP) group ($n = 41$), consisting of patients for whom there was no identifiable organic etiology to explain abdominal pain; and (b) the organic group ($n = 28$), consisting of patients whose medical evaluation had uncovered an organic cause that could account for abdominal pain. For the purposes of this study, organic causes were defined as those reflecting tissue pathology (damage, inflammation, structural change, abnormal growth). However, in planning the study it was not known what specific diagnoses would appear in the organic group. In fact, almost all of the patients in this group had ulcer or ulcer-related disorders. Diagnoses in this group included gastritis ($n = 9$), esophagitis ($n = 5$), peptic ulcer disease ($n = 4$), duodenitis ($n = 3$), reflux esophagitis with antral gastritis ($n = 1$), gastritis and duodenal ulceration ($n = 1$), reflux esophagitis versus peptic ulcer disease ($n = 1$), reflux versus lactose intolerance ($n = 1$), constipation with megacolon ($n = 1$), nodular lymphoid hyperplasia ($n = 1$), and salpingitis ($n = 1$).

The nature and extent of the medical evaluation for patients with abdominal pain was not influenced by study participation but rather was determined by each patient's primary physician. (The protocol for evaluation of pediatric abdominal pain is described by Greene & Walker, 1988.) Routine laboratory work was obtained for all patients. Additional tests and procedures were conducted at the discretion of the physician. Table I presents further details regarding the evaluation of both groups of abdominal pain patients. Most cases had been evaluated or treated previously by other practitioners in the region. One third of the patients in each group had a prior hospitalization for abdominal pain. If results of recent invasive diagnostic procedures were available, these procedures were generally not repeated.

A comparison group of well patients consisted of individuals who had presented to the pediatric clinics for routine examinations, such as a school or sports physical, or for an acute minor illness that was resolved at the time of the research interview. Subjects were recruited such that this group would have the same ratio of boys to girls and children to adolescents as the RAP group. Additionally, when it became clear that there were very few black patients in the RAP or organic groups, recruitment for the well group was

Table I. Evaluation of Abdominal Pain Patients[a]

	Recurrent abdominal pain group ($n = 41$) %	Organic group ($n = 28$) %
Hospitalized for evaluation	32	21
Evaluated by pediatric gastroenterologist	78	86
Radiographic studies (upper and/or lower GI)	27	32
Ultrasound	44	36
Endoscopy	22	64
CT Scan	5	7

[a]Percentages do not add up to 100 because some subjects in each group received more than one diagnostic procedure. Although abdominal pain was the primary complaint for all subjects, some had additional symptoms that influenced the nature and extent of medical evaluation.

Table II. Frequency of Subjects by Diagnostic Group, Age Group, and Sex

Subject	Well group	Recurrent abdominal pain group	Organic group
Children (age 8–11)			
Male	13	13	16
Female	9	9	4
Adolescents (age 12–17)			
Male	9	9	2
Female	10	10	6
Total	41	41	28

directed toward white patients in order to achieve similar proportions of subjects by race in each group (the final sample was primarily white, with 1 black patient in the RAP group, 3 in the organic group, and 3 in the well group).

Table II provides information on the age and sex of subjects in the three diagnostic groups. Demographic characteristics of the three groups were similar. Analysis of variance indicated no significant difference among the groups on the Hollingshead Index of Social Status (Hollingshead, 1975). The majority of participating families were in the middle class. Fathers (or father figures) were present in approximately 80% of the homes in each diagnostic group.

Father questionnaire data were received from 74 of the 90 children (82%) who had fathers (or father figures) in the home. Teacher data were received for 89 of the 110 subjects (81%).

Procedure

Parents of patients scheduled for evaluation of abdominal pain were typically contacted by telephone prior to their children's clinic appointments and invited to participate in the study. In some cases it was not possible to contact the families before the appointment and they were recruited at the clinic. Informed consent was obtained from both parent and child at the clinic. The research protocol was administered to the child and parents separately at the clinic and prior to completion of the medical evaluation and diagnosis. Parents self-administered the questionnaires after a brief explanation. An interviewer administered the questionnaires verbally to the children who responded by selecting items on printed cards that gave the response format for each questionnaire. When the father was not present at the clinic, his questionnaire was sent home and returned by mail.

Teachers were contacted by mail within approximately 1 month after the clinic visit. They were asked to complete the Child Behavior Checklist Teacher form describing the child's behavior in the previous 2 months.

The comparison group of well patients was obtained by contacting parents of children seen in the clinic for a well child visit or an acute minor illness. The majority of these patient families were interviewed in their homes.

Measures

Child Somatization Inventory. RAP is associated with multiple somatic symptoms suggestive of somatization disorder (Ernst et al., 1984). However, no formal criteria have been established for this disorder in children (Shapiro & Rosenfeld, 1987), and there are no published measures of child somatization. Thus, for the purposes of this research it was necessary to design an instrument to assess the extent of child somatization.

The Child Somatization Inventory includes symptoms from the somatization subscale of the Hopkins Symptom Checklist (Derogatis, Lipman, Rickels, Uhlenhuth, & Covi, 1974) and from the DSM-III criteria for somatization disorder (American Psychiatric Association, 1980). There are a total of 36 psychophysiological symptoms, many associated with recurrent abdominal pain (e.g., fatigue, nausea, dizziness, diarrhea). As is the case with any self-report measure of physical symptoms, it is not possible to evaluate whether there may be an organic basis for reported symptoms. The child rates the extent to which he or she experiences each symptom on a 4-point scale ranging from *not at all* to *a whole lot.* A total score is obtained by summing the ratings.

Functional Disability Inventory. This Inventory (Walker & Greene, 1988) assesses the child's physical and social functioning in the domains of school, home, recreation, and social interaction. The instrument lists 15 activities that are rated on a 5-point scale according to how difficult they were for the child to perform in the previous few days. A total score is obtained by summing the item scores. Both the forms for child self-report and mother report of child disability were used.

Pain Intensity. Children were asked to rate the intensity of pain experienced in the previous 2 weeks. The format for the rating was a 10-point visual analog scale (Scott & Huskisson, 1976). Children in the RAP and organic groups rated the intensity of abdominal pain. Children in the well group rated pain of any sort (e.g., headache, injury) experienced in the previous 2 weeks.

Spielberger State-Trait Anxiety Inventory for Children. The trait anxiety form of this self-report inventory was used to assess children's general level of anxiety. The instrument consists of 20 items that are rated on a 3-point scale ranging from *hardly ever* to *often* and are summed to obtain a total score. Total scores can range from 20 to 60. Evidence supporting the instrument's reliability and validity is provided by Spielberger (1973).

Child Depression Inventory. The CDI (Kovacs, 1980/1981; Kovacs & Beck, 1977) is a downward extension of the Beck Depression Inventory for adults (Beck, Ward, Mendelson, Mock, & Erbaugh, 1961). It is a child self-report instrument with 27 items scored on a 3-point scale. Each item represents a depressive symptom and is scored 0 for absence of the symptom and 2 for the most severe form of the symptom. Total scores range from 0 to 54. Mild depression is indicated by scores of approximately 9 or above, and moderate depression by scores of 16 or above. Studies of the psychometric properties of the CDI indicate good internal consistency, but test–retest reliability varies across populations and test–retest intervals (Saylor, Finch, Spirito, & Bennett, 1984). Validity studies demonstrate that the CDI has a high correlation with self-report measures of self-concept and can distinguish children with emotional distress from normal schoolchildren; however, the construct measured by the CDI may overlap somewhat with anxiety (Saylor et al., 1984).

Child Behavior Checklist. The CBCL (Achenbach & Edelbrock, 1983) provides a standardized description of children's problem behaviors during the previous 6 months as reported by their parents. It consists of 118 behavior problems each scored on a 3-point scale. There are two subscales. The Internalizing Behavior Problems scale reflects fearful, inhibited, overcontrolled behavior. The Externalizing Behavior Problems scale reflects aggressive, antisocial, undercontrolled behavior. Normalized T scores for the scales are standardized for child age and sex. These T scores were used in the present data analysis. The teacher form of the Child Behavior Checklist (Achenbach & Edelbrock, 1986) was also used.

Hopkins Symptom Checklist. This instrument is a self-report symptom inventory that is scored on underlying symptom dimensions that have been identified in factor analysis (Derogatis et al., 1974). Three dimensions (somatization, anxiety, depression) were used in this study to assess parent symptomatology.

RESULTS

The three diagnostic groups were compared on measures of symptomatology by means of a series of 3-way analyses of variance. The three factors were Diagnostic Group (RAP vs. Organic vs. Well), Age Group (Children vs. Adolescents), and Child Sex. Post hoc analyses used the Duncan Multiple Range Test.

Table III presents the means and standard deviations for each diagnostic group on the child variables. The RAP and Organic groups both scored significantly higher than the Well group on the Child Somatization Inventory but did not differ from each other, $F(2, 98) = 19.06$, $p < .001$. On the Functional Disability Inventory the RAP and Organic groups reported

Table III. Means and Standard Deviations for Child Characteristics

	Well (n = 41)		RAP (n = 41)		Organic (n = 28)	
Dependent variable	*M*	*SD*	*M*	*SD*	*M*	*SD*
Pain intensity	2.10	2.05	6.93[a]	2.51	7.18[a]	2.79
Somatization	7.93	9.98	20.34[a]	12.10	23.39[a]	12.76
Anxiety	31.17	5.74	36.02[a]	6.52	36.61[a]	7.68
Depression	7.00	4.35	10.24[a]	7.21	10.07[a]	6.31
Functional disability						
Child report	3.15	5.44	17.12[a]	12.92	15.00[a]	11.33
Mother report	2.26	5.75	17.41[a]	15.36	17.04[a]	15.02
Internalizing behavior						
Mother report	54.85	8.26	65.00[a,b]	7.75	60.25[a]	8.76
Teacher report[c]	53.61	10.23	57.19	11.43	56.32	8.52
Externalizing behavior						
Mother report	53.67	10.25	55.24	9.29	52.71	9.26
Teacher report[c]	54.46	10.50	52.58	8.50	51.40	6.50

[a]Significantly higher than the Well group ($p < .05$ or less).
[b]Significantly higher than Organic group ($p < .05$ or less).
[c]The number of teachers providing data for each group was as follows: Well group, $n = 28$; RAP group, $n = 36$; Organic group, $n = 25$.

more disability than the Well group but did not differ from each other, $F(2, 97) = 26.40$, $p < .001$ for child report, and $F(2, 96) = 21.03$, $p < .001$ for mother report. Finally, when asked to rate the intensity of recent pain, the RAP and Organic groups reported significantly greater recent pain than the Well group, $F(2, 97) = 55.04$, $p < .001$. There were no differences by age group or sex on any of these measures.

Turning to the measures of child anxiety and depression, children in the RAP and Organic groups scored significantly higher than Well children on the Spielberger Trait Anxiety Inventory and the Child Depression Inventory, $F(2, 98) = 8.96$, $p < .001$, and $F(2, 98) = 3.51$, $p < .05$, respectively. Further evidence of anxiety and depression in the RAP and Organic groups was found in the mothers' reports on the Internalizing scale of the Child Behavior Checklist. There was a significant difference among the groups, with mothers in the RAP group reporting more internalizing behavior in their children than reported by mothers in the Organic group, who in turn reported significantly more internalizing behavior than the Well group, $F(2, 96) = 15.12$, $p < .001$. Teachers, in contrast, reported no significant difference among the groups on internalizing behavior. Neither mothers nor teachers reported a significant difference among the groups on the Externalizing scale of the Child Behavior Checklist. Finally, there were no differences by age group or sex on measures of child adjustment.

With respect to parent symptomatology, the diagnostic groups differed on maternal anxiety, maternal depression, and maternal somatization,

Table IV. Mothers' Scores on Hopkins Symptom Checklist Subscales

	Well (n = 41)		RAP (n = 41)		Organic (n = 28)	
Subscale	M	SD	M	SD	M	SD
Anxiety	1.87	2.24	3.35[a]	3.53	2.07	2.29
Depression	3.72	3.49	6.45[a]	5.85	4.93	3.92
Somatization	3.67	2.42	7.27[a]	5.56	6.14[a]	4.02

[a]Significantly higher than the Well group ($p < .05$ or less).

$F(2, 96) = 2.93$, $p < .05$, $F(2, 96) = 3.49$, $p < .05$, and $F(2, 96) = 8.50$, $p < .001$, respectively. Means and standard deviations for mothers' scores are presented in Table IV. Post hoc analyses indicated significantly higher levels of maternal anxiety in the RAP group in comparison to the Well group, but no difference from the Organic group. Similarly, maternal depression was significantly greater for the RAP than the Well group, but neither group differed significantly from the Organic group. Mothers of both RAP and Organic patients reported significantly higher levels of somatization than mothers of Well patients. There was also a significant Diagnostic Group × Child Sex interaction effect for maternal somatization, $F(2, 96) = 6.87$, $p < .01$. Within the RAP group, somatization was significantly greater for mothers of girls ($M = 9.68$) than for mothers of boys ($M = 5.09$). The fathers' reports of anxiety, depression, and somatization did not differ by diagnostic group, age group, or child sex.

DISCUSSION

Results of the study contradict the common assumption that the basis of children's abdominal pain must be either organic or psychogenic. Others have argued that the absence of abnormal organic findings in children with recurrent abdominal pain does not necessarily indicate the presence of psychological disorder (Barr & Feuerstein, 1983; Levine & Rappaport, 1984; Whitehead & Schuster, 1985). Our own findings underscore that the presence of organic pathology associated with abdominal pain does not preclude coexisting emotional or behavioral problems. We found that both RAP and organic patients had significantly higher levels of anxiety and depression than well patients drawn from the same clinic population. This finding was supported both by the child's self-report and by the mother's report of the child's behavior during the previous 6 months. Furthermore, in a related study (Garber, Zeman, & Walker, 1988) results of a standardized psychiatric diagnostic interview (the K-SADS) with a subsample of the RAP and organic patients and their mothers indicated that more than 90% of patients in both groups met DSM-III-R criteria for a psychiatric diagnosis. Taken together these findings suggest that a large percentage of patients with both recurrent abdominal pain and ulcer-related conditions may have clinically significant emotional disorder.

An implication of these findings is that psychological evaluation of the sort undertaken here may not facilitate the physician's differential diagnosis of patients with abdominal pain, given that emotional distress is as likely in children with an organic etiology for abdominal pain as in those without. Nonetheless, psychological assessment is important because a significant number of children in both groups appear to be emotionally distressed and some may benefit from mental health intervention.

There are several plausible explanations for the present findings. First, it is important to note the nature of the organic group. It consisted primarily of patients with ulcer and ulcer-related conditions. It is possible that emotional distress plays a causal role in both recurrent abdominal pain and ulcer-related conditions. The present data, however, do not rule out the possibility that the child's anxiety and depression occurred as a reaction to repeated episodes of pain. One could also speculate that emotional distress resulted for different reasons in the two groups; in one group it may have been a cause, and in the other a consequence of abdominal pain. Results from our ongoing longitudinal research will contribute to untangling these issues of causality.

Regarding the teacher CBCL data, differences among the diagnostic groups did not reach significance. However, rank order of group means on the CBCL Internalizing scale was the same for teacher and mother data (see Table III). It is possible that distressed mothers in this study exaggerated their children's symptoms, resulting in higher CBCL scores from mothers than from teachers. However, it seems more likely that low teacher scores are due to teacher lack of awareness of subjective child symptoms of anxiety and depression. This would be especially so for children with more severe symptomatology because these children are likely to have extended school absences. Recent work on the use of multiple sources of information regarding children's psychiatric symptomatology suggests that children provide the single most important source of data (Reich & Earls, 1987). The fact that similar findings were obtained here from both child and mother data suggests that we can be reasonably confident in reporting more internalizing emotional and behavioral symptoms in abdominal pain patients than in well patients.

Turning to parent symptomatology, the present study yielded evidence of greater anxiety, depression, and somatization in mothers of RAP patients than in mothers of well patients. We cannot dismiss the possibility that distress in the RAP mothers was at least in part a stress reaction to having a child with RAP. Nonetheless, it seems likely that maternal distress played a role in the etiology or maintenance of the child's symptomatology. Other investigators, finding an association between maternal distress and child emotional and behavioral problems, have suggested that this link can be explained by the parenting style of distressed mothers, which may contribute to child adjustment difficulties (Forehand, Lautenschlager, Faust, & Graziano, 1986; Kochanska, Kuczynski, Radke-Yarrow, & Welsh, 1987). Similarly, the combination of emotional distress and multiple somatic complaints found in RAP mothers may influence mother–child interaction in a way that contributes to the child's somatic complaints.

There are several ways in which this might occur. First, maternal somatization could serve a modeling function for the child, who may learn illness behavior as a coping strategy. The finding of greater somatization in mothers of RAP girls than RAP boys suggests that a modeling process could be more central in the development of symptomatology for girls than boys. Others have demonstrated that maternal modeling influences girls' illness behavior (Whitehead, Busch, Heller, & Costa, 1986). Second, to the extent that maternal distress is stressful to the child it may create conditions for the development of RAP by giving rise to child distress. The child's distress may be manifest in both psychiatric and physical symptoms. However, if it occurs in the context of a mother with somatic preoccupations, then it is likely the family will focus on the child's physical symptoms and define the problem as medical in nature, neglecting the emotional component (cf. Pennebaker, 1982; Rodin, 1978). Finally, maternal anxiety and depression may influence mother–child interaction by interfering with the mother's capacity to reassure her child and increasing the likelihood that her concern will cause her to unintentionally reinforce the child's symptoms. The lack of association between father distress and child symptomatology deserves further study, but could be due in part to the tendency for fathers to be less involved in parenting.

It is likely that maternal distress played a role in the referral of RAP children for medical evaluation. Mothers tend to be the decision makers regarding family health service utilization (Turk, Litt, Salovey, & Walker, 1985), and psychological distress of the sort reported by the RAP mothers is associated with increased utilization (Gortmaker, Eckenrode, & Gore, 1982; Tessler, Mechanic, & Dimond, 1976). There may be many children in the community with symptoms of recurrent abdominal pain whose parents have not sought medical treatment or have been reassured by the negative findings produced at an initial evaluation. The present findings do not necessarily generalize to those children and their families but rather represent families of children who both have the symptoms of RAP and pursue extensive medical evaluations. In order to fully understand RAP, future research should also investigate subjects with abdominal pain who do not seek health care.

It is important to determine the normal frequency of unexplained abdominal pain in a healthy nonclinic population, and to identify factors specific to RAP that distinguish it from other disorders also associated with high health service utilization (cf. Drossman, Sandler, McKee, & Lovitz, 1982; Sandler, Drossman, Nathan, & McKee, 1984).

Recently, Costello et al. (1988) argued that emotional and behavioral problems in children are "the new hidden morbidity" in pediatrics. They presented evidence that mental health problems are present in a significant number of children visiting primary care pediatricians. Their data suggest that pediatricians underestimate the rate of psychiatric disorder, particularly anxiety and depression, in pediatric patients. The present findings of anxiety and depression in children with recurrent abdominal pain and ulcer-related conditions suggests that these disorders should be targeted in efforts to address "the new hidden morbidity."

REFERENCES

Achenbach, T. M., & Edelbrock, C. (1983). *Manual for the Child Behavior Checklist and Revised Child Behavior Profile.* Burlington: University of Vermont.

Achenbach, T. M., & Edelbrock, C. (1986). *Manual for the Teacher's Report Form and Teacher Version of the Child Behavior Checklist.* Burlington: University of Vermont.

American Psychiatric Association. (1980). *Diagnostic and statistical manual of mental disorders* (3rd ed.). Washington, DC: Author.

Apley, J. (1975). *The child with abdominal pains.* London: Blackwell.

Apley, J., & Naish, N. (1958). Recurrent abdominal pain: A field survey of 1,000 school children. *Archives of Diseases of Childhood, 33,* 165-170.

Barr, R. G., & Feuerstein, M. (1983). Recurrent abdominal pain syndrome: How appropriate are our basic clinical assumptions? In P. J. McGrath & P. Firestone (Eds.), *Pediatric and adolescent behavioral medicine* (pp. 13-27). New York: Springer.

Beck, A. T., Ward, C. H., Mendelson, M., Mock, J., & Erbaugh, J. (1961). An inventory for measuring depression. *Archives of General Psychiatry, 4,* 561-571.

Costello, E. J., Edelbrock, C., Costello, A. J., Dulcan, M. K., Burns, B. J., & Brent, D. (1988). Psychopathology in pediatric primary care: The new hidden morbidity. *Pediatrics, 82,* 415-424.

Derogatis, L. R., Lipman, R. S., Rickels, K., Uhlenhuth, E. H., & Covi, L. (1974). The Hopkins Symptom Checklist. *Behavioral Science, 19,* 1-15.

Drossman, D. A., Sandler, R. S., McKee, D. C., & Lovitz, A. J. (1982). Bowel patterns among subjects not seeking health care. *Gastroenterology, 83,* 529-534.

Ernst, A. R., Routh, D. K., & Harper, D. C. (1984). Abdominal pain in children and symptoms of somatization disorder. *Journal of Pediatric Psychology, 9,* 77-85.

Forehand, R., Lautenschlager, G. J., Faust, J., & Graziano, W. G. (1986). Parent perceptions and parent-child interactions in clinic-referred children: A preliminary investigation of the effects of maternal depressive moods. *Behavior Research and Therapy, 24,* 73-75.

Garber, J., Zeman, J., & Walker, L. S. (1988). Psychiatric status of children with recurrent abdominal pain. Presented at the annual meeting of the American Psychological Association, Atlanta, GA.

Gortmaker, S. L., Eckenrode, J., & Gore, S. (1982). Stress and the utilization of health services. *Journal of Health and Social Behavior, 23,* 25-38.

Greene, J. W., & Walker, L. S. (1988). *A protocol for the screening, diagnosis, and treatment of recurrent abdominal pain.* Unpublished manuscript, Vanderbilt University School of Medicine.

Hodges, K., Kline, J. J., Barbero, G., & Flanery, R. (1985). Depressive symptoms in children with recurrent abdominal pain and in their families. *Journal of Pediatrics, 107,* 622-626.

Hodges, K., Kline, J. J., Barbero, G., & Woodruff, C. (1985). Anxiety in children with recurrent abdominal pain and their parents. *Psychosomatics, 26,* 859-866.

Hollingshead, A. B. (1975). *Four factor index of social status.* Working paper, Department of Sociology, Yale University.

Hollingshead, A. B., & Redlich, F. C. (1958). *Social class and mental illness: A community study.* New York: Wiley.

Kochanska, G., Kuczynski, L., Radke-Yarrow, M., & Welsh, J. D. (1987). Resolution of control episodes between well and affectively ill mothers and their children. *Journal of Abnormal Child Psychology, 15,* 441-456.

Kovacs, M. (1980/1981). Rating scales to assess depression in school-aged children. *Acta Paedo Psychiatrica, 46,* 305-315.

Kovacs, M., & Beck, A. T. (1977). An empirical-clinical approach toward a definition of childhood depression. In J. Schulterbrandt & A. Raskin (Eds.), *Depression in childhood: Diagnosis, treatment, and conceptual models* (pp. 1-25). New York: Raven.

Levine, M., & Rappaport, L. (1984). Recurrent abdominal pain in school children. *Pediatric Clinics of North America, 31,* 969-991.

Liebman, W. (1978). Recurrent abdominal pain in children. *Clinical Pediatrics, 17,* 149-153.

McGrath, P. J., Goodman, J. J., Firestone, P., Shipman, R., & Peters, S. (1983). Recurrent abdominal pain: A psychogenic disorder? *Archives of Disease in Childhood, 58,* 888-890.

Pennebaker, J. W. (1982). *The psychology of physical symptoms.* New York: Springer.

Reich, W., & Earls, F. (1987). Rules for making psychiatric diagnoses in children on the basis of multiple sources of information: Preliminary strategies. *Journal of Abnormal Child Psychology, 15,* 601-616.

Rodin, J. (1978). Somatopsychics and attribution. *Personality and Social Psychology Bulletin, 4,* 531-540.

Routh, D. K., & Ernst, A. R. (1984). Somatization disorder in relatives of children and adolescents with functional abdominal pain. *Journal of Pediatric Psychology, 9,* 427-437.

Sandler, R. S., Drossman, D. A., Nathan, H. P., & McKee, D. C. (1984). Symptom complaints and health care seeking behavior in subjects with bowel dysfunction. *Gastroenterology, 87,* 314-318.

Saylor, F. S., Finch, A. J., Spirito, A., & Bennett, B. (1984). The Children's Depression Inventory: A systematic evaluation of psychometric properties. *Journal of Consulting and Clinical Psychology, 52,* 955-967.

Scott, J., & Huskisson, E. C. (1976). Graphic representation of pain. *Pain, 2,* 175-184.

Shapiro, E. G., & Rosenfeld, A. A. (1987). *The somatizing child: Diagnosis and treatment of conversion and somatization disorders.* New York: Springer.

Spielberger, C. D. (1973). *Manual for the State-Trait Anxiety Inventory for Children.* Palo Alto, CA: Consulting Psychologists Press.

Stone, R., & Barbero, G. (1970). Recurrent abdominal pain in childhood. *Pediatrics, 45,* 732-738.

Tessler, R. D., Mechanic, D., & Dimond, M. (1976). The effect of psychological distress on physician utilization: A prospective study. *Journal of Health and Social Behavior, 17,* 353-364.

Turk, D. C., Litt, M. D., Salovey, P., & Walker, J. (1985). Seeking urgent pediatric treatment: Factors contributing to frequency, delay, and appropriateness. *Health Psychology, 4,* 43-59.

Walker, L. S., & Greene, J. W. (1988). *Development and validation of a measure of functional disability for children and adolescents.* Paper presented at the Florida Conference on Child Health Psychology, Gainesville, FL.

Wasserman, A. L., Whitington, P. F., & Rivara, F. P. (1988). Psychogenic basis for abdominal pain in children and adolescents. *Journal of the American Academy of Child and Adolescent Psychiatry, 27,* 179-184.

Whitehead, W. E., Busch, C. M., Heller, B. R., & Costa, P. T. (1986). Social learning influences on menstrual symptoms and illness behavior. *Health Psychology, 5,* 13-23.

Whitehead, W. E., & Schuster, M. M. (Eds.). (1985). *Gastrointestinal disorders: Behavioral and physiological basis for treatment.* New York: Academic Press.

Zuckerman, B., Stevenson, J., & Bailey, V. (1987). Stomachaches and headaches in a community sample of preschool children. *Pediatrics, 79,* 677-682.

5

The Family Environment in Nonorganic Failure to Thrive: A Controlled Study[1]

Dennis Drotar and Debbie Eckerle
Case Western Reserve University School of Medicine and Cleveland Metropolitan General Hospital

Compared 48 families of nonorganic failure to thrive (NOFT) infants with those of 52 physically healthy infants of similar demographic characteristics using the Family Environment Scale (FES). Families of NOFT infants had more problematic relationships as indicated by lower scores on the Family Relationships Inventory (FRI) components of the FES, including lower Cohesion and Expressiveness, than families of physically healthy infants. Contrary to predictions, families did not differ in level of Conflict or Organization. Families of NOFT infants had lower intellectual and Cultural Orientation. These findings suggest that problematic intrafamilial relationships are associated with NOFT and may influence the psychological outcomes of children with this condition. Studies are needed to document the effects of family functioning on the physical growth and psychosocial development of NOFT children.

Nonorganic failure to thrive (NOFT) is a frequent pediatric condition that places young children at significant psychological and physical risk (Bithoney & Rathbun, 1983; Drotar & Sturm, 1988a; Hufton & Oates, 1977; Roberts

[1]This research was supported by MCJ 390557, Division of Maternal and Child Health, Bureau of Health Care Delivery & Assistance, The Cleveland Foundation, and National Institute of Mental Health, Prevention Research Center 30274.

& Maddux, 1982; Singer & Fagan, 1984). Although the etiology and longer term psychological outcomes of NOFT are not well understood (Drotar, 1988), clinical observations and research have indicated that this condition is associated with high levels of family stress and dysfunction (Bruenlin, Desai, Stone, & Swilley, 1983; Elmer, 1966; Evans, Reinhart, & Succop, 1972; Leonard, Rhymes, & Solnit, 1966; Patton & Gardner, 1962; Talbot, Sobel, Burke, Lindemann, & Kaufman, 1947). Dysfunctional family influences may have several consequences on the NOFT child's growth and development. For example, family problems may limit support for maternal caretaking, interfere with proper allocation of attention and nutrition to the child, and affect parents' ability to comply with recommended psychosocial interventions (Ayoub & Milner, 1985; Drotar & Malone, 1982; Drotar et al., 1985; Evans et al., 1972). For this reason, some clinicians believe that assessment of family functioning should be an integral part of treatment planning for NOFT children (Drotar & Malone, 1982; Drotar et al., 1985; Evans et al., 1972; Leonard et al., 1966). In some cases, family-centered psychosocial intervention is needed to address family problems that are serious enough to affect the NOFT child's physical growth and psychological development (Drotar et al., 1985).

Although the potential role of family influences in the etiology of NOFT has been recognized for some time (Talbot et al., 1947), controlled studies of family functioning in this population using objective measures are infrequent. Several studies have indicated that the families of NOFT infants have lower economic levels (Kanawati, Darwish, & McLaren, 1974), fewer extended family members available for help with child rearing (Bithoney & Newberger, 1987; Pollitt & Leibel, 1980), and greater social isolation (Bithoney & Newberger, 1987; Kotelchuck & Newberger, 1983) than families of comparison group children. In addition, family relationship problems have been implicated in the development of NOFT. Based on data from maternal interviews during pregnancy, Altemeier et al. (1979) found that family stresses differentiated families whose children eventually developed NOFT from those in which children developed normally. The majority of stresses associated with subsequent occurrence of NOFT involved problems in the relationship between the mother and the father of the infant she was carrying. Mothers of infants whose children eventually developed NOFT reported that they had significantly more arguments, separations, and reconciliations with the child's father than mothers whose children developed normally (Altemeier et al., 1979; Altemeier, O'Connor, Sherrod, & Vietze, 1985).

Although prior studies indicate that the families of NOFT infants have more problems than families of healthy children with comparable demographic characteristics, discrepant findings have also been reported. For example, Altemeier et al. (1985) found greater levels of reported conflict between mothers of NOFT infants and fathers, whereas Bithoney and Newberger (1987) noted that mothers of NOFT children reported fewer disagreements with their spouses. Such discrepant findings concerning family characteristics may reflect differences in sampling characteristics, timing of family assessments with respect to the onset and duration of NOFT, or measures of family functioning used by different investigators.

Additional research is needed to clarify discrepant findings concerning family functioning in NOFT. Moreover, the measurement of family functioning has been a salient methodological problem in previous research. Prior studies have utilized structured interviews with undemonstrated validity to assess family functioning. Measures have usually involved descriptive information concerning family life (e.g., presence or absence of conflict rather than comprehensive assessment of clinically relevant dimensions of the family environment). Comprehensive, objective measurement is needed to adequately document similarities and differences between the family environments of NOFT infants versus those of comparison group infants.

The purpose of the present study was to compare the families of NOFT infants with those of physically healthy infants from similar socioeconomic backgrounds using an objective measure, the Family Environment Scale (FES) (Moos & Moos, 1976, 1981). Because NOFT is often associated with risk factors such as economic disadvantage which might be expected to influence the quality of family environments (Bruenlin et al., 1983), a comparison group was included to control for the influence of various child and family characteristics. Prior research and clinical observations suggested the hypothesis that families of NOFT infants would have more problematic intrafamilial relationships than comparison group families. Specifically, we hypothesized that families of NOFT infants would demonstrate greater conflict, less mutual support (Cohesion), and less adequate emotional expression (Expressiveness) on the FES than families of comparison group infants (Altemeier et al., 1985; Bithoney & Newberger, 1987; Drotar et al., 1985). Based on clinical observations that have suggested that families of NOFT infants are chaotic and poorly organized (Bruenlin et al., 1983; Drotar et al., 1985), we also predicted that the family environments of NOFT infants would demonstrate lower Organization than those of comparison group infants.

METHOD

Subjects (NOFT)

In accord with standard pediatric diagnostic practice (Bithoney & Rathbun, 1983) children were diagnosed as NOFT if they demonstrated: (a) weight at or below the 5th percentile based on norms (Hammill et al., 1979); (b) absence of major organic conditions that could directly affect the child's capacity to gain weight and/or cognitive development as indicated by physical and laboratory examination, including complete blood count and urinalysis: (c) demonstration of weight gain in the hospital (Schmitt, 1978); and (d) decrease in rate of weight gain from within normal limits at birth to below the 5th percentile. Children who demonstrated slow but constant patterns of growth consistent with constitutional growth deficiency were excluded. Children with below-normal growth potential were also excluded by requiring that growth parameters (height, weight, and head circumference) be appropriate for gestational age at birth and a birth weight of at least 1,500 grams. Three criteria increased sample homogeneity and simplified data collection: (a) age between 1 and 9 months of age; (b) absence of child abuse (three children were excluded for this reason): and (c) geographic proximity (within an hour's distance) from the hospital.

Subjects were recruited from children hospitalized for NOFT at one of seven area hospitals. The study coordinator reviewed charts and referrals to make sure that children met the above criteria for NOFT. A total of 88 children met study criteria. Eight families did not choose to participate in the study, leaving a total of 77 families who initially consented. Of this group, 29 families were not included because they could not be located, dropped out of the study, or did not complete the FES. The present NOFT sample included a total of 48 families. Mothers filled out the FES as a part of baseline assessment conducted within 1 month after the child's hospitalization. Nonparticipants did not differ in child or family demographic characteristics from those families who elected to participate. No differences were found in demographic characteristics including family size, income, number of children, maternal age, and education, birth order, and age of intake between families of NOFT children who completed the FES and those who did not.

Comparison Group

A comparison group of families of physically healthy infants was recruited from similar pediatric clinics and hospitals as the NOFT children. Comparison group families were recruited to resemble the NOFT sample in child characteristics (age at intake, sex, race, birth order, and gestational age), maternal characteristics (education and age), and family characteristics (family size, income, and structure). Comparable to the NOFT group, comparison group subjects weighed at least 1,500 grams at birth and had growth parameters (height, weight, and head circumference) at birth that were appropriate for their gestational age.

A total of 91 families of physically healthy infants with comparable demographics to the NOFT sample were approached for their consent. Fifteen mothers did not give their consent. Twenty-four of the 76 families who initially participated were not included in this report because they could not be located, dropped out of the study, or did not complete the FES. The comparison group sample included 52 families. Nonparticipants did not differ in child and family characteristics from those who participated. In addition, there were no significant differences in child or family demographic characteristics between comparison group families who completed the FES versus those who did not.

Sample Demographic Characteristics

The child and family characteristics of the two groups are shown in Table I. Chi-square analyses and *t* tests indicated no significant differences in child or family demographic (age, sex, race, birth order, prematurity, maternal age and education, Aid to Dependent Children status, family size and constellation). Families in the NOFT (n = 48) and comparison group (n = 52) were economically disadvantaged. The majority of families of NOFT

Table I. Means, Standard Deviations, and Frequencies of Family and Child Characteristics

	Nonorganic failure to thrive		Comparison group	
	M	*SD*	*M*	*SD*
Family characteristics				
No. of adults	2.5	1.5	2.2	1.1
No. of children	2.5	1.3	2.2	1.0
Maternal age	21.7	3.4	22.1	4.1
Maternal education	11.0	1.9	11.5	1.6
Job class	6.3	1.4	6.1	1.9
ADC recipient	38	1.4	41	1.9
Not receiving income from jobs	10		11	
Family constellation				
Nuclear	31		25	
Mother alone	6		10	
Extended	11		17	
Child characteristics				
Age at intake	4.7	2.8	5.0	2.7
Birth order	2.4	1.2	2.1	1.0
Male	32		34	
Female	16		18	
White	22		16	
Black/Hispanic	26		36	
Prematurity	11		10	

and comparison group infants received Aid to Dependent Children (ADC). Mothers in both samples were relatively young (M = 22) and had more than two children on the average.

Instruments

Family Environment Scale (FES). The FES, a 90-item scale, includes three domains: interpersonal relationships, personal growth, and family organization and structure (Holahan & Moos, 1981, 1983; Moos & Moos, 1976). Originally standardized on 285 families from different areas of the country, the FES has been shown to discriminate families whose members demonstrate psychological problems from those who do not (Moos & Moos, 1981). Internal consistencies (.64 to .78) and test–retest reliabilities (.68 to .91) over a 4-month interval have been reported (Moos & Moos, 1981). Four FES subscales were relevant to our major hypotheses: Cohesion assessed the degree to which family members are helpful and supportive of each other. Expressiveness involved the degree to which family members are encouraged to act openly and express their feelings directly. Conflict measured the extent to which open expression of anger and conflictual interactions are characteristic of the family. Finally, Organization assessed the importance of order and organization in the structuring of family activities and financial planning and the clarity of family roles and responsibilities. No differences were predicted between the NOFT and comparison group families on the other FES subscales. However, the entire scale was included to provide an descriptive profile of family environments in the NOFT versus comparison groups. This descriptive profile is of clinical interest because there is limited empirical information concerning the family environments of NOFT infants using objective instruments. Additional FES scales included Independence, the extent to which family members are encouraged to be self-sufficient; Achievement Orientation, the extent to which family activities fit in an achievement oriented framework; Intellectual and Cultural Orientation, family concern with intellectual and cultural activities; Active-Recreational, family participation in recreation and sports; Moral-Religious Emphasis, the degree to which religious activities are emphasized; and Control, family emphasis on rules and procedures.

Family Relationships Inventory (FRI). The majority of the hypothesized differences between the families of the NOFT and comparison groups reflected the relationship dimensions of the FES. For this reason, the Family Relationships Inventory (FRI; Holahan & Moos, 1981, 1983) was included to asses the quality of family relationships in a single measure. The FRI, a 27-item index of the quality of social relationships, is based on the three subscales, Cohesion, Conflict, and Expressiveness that constitute the relationship domain of the FES. The scoring of the Conflict subscale was reversed to that all subscales would have scores in the same direction. At an item level the FRI measured the perceived quality of family social support including such items as "family members really help and support one another."

RESULTS

Consistent with the hypothesis that the families of NOFT infants would demonstrate less optimal relationships than a comparison group, the two groups differed on the FRI. Families of NOFT infants had lower FRI scores (M = 15.92, SD = 5.57) than the comparison group (M = 18.67, SD = 3.50), $t(98) = -3.02$, $p < .001$. Average standard scores for the subscales of the FRI were 48.53, SD = 10.51, for the NOFT group and 53.98, SD = 6.69, for the comparison group, $t(98) = -3.22$, $p < .001$.

The means and standard deviations of FES standard scores (M = 50, SD = 10) are shown in Table II. As predicted, families of NOFT infants demonstrated lower levels of Cohesion (M = 47.8 vs. M = 54.3), $t(98) = -3.04$, $p < .01$, and lower levels of Expressiveness (M = 44.8 vs. 51.1), $t(98) = -2.61$, $p < .01$, than families of comparison group infants. Although the families of NOFT infants had higher levels of Conflict (M = 45.3) than comparison group families (M = 42.4), this difference was not significant, $t(98) = 1.32$, ns. Contrary to prediction, families of NOFT infants (M = 50.3) did not differ in Organization from those of comparison groups (M = 52.3), $t(98) = 0.99$, ns. Although this finding was not predicted, families of NOFT infants had lower Intellectual and Cultural Orientation

Table II. FES Scores for Families of NOFT and Comparison Group Infants

FES subscale	NOFT scaled score		Comparison group scaled score		
	M	SD	M	SD	t
Cohesion	47.8	12.7	54.3	8.1	-3.04^b
Expressiveness	44.8	13.6	51.1	10.6	-2.61^b
Conflict	45.3	11.3	42.4	10.2	1.32
Independence	46.4	14.6	50.7	12.3	1.63
Achievement-Orientation	51.5	9.2	52.6	9.2	0.58
Intellectual-Cultural Orientation	40.9	9.8	45.3	9.5	-2.34^a
Active Recreational-Orientation	38.9	14.7	40.6	13.6	0.60
Moral Religious-Emphasis	54.7	8.0	57.0	7.0	1.53
Organization	50.3	10.2	52.3	9.8	0.99
Control	49.8	10.5	51.1	9.2	0.64

$^a p < .05$.
$^b p < .01$.

(M = 40.9) than families of comparison group infants (M = 45.3), $t(98) = -2.34$, $p < .05$.

The number of families with lower scores (more than 1 standard deviation below the mean of the standardization sample) on the FES reflected the group differences. Fifteen families of NOFT infants (31.2%) had scores of less than 40 on the Cohesion scale compared to only 3 (7.4%) of those in the comparison group, $\chi^2(1, N = 100) = 8.58$, $p < .01$. In addition, a greater number (18) of families (33.3%) of NOFT children had scores below 40 on Expressiveness than families (7 or 13%) of comparison group infants $\chi^2(1, N = 100) = 6.46$, $p < .05$. Of the families of NOFT infants, 24 (50%) had scores below 40 on Intellectual and Cultural Orientation compared with 18 (35.2%) of the families of comparison group infants $\chi^2(1, N = 100) = 1.83$, ns.

DISCUSSION

As perceived by mothers, the family environments of NOFT infants were characterized by less adaptive relationships (especially lower expressiveness and cohesion) than those of physically healthy infants. Our findings are consistent with studies that have described more problematic relationships in families of NOFT infants compared with controls (Altemeier et al., 1979, 1985). On the other hand, contrary to prediction, no differences were found in family conflict or organization. The problematic organization and conflicts attributed to families of NOFT infants in uncontrolled clinical observations may reflect the influence of stresses associated with economic disadvantage and other risk factors. Family problems may not be as evident when family and child demographics are controlled as in the present study. It is also possible that the mothers of NOFT children may minimize or fail to recognize the degree of conflict or organizational problems that exist in their families.

Although this result was not predicted, mothers of NOFT infants reported less family involvement in cultural and intellectual activities than comparison group families. This finding is difficult to interpret but coincides with findings that mothers of NOFT infants provide less optimal intellectual stimulation to their children than mothers of comparison group children (Casey, Bradley, & Wortham, 1984).

Our cross-sectional study design does not allow us to make causal inferences concerning the origins of the differences in family relationships between NOFT and comparison group infants. However, data from several sources indicate that dysfunctional intrafamilial relationships can disrupt maternal child-rearing competence (Belsky, 1984; Wahler, 1980) and increase the likelihood of child maltreatement in some cases (Garbarino, 1977).

Problematic family relationships, especially cohesion and expressiveness, may have contributed to NOFT, by affecting maternal self-esteem and abilities to provide adequate attention and/or food to their children (Drotar & Sturm, 1988b; Drotar et al., 1985). One alternative explanation is that the less adaptive family environments of NOFT infants were a product of the stresses associated with the child's condition, medical diagnosis, or hospitalization. Evidence that FES scores are relatively stable (Moos & Moos, 1976, 1981) and that family problems precede the diagnosis of NOFT (Altemeier et al., 1979, 1985) suggests that it is more likely that the differences in family environments found in this study predated the diagnosis of NOFT. Assessment of the family environment prior to the development of NOFT or at the point of initial growth deceleration might help to clarify the direction of family influence. In addition, a control group of infants who are hospitalized for organic FTT or comparable physical problems is needed to assess the influence of stresses related to hospitalization on family environment.

The degree of similarity between the family environments of NOFT versus comparison group infants as both an interesting and unexpected finding. As compared with those of physically healthy infants, the family environments of NOFT infants were characterized by specific rather than generalized deficiencies. Differences in family environments were apparent in the relationship domain of the FES but not in personal growth or organizational dimensions (Holahan & Moos, 1983). The relatively few differences in the family environments between NOFT and comparison groups may reflect the fact that the two groups were closely matched on a relatively large number of several child and family risk factors. The failure to identify seriously dysfunctional family environments as measured by the FES also coincides with clinical observations of significant variation in psychological and family risk factors associated with NOFT (Chatoor & Egan, 1983; Pugiliese, Weyman-Daum, Moses, & Lifshitz, 1987; Woolston, 1985). In some cases, NOFT may stem directly from family relationship problems that are serious enough to disrupt the maternal-child relationship and feeding patterns (Drotar & Sturm, 1987). In other cases, NOFT may reflect parental underestimation of the child's needs for caloric intake which relates directly to specific health beliefs (Pugiliese et al., 1987) or financial problems (Frank, Allen, & Brown, 1985) rather than family dysfunction. It is possible that the present sample may have included a relatively large number of children whose NOFT was a product of various types of underfeeding rather than serious family dysfunction.

Limitations

The sampling characteristics and methodological limitations of this study should guide the interpretation of the findings. Identified at a young age (5 months on the average), this sample of NOFT infants was selected on the basis of research criteria rather than clinical referral. Families selected in this manner might be expected to demonstrate more adaptive family environments than those selected from NOFT children referred for treatment of psychological problems or to protective service agencies for evaluation of neglect or abuse. For this reason, the present selection criteria might be expected to limit the detection of differences between families of NOFT versus comparison infants. As a consequence, the differences that were found may be considered robust.

Sample attrition may have biased our findings. More than one third of families of NOFT and physically healthy children who were potentially eligible for the study did not complete the FES. The demographic characteristics of families who completed the FES did not differ from families who did not complete this measure. However, it is quite possible that the dropouts in the NOFT group may have experienced more family disruption than the dropouts in the comparison group. Finally, the present assessment of family environment was based entirely on maternal report. Maternal reports may reflect a unique perspective concerning the family environment and may be influenced by personal feelings of stress. On the other hand, maternal perceptions of the family environment are important in their own right because of the potential influence on maternal self-esteem and child-rearing competence (Belsky, 1984). However, we anticipate that reports of other family members or direct observational measures might yield different findings. For example, observers might detect signs of conflict or other family problems that are ignored or minimized by the mothers of NOFT infants. Unfortunately, it was not feasible to gather data from alternative family assessments.

Clinical and Research Implications

Our findings suggest that it might be useful to consider such qualities of family relationships as cohesion (mutual support) and expressiveness in planning psychosocial interventions for NOFT infants. Instruments such as the FES or other objective measures of family functioning (Lewis, Beavers, Gossett, & Phillips, 1976; Olson, Sprenkle, & Russell, 1979) might be used to identify specific family problems that provide a focus for intervention. In some cases, family members may need professional help to provide more effective support to the NOFT child's mother and express their feelings more openly (Drotar et al., 1985; Drotar & Sturm, 1988b). Relationship problems may also interfere with family members' abilities to comply with recommended psychosocial intervention for their NOFT children. Clinical management of NOFT might be enhanced by encouraging family members to discuss their perceptions of the NOFT child's condition and expectations concerning treatment (Drotar & Sturm, 1988b).

Our findings suggest several interesting directions for future research concerning family influences in NOFT. Conceptual models of family influence proposed by developmental psychologists (Parke, 1979; Parke, Power, & Gottman, 1979; Siegel & Parke, 1987) suggest that alternative pathways of family influences on the development of NOFT should be considered. For example, family relationship difficulties may influence the child's growth by affecting the availability and allocation of food, the consistency and organization of child care, and/or by exposing the child to parental conflict (Drotar & Sturm, 1987). Alternatively, the quality of family relationships may affect the NOFT child indirectly by disrupting maternal caretaking competence (Sherrod, O'Connor, Altemeier, & Vietze, 1985). In a study of normal children, Pedersen, Anderson, and Cain (1980) demonstrated that the quality of the marital relationship affected mother–infant interaction during feeding. Similar processes may operate in families of NOFT infants in which more serious family dysfunction limits maternal energy, consistency of response, or ability to monitor the child's nutrition (Drotar & Sturm, 1987).

The effect of the family environment on the NOFT child's physical and psychological status and prognosis is another interesting research question. Future studies of family communication, social support, or decision making should provide useful information concerning family variables that influence the NOFT child's psychological adaptation and prognosis. Objective measures of family functioning might be used to identify specific family risk patterns or profiles that correspond to etiological subtypes or patterns of behavioral disturbance among NOFT children (Ayoub & Milner, 1985). Finally, the influence of family functioning and communication on family participation in and responsiveness to recommended medical and psychosocial intervention should be assessed.

REFERENCES

Altemeier, W. A., O'Connor, S. M., Sherrod, K. B., & Vietze, P. M. (1985). Prospective study of antecedents for nonorganic failure to thrive. *Journal of Pediatrics, 103,* 360-368.

Altemeier, W. A., Vietze, P., Sherrod, K. B., Sandler, H. M., Falsey, S., & O'Connor, S. (1979). Prediction of child maltreatment during pregnancy. *Journal of the American Academy of Child Psychiatry, 18,* 205-219.

Ayoub, C. C., & Milner, J. S. (1985). Failure to thrive: Parental indicators, types, and outcomes. *Child Abuse and Neglect, 9,* 491-499.

Belsky, J. (1984). The determinants of parenting: A process model. *Child Development, 55,* 83-96.

Bithoney, W. G., & Newberger, E. H. (1987). Child and family attributes of failure to thrive. *Journal of Developmental and Behavioral Pediatrics, 8,* 32-37.

Bithoney, W. G., & Rathbun, J. M. (1983). Failure to thrive. In M. B. Levine, W. C. Carey, A. D. Crocker, & R. J. Gross (Eds.), *Developmental behavioral pediatrics* (pp. 557-572). W. B. Saunders: Philadelphia.

Bruenlin, D. C., Desai, V. J., Stone, M. E., & Swilley, J. (1983). Failure to thrive with no organic etiology: A critical review. *International Journal of Eating Disorders, 2,* 25-49.

Casey, P. M., Bradley, R. H., & Wortham, B. (1984). Social and non-social home environments of children with non-organic failure to thrive. *Pediatrics, 73,* 348-353.

Chatoor, I., & Egan, J. (1983). Nonorganic failure to thrive and dwarfism due to food refusal: A separation disorder. *Journal of American Academy of Child Psychiatry, 22,* 294-301.

Drotar, D. (1988). Failure to thrive. In D. K. Routh (Ed.), *Handbook of pediatric psychology* (pp. 71-107). New York: Guilford.

Drotar, D., & Malone, C. A. (1982). Family-oriented intervention in failure to thrive. In M. Klaus & M. O. Robertson (Eds.), *Birth interaction and attachment* (Vol. 6, pp. 104-112). Skillman, NJ: Johnson and Johnson Pediatric Round Table.

Drotar, D., & Sturm, L. A. (1987). Paternal influences in non-organic failure to thrive: Implications for psychosocial management. *Infant Mental Health Journal, 8,* 37-50.

Drotar, D., & Sturm, L. (1988a). Prediction of intellectual development at age three in children with early histories of nonorganic failure-to-thrive. *Journal of Pediatric Psychology, 13,* 281-295.

Drotar, D., & Sturm, L. (1988b). The role of parent-practitioner communication in failure to thrive. *Family Systems Medicine, 6,* 42-53.

Drotar, D., Woychick, J., Mantz-Clumpner, C., Brickell, C., Negray, J., Wallace, M., & Malone, C. A. (1985). The family context of failure to thrive. In D. Drotar (Ed.), *New directions in failure to thrive. Implications for research and practice* (pp. 295-310). New York: Plenum Press.

Elmer, E. (1966). Failure to thrive: The role of the mother. *Pediatrics, 25,* 717-725.

Evans, S. L., Reinhart, J. B., & Succop, R. A. (1972). Failure to thrive: A study of 45 children and their families. *Journal of the American Academy of Child Psychiatry,* 1972, *11,* 440-459.

Frank, D. A., Allen, D., & Brown, J. L. (1985). Primary prevention of failure to thrive: Social policy implications. In D. Drotar (Ed.), *New directions in failure to thrive: Implications for research and practive* (pp. 337-358). New York: Plenum Press.

Garbarino, J. (1977). The human ecology of child maltreatment: A conceptual model for research. *Journal of Marriage and the Family, 39,* 721-735.

Hammill, P. V. V., Drizd, T. A., Johnson, C. L., Reed, R. B., Roche, A. F., & Moore, W. M. (1979). Physical growth: National Center for Health Statistics percentages. *American Journal of Clinical Nutrition, 32,* 607-629.

Holahan, C. J., & Moos, R. H. (1981). Social support and psychological distress: A longitudinal analysis. *Journal of Abnormal Psychology, 90,* 365-370.

Holahan, C. J., & Moos, R. H. (1983). The quality of social support: Measures of family and work relationships. *British Journal of Clinical Psychology, 22,* 157-162.

Hufton, I. W., & Oates, R. K. (1977). Non-organic failure to thrive: A long-term follow-up. *Pediatrics, 59,* 73-79.

Kanawati, A. A., Darwish, O., & McLaren, D. S. (1974). Failure to thrive in Lebanon. III: Family income, expenditure and possession. *Acta Paediatrica Scandinavia, 63,* 849-854.

Kotelchuck, M., & Newberger, E. H. (1983). Failure to thrive: A controlled study of family characteristics. *Journal of the American Academy of Child Psychiatry, 22,* 322-328.

Leonard, M. F., Rhymes, J. P., & Solnit, A. J. (1966). Failure to thrive in infants: A family problem. *American Journal of Diseases of Children, 111,* 600-612.

Lewis, J. M., Beavers, W. R., Gossett, J. T., & Phillips, V. A. (1976). *No single thread: Psychological health in family systems.* New York: Brunner/Mazel.

Moos, R. H., & Moos, B. S. (1976). A typology of family social environments. *Family Process, 15,* 357-371.

Moos, R. H., & Moos, B. S. (1981). *Family Environment Scale Manual.* Palo Alto, CA: Consulting Psychologist Press.

Olson, D. H., Sprenkle, D., & Russell, C. (1979). Circumplex model of marital and family systems. I: Cohesion and adaptability dimensions, family types and clinical applications. *Family Process, 18,* 3-28.
Parke, R. D. (1979). Perspectives on father-infant interaction. In J. D. Osofsky (Ed.), *Handbook of infant development* (pp. 549-590). New York: Wiley.
Parke, R. D., Power, T. G., & Gottman, J. M. (1979). Conceptualizing and quantifying influence patterns in the family triad. In M. E. Lamb, S. J. Suomi, & G. R. Stephenson (Eds.), *Social interaction analysis* (pp. 231-253). Madison: University of Wisconsin Press.
Patton, R. G., & Gardner, L. I. (1962). Influences of family environment on growth: The syndrome of maternal deprivation. *Pediatrics, 30,* 957-962.
Pedersen, F. A., Anderson, B. J., & Cain, R. C. (1980). Parent-infant and husband-wife interaction observed at age 5 months. In F. A. Pedersen (Ed.), Father-infant relationship. Observational studies in the family setting (pp. 71-86). New York: Praeger.
Pollitt, E., & Leibel, R. (1980). Biological and social correlates of failure to thrive. In L. Greene & F. E. Johnson (Eds.), *Social-biological predictors of nutritional status, physical growth, and neurological development* (pp. 173-200). New York: Academic Press.
Pugiliese, M. T., Weyman-Daum, M., Moses, N., & Lifshitz, P. (1987). Parental health beliefs as a cause of non-organic failure to thrive. *Pediatrics, 80,* 175-181.
Roberts, M. C., & Maddux, J. E. (1982). A psychosocial conceptualization of nonorganic failure to thrive. *Journal of Clinical Child Psychology, 11,* 216-226.
Schmitt, B. (Ed.). (1978). *The child protection team handbook.* New York: STM Press.
Sherrod, K. B., O'Connor, S., Altemeier, W. A., & Vietze, P. (1985). Toward a semispecific, multidimensional, threshold model of maltreatment. In D. Drotar (Ed.), *New directions in failure to thrive: Implications for research and practice* (pp. 89-107). New York: Plenum Press.
Siegel, I. E., & Parke, R. D. (1987). Structural analysis of parent-child research models. *Journal of Applied Developmental Psychology, 8,* 123-137.
Singer, L. T., & Fagan, J. F. (1984). The cognitive development of the failure to thrive infant. A three-year longitudinal study. *Journal of Pediatric Psychology, 9,* 363-383.
Talbot, N. B., Sobel, E. H., Burke, B. S., Lindemann, E., & Kaufman, S. B. (1947). Dwarfism in healthy children: Its possible relation to emotion, nutritional and endocrine disturbances. *New England Journal of Medicine, 236,* 783-793.
Wahler, R. G. (1980). The insular mother: Her problems in parent-child treatment. *Journal of Applied Behavior Analysis, 13,* 207-219.
Woolston, J. (1985). Diagnostic classification: The current challenge in failure to thrive syndrome research. In D. Drotar (Ed.), *New directions in failure to thrive: Implications for research and practice* (pp. 225-234). New York: Plenum Press.

6

AIDS and Hemophilia: Implications for Interventions with Families[1]

Patrick J. Mason
Department of Pediatrics and Department of Psychiatry and Behavioral Sciences, University of Oklahoma Health Sciences Center

Roberta A. Olson
Department of Psychiatry and Behavioral Sciences, University of Oklahoma Health Sciences Center

Jennifer G. Myers
Civil Aeromedical Institute, Federal Aviation Administration, Oklahoma City, Oklahoma

Heather C. Huszti
Department of Pediatrics and Department of Psychiatry and Behavioral Sciences, University of Oklahoma Health Sciences Center

Mary Kenning
University of Nebraska

Informational needs of hemophiliacs must first be assessed to develop effective educational and prevention programs. A survey of 132 hemophilia patients and family members was conducted to determine the information needs, the preferred source of information and the patients' knowledge of AIDS. Results indicated that the major source of information for the pa-

[1]We thank Felicia Kiplinger and Carla Horton for their help in preparing this manuscript. We especially acknowledge the time the effort of the families who participated in this study. This study was funded in part by the Hemophilia Grant from Maternal and Child Health (MCJ-130061-41045), Sharon Barrett, Director

tients was the media; the preferred source was the hemophilia treatment center. Most patients wanted more information about the treatment of AIDS and how to cope with the stresses of AIDS. Although patients indicated that they had received sufficient information about the sexual transmission of AIDS, answers to knowledge questions indicated important misconceptions. Results are discussed with respect to the development of educational and prevention programs for hemophiliacs and their families.

Hemophilia is a sex-linked hereditary blood coagulation disease that affects approximately 20,000 males in the United States. Persons with hemophilia lack necessary clotting proteins in their blood, which can result in painful hemorrhaging in major muscle groups and large joints. Repeated hemorrhaging in the joints can result in permanent crippling, and cerebal hemorrhaging can cause death. The primary treatment for bleeding episodes is the intravenous infusion of the missing clotting factor. In the 1960s it was discovered that the missing factor could be separated from whole blood and conveniently stored as a powdered concentrate that is mixed with sterile water prior to infusion (Pool & Shannon, 1965). This discovery enabled people with hemophilia to treat themselves at home in a more timely fashion, thus lengthening the life-span and enhancing the quality of life for the person with hemophilia.

Regional Hemophilia Diagnostic and Treatment Centers were established by a Block Services Grant Act that is administered by Division of Maternal and Child Health (Department of Health and Human Services). The Hemophilia Program was established to provide comprehensive health care to persons with hemophilia and their families. Studies that precipitated the development of the Hemophilia Program found that families with hemophilia had a number of unmet medical and psychosocial needs (Hilgartner, Aledor, & Giardina, 1985). Local physicians were unable to treat hemophilia adequately or respond to medical emergencies resulting from hemorrhaging. Families also were not receiving the guidance they needed in determining activities children with hemophilia could participate in, nor were they informed of the probabilities involved in giving birth to a second child with hemophilia. Thus, the goals and activities of the Hemophilia Centers were identified as (a) to improve the quality of hematological and orthopedic care, (b) to provide parents of children with hemophilia preventative counseling in the areas of child-rearing and safe physical activities, and (c) to provide genetic counseling to adolescents and adults with hemophilia.

Hemophilia has long been associated with a number of psychosocial difficulties for both the patient and their family members (Varni & Wallander, 1988). The discovery of cases of Acquired Immune Deficiency Syndrome (AIDS) and its possibility of transmission through blood and blood products created new problems for the hemophiliac and his family. A nationwide survey of regional Hemophilia Treatment Centers indicated that in 1985, 88% of pediatric and 94% of adult Factor VIII patients were seropositive (Jason, Stehr-Green, Holman, Evatt, & Hemophilia-AIDS Collaborative Study Group, 1988). For Factor IX deficient patients, 65% of pediatric and 43% of adults were seropositive. Since 1986, all blood products have been screened for the AIDS virus and inactivation processes have been employed so that the spread of AIDS through this means has been virtually eliminated. However, hemophiliacs who are currently infected with the AIDS virus, and their families, are now faced with potential new medical and psychosocial problems associated with this life-threatening condition.

HIV infection can add a variety of additional psychosocial stressors to hemophiliacs and their family members (Mason & Olson, in press). There is widespread social stigmatization associated with HIV infection and fears of job, school, community, and insurance discrimination are not unfounded (Backer, 1988; Kelly, St. Lawrence, Smith, Hood, & Cook, 1987; Tross & Hirsch, 1988). Parents must decide when and how to tell their infected child of his illness (Olson, Huszti, Mason, & Seibert, 1989). Sexually active seropositive hemophiliacs must alter their sexual behavior in order to prevent transmitting HIV to their partners (Mason, Olson, & Parish, 1988). Finally, as with all members of high-risk groups, hemophiliacs encounter multiple losses, including the deaths of family members and fellow patients from HIV-related diseases.

Previous research with terminally ill adults and children has suggested these individuals benefit from having an accurate understanding of their illness, as well as cognitive and emotional skills to cope with an uncertain future (Koocher, 1986; Kellerman, Rigler, & Siegel, 1977; Mishel, Hostetter, King, & Graham, 1984).

Few studies exist that have specifically addressed the potential needs of hemophiliacs and their families in dealing with AIDS. Agle, Gluck, and Pierce (1986) assessed emotional and behavioral reactions of persons with hemophilia and their families to the AIDS threat by surveying families enrolled in comprehensive hemophilia centers in Ohio, California, Massachusetts, and Washington. Agle et al. found that hemophiliacs were distressed about the possibility of HIV transmission and were at risk for developing psychological and social problems. The risk was inferred from respondents' level of distress. Parents of hemophiliacs reported significantly greater levels of concern, anger, and unhappiness than did hemophiliacs or their spouses. A critical finding was that the treatment of bleeding episodes was being affected, even though the risk for being exposed to HIV through blood products has been virtually eliminated. Hemophiliacs and parents of hemophiliacs reported treating fewer bleeding episodes per month after they had learned about AIDS and its association with hemophilia. The failure to treat bleeding episodes endangered the health of these children and adults with hemophilia. Additionally, approximately 7% of the parents reported that they were reluctant to be physically close to their sons because of fear of transmission of AIDS. These results suggest that interventions may be necessary to prevent medical and psychological problems arising from fear of exposure to the AIDS virus.

Assessment of knowledge of AIDS provides a second type of indicator of needs among the hemophiliacs and their families. Lack of knowledge regarding particular aspects of the treatment and transmission of AIDS suggests areas of information that should be targeted for dissemination to families with hemophilia. Distress or concerns may be reduced by providing such information. A national sample of 107 adult hemophiliacs were surveyed to examine their knowledge of HIV testing and AIDS (Hargraves et al., 1987). The respondents knew that homosexuals and intravenous drug users were at high risk for contracting AIDS. The majority of respondents also understood that a seropositive test result indicated the individual had been infected with HIV. However, a significant percentage of the respondents did not know that spouses of AIDS patients (29%) were at risk for contracting AIDS. These results indicated a need for further education concerning the risk of HIV exposure through sexual contact with HIV-infected hemophiliacs.

Little research exists on which to base a comprehensive program of prevention and intervention regarding AIDS for persons with hemophilia and their families. These studies by Agle et al. (1986) and Hargraves et al. (1987) separately suggest that hemophiliacs and their families have psychological and informational needs. However, the needs are not clearly identified, nor have the needs of family members been addressed separately. Too often educational programs and services are developed for specific populations without first assessing the actual needs of the population. If programs do not address the needs of their target population, they will not be be effective regardless of how well the program may be designed. The current study addressed these issues by surveying hemophilia patients and their families enrolled in a hemophilia treatment center. Respondents were asked to identify (a) their sources of information about AIDS-related topics, (b) those sources which provided the most useful information, (c) their preferred sources of additional information, and (d) the amount of information they had received for AIDS-related topics. An objective index of individuals' knowledge of the treatment and transmission of AIDS knowledge was also obtained.

METHOD

Subjects

The sample consisted of parents of children with hemophilia (57%), spouses of hemophiliacs (11%), and hemophiliacs over 13 years old (32%) enrolled in a Southwestern regional comprehensive hemophilia treatment center. All patients and their family members of the hemophilia treatment center were eligible to participate. Patients and family members were contacted by mail and telephone to explain the purpose of the study. Written informed consent was obtained from every participant prior to mailing the questionnaires. The first author was the only person who could match participants' identities to the numbered, confidential questionnaires. The first author had previous knowledge of each participations' HIV status because he was the psychologist assigned to the hemophilia center. Thus, confidentiality was maintained and APA's guidelines for conducting human subject research related to AIDS were followed. A total of 132 of a possible 165 individuals responded to the questionnaire, resulting in a return rate of 80%. The sample represents approximately 70% of the population regularly served by the hemophilia center. There were no systematic differences in demographics between patients who completed and return the questionnaires, and those who did not. Demographic information and HIV antibody status are presented in Table I.

Procedure

Families were first contacted by phone or mail to solicit participation in the study. Only one family declined to participate at this stage of contact. Individuals were offered $5 for their participation. A Susan B. Anthony dollar was sent with the questionnaire; the remaining $4 was sent following receipt of the questionnaire. Questionnaires were distributed in the spring of 1986. A follow-up mailing was sent 10 days after the questionnaire had been sent, reminding participants to return the questionnaire if they had not already done so.

Instruments

Demographic Information. Patients and family members were asked to provide age, diagnosis, (Factor VIII or IX), severity of factor deficiency

Table I. Subject Characteristics of Sample ($N = 132$)

Variable	n		% of total
Type of subjects			
Mother of patient	46		35
Father of patient	29		22
Spouse of patient	15		11
Patient over 18 ($n = 29$)			
Patient under 18 ($n = 13$)			
Patient total	42		32
Age of subjects			
13–21 years	19		14.2
22–35 years	61		46.2
36–60 years	52		39.4
Education of parents			
Completed high school	66		89%
Some college course work	43		57%
HIV antibody status of patient ($n = 74$)	Positive	Negative	Don't remember
	56%	38%	6%

(mild, moderate, or severe), and whether they had been tested for HIV antibodies and the results of that test. Consequently, HIV status was disclosed voluntarily. Family members were asked to respond to the above questions giving information about their relative with hemophilia.

HIV Needs Assessment for Hemophiliacs (HNAH). The HNAH was designed to assess respondent's sources and needs for information on 10 topics related to AIDS and hemophilia. The 10 topics were AIDS, patient testing for AIDS, blood donor testing, home infusion safety, HIV, sexual relations and AIDS, preventing the spread of AIDS, dealing with the attitudes of others about AIDS, and coping with the stress of AIDS. For each topic respondents were asked to identify (a) the sources of their information, (b) the sources that gave the most information, and (c) the sources of information that they prefer for receiving additional information. Respondents were instructed to check one or more of the sources listed (hemophilia clinic, National Hemophilia Foundation Newsletter, TV or written media, family or friends, National Hemophilia Foundation meeting, or special workshops) including an option to list a source not identified in the list. Respondents could indicate that they had never heard of the topic or that they did not want information on the topic. Finally, respondents were also asked to rate the amount of useful information they had received on each topic using a 5-point scale: *definitely too little, maybe too little, just right, maybe too much*, and *definitely too much.*

AIDS Knowledge Assessment (AKA). The AKA (Hargraves et al., 1987) was designed by the Centers for Disease Control and the National He-

Table II. Sample Question and Answer Format of the AIDS Knowledge Assessment (AKA)[a]

	Definitely yes	Probably yes	Don't know	Probably no	Definitely no
1. A person with antibodies to the AIDS agent (someone who is antibody-positive):					
(a) has AIDS	—	—	—	—	—
(b) is protected from AIDS	—	—	—	—	—
(c) has come in contact with the AIDS agent	—	—	—	—	—
(d) can give AIDS to someone else	—	—	—	—	—
(e) can still have the AIDS agent in his/her blood	—	—	—	—	—

[a]Permission to use the AKA may be obtained by contacting Dr. J. Jason, Center for Disease Control, Division of Host Factors, Atlanta, GA 30333.

mophilia Foundation to assess hemophilia patients' knowledge about (a) the cause of AIDS, (b) high-risk groups for contracting AIDS, (c) transmissibility of HIV, (d) treatment for AIDS, and (e) the meaning of HIV antibody status results. The questionnaire contains 14 items to which participants responded by marking "Definitely yes," "Probably yes," "Unsure," "Probably no," or "Definitely no." Some items contained multiple possible answers, each of which was also responded to using the answer categories above. An example of this type of question is found in Table II. A similar version of the AKA for use with nonhemophiliacs was administered to 98 high school students and 100 college students. The internal consistency was .75 using Cronbach's alpha (Huszti, Clopton, & Mason, in press).

RESULTS

Information Needs

The media (TV, newspapers, magazines) were cited by the largest percentage of respondents as sources of information for half of the 10 topics: AIDS, treatment of AIDS, preventing the spread of AIDS, sexual relations and AIDS, and dealing with attitudes of others about AIDS. The hemophilia center was the source of information for a majority of respondents regarding patient testing for AIDS, blood donor testing for AIDS, home infusion safety, and HIV (see Table III). A similar pattern of of responses was found for identification of sources that provided the *most information*. The media provided the most information about AIDS, its treatment and transmission, while the hemophilia treatment center addressed AIDS-related top-

Table III. Sources of AIDS Information by Percentage of Responses (N = 125)[a]

Topic category	Media	Hemophilia center	National Hemophilia Foundation	Special meeting
AIDS in general				
AIDS	93	51	31	6
Treatment for AIDS	59	23	9	3
AIDS and hemophilia				
Patient testing for AIDS	33	73	10	2
Blood donor testing/AIDS	26	63	22	2
Home infusion safety	3	72	6	5
HTLV-III (HIV)	29	63	23	2
AIDS and sex				
Preventing spread of AIDS	54	46	19	5
Sexual relationships and AIDS	70	34	19	3
AIDS and stress				
Dealing with attitudes of others about AIDS	44	24	7	3
Coping with stress and AIDS	41	53	15	4

[a]Multiple responses were allowed, thus categories do not add to 100%.

ics specific to the hemophiliac and his family. Few respondents (5% or less) selected any of the other alternatives as a source of information.

Although the media were an important source of information for a large percentage of individuals, two thirds or more of the respondents preferred the hemophilia center as a *source of additional information* for all the topics presented. In addition, approximately one third or more of the respondents also preferred the National Hemophilia Foundation Newsletter as a source of additional information on all of the topics.

The final question for each topic on the HNAH asked respondents to rate the amount of useful information they had received. This question was used to indicate respondents' perceived need for more information about each topic. Respondents who indicated they had received either "Definitely too little" information or "Maybe too little" information were categorized as needing additional information. The percentages of respondents who indicated a need for additional information for each category of AIDS-related topics are found in Table IV. Overall, a majority of respondents expressed needs for more information on all of the topics except for the following: (a) sexual relations and AIDS and (b) home infusion safety. The majority of respondents reported receiving too little information about (a) the treatment of AIDS (87%), (b) dealing with the attitudes of others about AIDS (84%), and (c) coping with stress and AIDS (87%).

This pattern of needs is essentially the same across parents, patients, and spouses although some interesting differences also emerged. A higher

Table IV. Percentages of Subjects Perceived Need for Additional AIDS-Related Information

Topic category	Need %	%
AIDS in general		79
AIDS	71	
Treatment for AIDS	87	
AIDS and hemophilia		63
Patient testing for AIDS	70	
Blood donor testing/AIDS	65	
Home infusion safety	45	
HTLV-III (HIV)	75	
AIDS and sex		57
Preventing spread of AIDS	65	
Sexual relationships and AIDS	49	
AIDS and stress		86
Dealing with attitudes of others about AIDS	84	
Coping with stress and AIDS	87	

percentage of spouses of patients expressed a need for additional information about sexual relations and AIDS (62%) than did patients (53%), fathers of patients (57%), or mothers of patients (38%). In comparison to the other groups, a higher percentage of spouses also felt they had received too little information on preventing the spread of AIDS and the topic of AIDS in general.

A one-way multivariate analysis of variance (MANOVA) was computed to determine differences in responses between mothers, fathers, spouses, and patients using all 10 AIDS-related topics as the dependent variables. Additionally, a MANOVA was performed using known patient HIV status (positive or negative as supplied by the patient) as the independent variable and the 10 topics as the dependent variables. Neither analysis demonstrated significant differences among the groups tested.

AIDS Knowledge Assessment (AKA)

The internal consistency of the AKA was calculated using all 37 items on the questionnaire (Cronbach's alpha = .81). However, the statistic was based on only two thirds of the sample because of the large amount of missing data. Respondents appeared to be confused by the format of the questionnaire, which required responding to all alternative answer for particular questions (see Table II). Despite some participant confusion over the format of the questionnaire, the AKA was utilized in this study because it has been used with other populations of hemophiliac patient and family members (Hargraves et al., 1987), allowing for a direct comparison of knowledge level of AIDS across different hemophilia populations.

A one-way analysis of variance (ANOVA) was computed to investigate the differences between mothers', fathers', spouses', and patients' total scores on the AKA. No significant differences between groups were found, $F(3, 83) = 1.67$, $p = .18$. Furthermore, no significant differences on the AKA were found between respondents who had an HIV antibody-positive family member and those who did not.

In order to compute the percentage of respondents who answered correctly, incorrectly, or do not know, the five-point scale of the AKA was collapsed. The results revealed that 50% of the respondents did not know whether sexual partners of hemophiliacs were considered a risk for AIDS; 21% incorrectly assumed that children of hemophiliacs were at risk for AIDS and 24% were not sure. Many respondents were either incorrect or unsure if AIDS could be spread by eating utensils (38%), kissing (50%), or saliva (73%). Table V provides a summary of the percentages of inaccurate responses to the AKA.

Table V. Percentages of Inaccurate Responses to AIDS Knowledge Assessment Questionnaire ($N = 125$)

Topic	Correct answer	% of cases incorrect	% of cases don't know
Cause of AIDS			
Bacteria	no	18	27
Risk groups			
Sexual partners of hemophiliacs	yes	33	17
Health care workers	no	33	17
Children of hemo fathers	no	21	24
Spread of AIDS			
Eating utensils	no	20	18
Kissing	no	29	21
Saliva	no	42	29
Hemophilia – infusion safety			
Heat – treated vs. not – heat treated concentrate	yes	0	16
Avoid infusion for bleeds	no	14	12
Treatment of AIDS			
Medical care can help	yes	16	31
Cure from AIDS	no	6	35
Implications of seroposition test			
Has AIDS	no	11	34
Protected from AIDS	no	7	27
Been exposed to AIDS agent	yes	4	22
Can give AIDS	yes	15	45
Still has AIDS agent in blood	yes	3	28

Fourteen percent of the respondents were incorrect in assuming it was better to avoid treating some joint bleeds (hemorrhages) to decrease the risk of AIDS. Sixteen percent were not sure if heat-treated blood concentrate was safer than non-heat-treated concentrate.

Questions designed to assess knowledge about the implications of a seropositive test result revealed that a significant minority of respondents did not know if a positive result meant that person had AIDS (34%), was protected from AIDS (27%), had been exposed to the AIDS agent (22%), could give AIDS to someone else (45%), or still had the AIDS agent in his blood (28%).

The relationship between respondents' objective index of AIDS-related knowledge (AKA) and their perceived need for additional information (HNAH) was examined by computing Pearson product correlation coefficients between the summary scores on the AKA with each of the perceived need scores on the 10 AIDS-related topics on the HNAH. None of the resultant coefficients were statistically significant and they ranged from $-.04$ to $.17$. The correlation coefficient for the summary score on the AKA and the summary score for perceived need on the HNAH was $r = .08$, $p = .21$. Respondents' level of AIDS knowledge was not significantly related to their perceived need for additional AIDS information.

DISCUSSION

The results of this study indicated that most hemophiliacs and their family members were receiving their information about the treatment and transmission of AIDS from the media. Respondents received information about other aspects of AIDS specific to hemophilia (e.g., blood donor testing) through the hemophilia center. However, a majority of the respondents preferred to receive additional information on all topics from the hemophilia center. The need for additional information about AIDS and the AIDS knowledge level of hemophiliacs and their family members were not affected by HIV status. It is possible that the length of time since being informed of HIV status may effect knowledge levels or the need for information, but because HIV status itself made no difference in these two variables, length of time since diagnosis of HIV infection was not included as a variable.

Respondents' desires to receive information from a hemophilia center may reflect a level of trust and credibility that has been established between the patients' families and the hemophilia center. Many of these families have long-standing ties with the hemophilia center. In addition, hemophiliacs and their families are probably less likely to seek out information from relatives and friends who may typically serve as information resources for other parenting and life-style issues because of the stigma associated with AIDS. The fact that respondents desired additional information from the hemophilia center, yet were receiving the most useful information on some of the topics from the media, suggests that hemophilia centers should increase the amount and types of information they provide to their patients. Hemophilia centers throughout the United States are implementing new strategies to meet these needs (see Mason et al., 1988).

The needs of information reported by respondents centered around treatment of AIDS, attitudes of others, and stress. Each of these needs suggests a slightly different approach. Treatment issues can be handled through the dissemination of factual information and face-to-face discussion. Respondents' concerns regarding the attitudes of others about AIDS requires targeting the community for intervention, as well as the patient. Educational programs for children and adults about AIDS and its transmission can shape the attitudes of these individuals (Huszti et al., in press) and help to reduce the stigma and subsequent psychological impact on hemophiliacs and their families.

The largest needs for information were reported for treatment of AIDS, dealing with the attitude of others regarding AIDS, and psychological needs associated with the threat of AIDS. Although fewer respondents wanted additional information on sexual relations and AIDS, scores on the AIDS Knowledge Assessment revealed that approximately half of those surveyed had inaccurate knowledge of the risks associated with sexual contact with hemophiliacs and the meaning of seropositive test results. Overall, no relationship was found between knowledge scores and needs for information.

The finding that 50% of the respondents did not know that sexual partners of hemophiliacs were at risk for AIDS indicates that there is a need for additional information regarding the transmissibility of HIV with this population. However, the topic "sexual relations and AIDS" was least endorsed as an information need for most of the respondents. Rather, AIDS topics related to managing stress and more general AIDS-related topics were the most often identified areas for further information. Perhaps the respondents felt that the information they had was accurate, or they were simply reluctant to indicate that they needed additional information in this area. Another interpretation of these findings is that patients and their families are currently more interested in receiving information to help them better "cope and hope" with the fears and social stigma associated with AIDS.

Another possible explanation is that hemophiliacs may wish to distance themselves from any connection with the homosexual high-risk group and that a focus on changing sexual practices is too similar to the changes made by the homosexual/bisexual population. Even more likely is that the characteristic coping patterns that hemophiliacs have used to deal with the consequences of their chronic disease, such as a denial of pain and a determination that their disease will not stop their participation in all activities, are being used to deal with their HIV infection (Mason et al., 1988). This explanation is supported by the fact that there were no differences in the knowledge levels of HIV-positive and HIV-negative patients. Both types of patients had acquired an equivalent degree of AIDS knowledge. Unfortunately, these coping patterns are not effective when applied to the prevention of the further spread of HIV infection to sexual partners. Prevention requires the acquisition of knowledge about the sexual transmission of HIV and of new behaviors that decrease the likelihood of HIV transmission, such as the use of condoms.

Because sexual transmission of HIV remains a critically important health issue, safe sexual practices must be communicated to this high-risk group in a way that results in patients comprehending the information and complying with the recommendations. These results highlight the necessity of conducting needs assessments prior to implementing new educational or treatment programs. Although the results of the AKA strongly suggest the need for additional information about sexual transmission of HIV, the results of the needs assessment indicate hemophiliacs do not recognize that need. Consequently, it is likely the programs stressing sexual information will not be widely utilized by the hemophilia population. Efforts need to be made to help hemophiliacs recognize their need for additional information about sexual transmission before patient education can be successful.

The lack of relationships between knowledge and needs can be accounted for by the high percentages of respondents requesting additional information on AIDS-related topics. Regardless of what the respondents already knew, they wanted more information. The threat of AIDS and the desire to be knowledgeable of all aspects of AIDS was present whether the HIV antibody status was positive or negative, suggesting that all hemophiliacs and their families are affected in some way by the disease.

Although the AKA and Needs Assessment were administered in March 1986, more recent testing of additional hemophiliacs in a different setting using the AKA suggest that knowledge has not significantly increased over the past 2 years (VanVoorhess, Cruz, Bordeaux, & Mason, 1989).

The results of this needs assessment suggest that federally funded programs designed to reduce the spread of HIV and encourage safer sexual practices must include instructive and supportive coping skills training to deal with the stresses associated with the threat of AIDS and HIV infection. By being an "empathic helper" (Thoits, 1986), more effective support can be provided that may lead to positive changes in behavior. Additionally, these programs must recognize and address the stresses associated with hemophilia that are separate from HIV-related issues.

Needs assessments should be an integral part of the development of new programs. Periodic needs assessments should be performed to determine if additional services are needed. For example, a recent needs assessment of homosexual/bisexual males suggests that the majority want additional informational about ways to improve their immune system functioning (Lovejoy, Moran, & Paul, 1988). Baseline information assessing perceived needs and knowledge are essential to evaluate the intensive ongoing patient–family educational programs that have been initiated through multimillion dollar federal funding of hemophilia prevention programs.

REFERENCES

Agle, D., Gluck, H., & Pierce, G. F. (1986). The risk of AIDS: Psychologic impact on the hemophilic population. *General Hospital Psychiatry, 9,* 11-17.

Backer, T. E. (1988). Managing AIDS at work: Psychology's role. *American Psychologist, 43,* 983-987.

Eiser, C., Eider, J. R., & Lang, J. (in press). How adolescents compare AIDS with other diseases: Implications for prevention. *Journal of Pediatric Psychology.*

Hargraves, M. A., Jason, J. M., Chorba, T. L., Holman, R. C., Dixon, G. R., Eastham, C. J., Brownstein, A. P., Heine, P., Agle, D. P., & Evatt, B. L. (1987). Hemophiliac patients' knowledge and educational needs concerning AIDS. *American Journal of Hematology, 26,* 115-134.

Herek, G. M. & Glunt, E. K. (1988). An epidemic of stigma: Public reactions to AIDS. *American Psychologist, 43,* 886-891.

Hilgartner, M. W., Aledort, L., & Giardina, P. J. V. (1985). Thalassemia and hemophilia. In N. Hobbs & J. M. Perrin (Eds.), *Issues in the care of children with chronic illness* (pp. 299-323). San Francisco: Jossey-Bass.

Huszti, H. C., Clopton, J. R., & Mason, P. J. (in press). Effects of AIDS education programs on adolescents' knowledge and attitudes. *Pediatrics.*

Jason, J. M., Stehr-Green, J., Holman, R. C., Evatt, B. L., & Hemophilia–AIDS Collaborative Study Group. (1988). Human immunodeficiency virus infection in hemophilic children. *Pediatrics, 82,* 565-570.

Kellerman, J., Rigler, D., & Siegel, S. E. (1977). Psychological effects of isolation in protected environments. *American Journal of Psychiatry, 134,* 563-568.

Kelly, J. A., St. Lawrence, J. S., Smith, S., Hood, H. V., & Cook, D. J. (1987). Stigmatization of AIDS patients by physicians. *American Journal of Public Health, 77,* 789-791.

Koocher, G. P. (1986). Psychosocial issues during the acute treatment of pediatric cancer. *Cancer, 58,* 468-472.

Lovejoy, N. C., Moran, T. A., & Paul, S. (1988). Self-care behaviors and informational needs of seropositive homosexual/bisexual men. *Journal of Acquired Immune Deficiency Syndromes, 1,* 155-161.

Mason, P. J., & Olson, R. A. (in press). Psychosocial aspects of AIDS and HIV infection in pediatric hemophilia patients. In J. Seibert & R. Olson (Eds.), *Children, adolescents, and AIDS.* Lincoln: University of Nebraska Press.

Mason, P. J. Olson, R. A., & Parish, K. L. (1988). AIDS, hemophilia and prevention efforts within a comprehensive care program. *American Psychologist, 43,* 971-976.

Mishel, M. H., Hostetter, T., King, B., & Graham, V. (1984). Predictors of psychosocial adjustments in patients newly diagnosed with gynecological cancer. *Cancer Nursing, 7,* 291-299.

Olson, R. A., Huszti, H. C., Mason, P. J., & Seibert, J. M. (1989). Pediatric AIDS/HIV infection: An emerging challenge to pediatric psychology. *Journal of Pediatric Psychology, 14,* 1-21.

Pool, J. G., & Shannon, A. E. (1965). Production of high-potency concentrates of antihemophilic globulin in a closed bag system: Assay in vitro and in vivo. *New England Journal of Medicine, 273,* 1443-1447.

Thoits, P. (1986). Social support as coping assistance. *Journal of Consulting and Clinical Psychology, 54,* 416-423.
Tross, S., & Hirsch, D. A. (1988). Psychological distress and neuropsychological complications of HIV infection and AIDS. *American Psychologist, 43,* 929-934.
VanVoorhess, C. J., Cruz, M. C., Bordeaux, J., & Mason, P. J. (1989). Demographic differences in accuracy of AIDS knowledge. Manuscript submitted for publication.
Varni, J. W., & Wallander, J. L. (1988). Pediatric chronic disabilities: Hemophilia and spina bifida as examples. In D. K. Routh (Ed.), *Handbook of pediatric psychology* (pp. 190-221). New York: Guilford.

7

Family Variables and Disease Management in Juvenile Rheumatoid Arthritis

John M. Chaney and Lizette Peterson
University of Missouri–Columbia

Examined the relationship between family functioning and regimen knowledge, medication compliance, and disease activity for children with juvenile rheumatoid arthritis. A strong relationship was found across several measures of family functioning and a self-monitoring index of medication compliance. Family functioning was not related to regimen knowledge or disease activity. The implications of these findings for the continued study of chronically ill children are discussed.

Juvenile rheumatoid arthritis (JRA) is a type of chronic arthritis that manifests itself prior to the age of 16. Roughly 5,000 new cases of JRA are diagnosed annually, making it the most common childhood connective tissue disease (Phillips, 1981). JRA represents a heterogeneous illness that can be divided into three distinct onset types: (a) systemic-onset; (b) polyarticular-onset; and (c) pauciarticular-onset. There exists a great deal of variability both between and within the disease subtypes regarding age at onset, clinical manifestation, and disease course—which can include periods of acute exacerbation and unpredictable remissions (Brewer et al., 1977; Wedgwood & Schaller, 1977).

Comprehensive approaches to the treatment of JRA have been suggested (Rennebohm & Correll, 1984; Singsen, Johnson, & Bernstein, 1979) that include a broad spectrum of services (e.g., physical and occupational therapies, psychological and social services) in addition to pharmacologic management. The ultimate goals of such approaches would be the culmination of efforts to minimize inflammation and to maximize physical and psychosocial functioning (Hunder & Bunch, 1982; Sullivan, 1982).

Pharmacologic management of JRA is largely an additive process, and the effectiveness of a medication regimen is chiefly determined by clinical trials of a particular drug. Decisions to alter and/or augment therapy for a given child are based on the success or failure of a given trial. The initial drug of choice is acetylsalicylic acid (aspirin), but other nonsteroidal anti-inflammatory drugs (NSAIDs) are also used in JRA (e.g., tolmetin sodium, naproxin). Patients typically receive an initial trial of aspirin, but responses vary considerably and a legitimate trial requires maintenance of the drug at therapeutic levels for several weeks (Wedgwood & Schaller, 1977).

If no satisfactory response is achieved with salicylates or another NSAID over a period of several months, more aggressive treatment is implemented. This usually involves the introduction of gold salt (a slower acting antirheumatic drug; SAARD), hydroxychloroquine (a slow-acting antimalarial drug), and as a last resort corticosteroids. Each progression up the therapeutic ladder, or "pyramid" (Deyo, 1982, p. 234) involves an increase both in the invasiveness of the regimen (e.g., parenteral injections of gold salt) and/or toxicity of the medication (e.g., hydroxychloroquine, corticosteroids).

Without considering the integrity of administration (or actual amount received) of the treatment during clinical trials, failure to achieve therapeutic response may be erroneously attributed to the ineffectiveness of the regimen or of a particular drug. Further, there is some evidence that the use of NSAIDs can serve to decrease the need for corticosteroids in the medication regimen (Blechman & Zane, 1976). This suggests that more attention should be focused on compliance to the regimen, particularly in the early stages of therapy before initiating more aggressive treatment (cf. Anderson, Bradley, Young, McDaniel, & Wise, 1985). Feinstein (1979) illustrated the manner in which disparate rates of compliance can yield a false dissimilarity in the apparent efficacy of two pharmacologically equal drugs. Thus, it appears that increasing compliance to medication regimens could assist in establishing the efficacy of pharmacological treatments for JRA.

With the exception of a few studies (e.g., Litt & Cuskey, 1981; Litt, Cuskey, & Rosenberg, 1982; Rapoff, Lindsley, & Christophersen, 1984; Rapoff, Purviance, & Lindsley, 1988), little attention has been given to medication regimen compliance in JRA. Additionally, the primary social context in which disease management occurs, the family, has been largely ignored. If, as suggested, a comprehensive approach to managing JRA (e.g., Singsen et al., 1979) is to be adopted, then an examination of the role that family relations plays appears to be crucial.

Researchers investigating other chronic illnesses have provided evidence to suggest that family relations play an important role in compliance and disease management (e.g., Anderson, Miller, Auslander, & Santiago, 1981; Fehrenbach & Peterson, 1989; Hanson, Henggeler, Burghen, & Moore, in press; Korsch, Fine, & Negrete, 1978; Koski & Kumento, 1977). Further, it has been suggested that family factors may directly impact disease activity, independent of adherence (Hanson, Henggeler, & Burghen, 1987a, 1987b).

Comprehension of the regimen also appears to play a necessary, but not sufficient, role in determining (non)compliance (Podell, 1975). However, this relationship is not unequivocal, suggesting that other factors (perhaps family relations) may mediate the association between regimen knowledge and regimen implementation.

The purpose of the present study was to examine the relationship of family factors with disease management in JRA. The Circumplex Model of Marital and Family Systems (Olson, Sprenkle, & Russell, 1979) was chosen to derive the important family variables. This family conceptualization incorporates many of the variables (i.e., cohesion and adaptability, family satisfaction, family stress and coping) demonstrating utility in previous research with chronically ill children (e.g., Hanson et al., 1987a, 1987b; Minuchin, Rosman, & Baker, 1978).

METHOD

Subjects

Subjects were 16 female and 9 male JRA patients, ages 7–17, and their parents from a pediatric rheumatology clinic. Of 27 families requested to participate, 25 (approximately 96%) agreed to take part in the study. One family refused to participate due to time constraints and another family declined for personal reasons. The mean age for the group was 12.5 years, ranging from 7.75 to 17.75 years of age. Forty-four percent of the sample had pauciarticular-onset JRA, 44% had polyarticular JRA, and 12% had systemic-onset JRA. Eighty-eight percent of the families were intact; 12% were divorced. The average socioeconomic level of the families was 47 (Hollingshead social class = IV; Hollingshead & Redlich, 1958), with scores ranging from 11 to 65, indicating that families ranged from lower to upper socioeconomic classes

Procedure

During a routine medical visit with the physician, the measures of disease activity were taken. All physical examinations were performed by the same pediatric rheumatologist to minimize rater variability. The rheumatologist was uninformed of the self-report measures. Following the visit, the patient and his/her parent(s) were asked to participate in the study. If verbal consent was obtained, the patient and his/her parent(s) were instructed in the completion of the self-report measures, were separated until the measures were completed, and were then jointly trained by the primary investigator in the self-monitoring and recording of medication compliance. The interviewer was uninformed of the patients' level of disease activity.

Because of the possibility that the instruments exceeded the reading level of many of the subjects, questionnaires were read aloud to all children. The total length of contact time with each family was approximately 1¼ hours. Parents not present at the time of the initial contact were asked to complete the measures at home and return them by mail in an addressed, postage-paid envelope. Preaddressed, stamped compliance records were also mailed in weekly by the families.

Measures

Disease Activity

Disease activity was assessed by the pediatric rheumatologist across a number of disease parameters: (a) number of swollen joints, (b) number of tender joints, (c) number of joints that are painful or have limited range of motion; and (d) duration (in minutes) of morning stiffness. Consistent with Brewer and Giannini (1982), the number of joints was treated as the primary index of disease activity. Joint counts in each category were summed to yield the overall disease activity measure. A moderate coefficient alpha (.55) was determined for this measure. Duration of morning stiffness was analyzed separately. In addition, physician, patient, and parent 0–10 Likert scale estimates of disease activity were collected.

Knowledge of the Regimen

Each available member of the child–mother–father triad was measured separately on a medication quiz for his/her knowledge of the medication regimen in five areas: (a) name of the medication, (b) purpose of the medication, (c) amount of the drug to be taken in each dose, (d) total number of daily doses, and (e) time of administration of each dose. These items were assessed for accuracy via medical records and physician reports. Items were scored in a dichotomous fashion (i.e., yes–no) and were summed to yield a knowledge score for each available member. Interview reports determined the person responsible for regimen implementation, and that person's score was treated as the primary measure of regimen knowledge. A coefficient alpha of .82 was calculated for the primary knowledge measure.

Compliance

Compliance was measured in two ways. First, family members (parents and patients) were asked to estimate the patient's typical compliance (number of doses taken) for an average week. This global measure of the patient's weekly compliance was calculated by dividing the number of estimated doses taken by the actual number of prescribed doses. The compliance estimate of the person responsible for regimen implementation was utilized as the global compliance estimate.

A self-monitoring, weekly medication diary was also utilized. The parent(s) and the child recorded the number of doses as the medication was taken by the patient over a 3-week period. Diaries were prepared by the interviewer to reflect the number of prescribed medications, number of prescribed daily doses, and prescribed time for daily doses.

A percentage compliance score was calculated by dividing the number of doses reported to have been administered by the number of prescribed doses and was considered the primary measure of compliance. Forty-one percent of the families ($n = 9$) returned all diaries, 36% ($n = 8$) returned two, 5% ($n = 1$) returned one diary, and 18% ($n = 4$) failed to return diaries. Thus, a total of 18 families (82%) were included in the analysis regarding compliance.

Family Adaptability and Cohesion

These dimensions were assessed by the Family Adaptability and Cohesion Evaluation Scales III (FACES III; Olson, Portner, & Lavee, 1985). FACES III is a 20-item self-report instrument that yields two orthogonal dimensions, cohesion and adaptability (Olson et al., 1985). Internal consistency and test-retest reliability has been demonstrated by Olson (1986).

Consistent with Olson et al. (1983), the parent and adolescent scores obtained on this scale were regarded as the primary data on cohesion and adaptability. The cohesion dimension ranges from extremely low levels of cohesion (disengaged) to extremely high levels (enmeshed). Adaptability ranges from extremely low (rigid) to extremely high (chaotic). Scores near the center represent optimum levels of these dimensions. Family mean and distance from center (DFC) scores were calculated to determine family levels of reported adaptability and cohesion as well as each family's relative position from the center of the circumplex (Olson et al., 1985).

Because there was no known scale to assess young children's perceptions of family functioning, subjects under the age of 12 were administered a modified version of the FACES III created for the present study (FACES III-K). The FACES III-K employed simpler terminology and utilized a "structured alternative format" (cf. Harter, 1982), thus preserving the information and method of scoring similar to that of the original FACES III.

Primary analyses considered only adult FACES III scores when the child was under the age of 12 and utilized both adult and adolescent scores when the child was 12 or older. However, exploratory analyses utilized DFC scores on the FACES III-K scale in the same fashion as the adolescent scores.

Family Satisfaction

Parents, and subjects 12 and over, completed the 14-item, self-report Family Satisfaction questionnaire (Olson & Wilson, 1985) which measures individual's degree of satisfaction with the family's current level of functioning on the cohesion and adaptability dimensions. Acceptable levels of internal consistency and test–retest reliability are reported by Olson et al. (1985). Because Olson and his colleagues reported that the measure is unidimensional, total scores were used to determine each person's level of overall satisfaction.

As with the FACES III measure, there was no comparable family satisfaction scale for younger children. Therefore, utilizing the format mentioned above, a scale was designed for the present study that assessed younger children's self-reported family satisfaction (Family Satisfaction-K).

Family Coping

Family coping strategies were assessed by the Family Crisis Oriented Personal Evaluation Scales (F-COPES; McCubbin, Larsen, & Olson, 1985). The F-COPES is a 30-item self-report scale that was completed by the parents. Acceptable test–retest and internal consistency has been demonstrated by Olson et al. (1985). Parents' scores were analyzed separately (cf. Olson et al., 1983).

Family Life Events

The Family Inventory of Life Events and Changes (FILE; McCubbin, Patterson, & Wilson, 1985) instrument was administered to the parents. The FILE is a 70-item questionnaire that assesses the family's life stress. Acceptable levels of internal consistency and test–retest reliability are provided by Olson et al. (1985). Items endorsed by either parent were counted as a stressor for both and were combined to constitute the measure of family stress.

RESULTS

The primary analyses focused on the relationship between family variables and medication compliance. Partial correlational analyses were conducted to determine the nature of the relationship between the family variables, regimen knowledge, compliance, and disease activity. Exploratory analyses examined the relationship among (a) original scales and those created for the present study, (b) the various estimates of compliance, and (c) the global indices of disease activity and objective measures of disease activity.

Pearson product-moment correlations were calculated to determine the relationships between the various family measures and the compliance measures (means for all of these variables are found in Table I). As seen in

Table I. Means and Standard Deviations of Dependent Measures

Dependent measures	*M*	*SD*
Family adaptability	23.7	3.3
Family cohesion	39.3	4.9
Father coping	73.2	20.7
Mother coping	84.9	17.1
Father satisfaction	42.7	8.2
Mother satisfaction	44.6	8.2
Child satisfaction	43.5	10.8
Family life events	16.6	9.3
Disease activity	19.2	20.6
Minutes of morning stiffness	10.6	16.4
% compliance (medication diary)	87.9	11.9
% compliance (global estimate)	96.0	5.7
Regimen knowledge	4.6	0.7

Table II. Correlations Between Family Variables and Medication Regimen Compliance

Family variable	Compliance
Family distance from center (FACES III)	$-.54^{b}$
Family mean adaptability (FACES III)	$-.16$
Family mean cohesion (FACES III)	.32
Family inventory of life events and changes (FILE)	$-.61^{d}$
Family satisfaction (mother)	.05
Family satisfaction (father)	$.61^{c}$
Family satisfaction (child)	.24
Family crisis-oriented personal evaluation scales (mother)	$.49^{a}$
Family crisis-oriented personal evaluation scales (father)	.35

$^{a}p < .03$.
$^{b}p < .02$.
$^{c}p < .01$.
$^{d}p < .006$.

Table II, the results showed several significant correlations between the family variables and percentage compliance on the compliance diary. No significant relationships were found for the family variables and the global estimate of compliance.

The negative relationship between the family DFC scores and the primary measure of compliance, $r(16) = -.54$, $p < .02$, indicated that more extreme families (i.e., those further from the center of the circumplex model) were associated with lower levels of medication compliance. This nonlinear association was further highlighted by the lack of significant correlations between both family mean adaptability and cohesion scores and regimen compliance.

To further investigate the relationship between percentage compliance and adaptability and cohesion, both dimensions were placed into quadratic regression equations. To reduce multicollinearity (Neter, Wasserman, & Kutner, 1983), the mean scores utilized were deviation mean scores (i.e., the group family mean scores on these two dimensions were subtracted from each family's mean score on the same dimension). Family mean cohesion and adaptability were entered first into the respective models, then the quadratic terms were entered. The results indicated that the quadratic term for cohesion produced a significant model for predicting percentage compliance, $R = .47$, $F(2, 13) = 4.9$, $p < .03$. The quadratic term for adaptability approached significance, $R = .27$, $F(2, 13) = 1.99$, $p < .08$. Because the linear terms in both equations accounted for no significant additional variance in the models, the same analyses were performed with only the quadratic terms in the models to predict percentage compliance. The results were similar to the initial curvilinear tests. For cohesion, $R = .40$, $F(1, 13) = 7.95$, $p < .01$, and for adaptability, $R = .26$, $F(1, 13) = 4.24$, $p < .06$.

Family life events demonstrated a negative relationship with compliance, $r(16) = -.61$, $p < .006$. Thus, families who endorsed a greater number of life stressors reported lower levels of medication compliance. Conversely, two family variables exhibited positive correlations with medication compliance; specifically, mothers' coping, $r(16) = .49$, $p < .03$, and fathers' satisfaction, $r(13) = .61$, $p < .01$. These correlations indicated that mothers who endorsed a greater number of coping behaviors were associated with higher levels of children's adherence. Further, fathers who reported higher levels of family satisfaction had children who demonstrated better compliance with the medication regimen. All of these relationships were in the predicted direction.

Family Functioning and Medication Compliance as Mediators

Pearson product-moment correlations and partial correlations were performed to test whether (a) family relations mediated the relationship between regimen knowledge and compliance, and (b) medication compliance mediated the relationship between family functioning and disease activity. The original correlation between primary regimen knowledge scores and percentage compliance revealed a nonsignificant relationship, $r(16) = .21$, $p > .05$. This may have been due in part to a ceiling effect demonstrated by the regimen knowledge variable. The maximum possible score for the variable was 5; the mean regimen knowledge score observed was 4.59, with a restricted range of 3 to 5. The individual partial correlations, controlling for the effects of family functioning, revealed no significant partial correlations.

The zero-order correlations between all family variables and disease activity were nonsignificant. Similarly, when compliance was partialed out of the relationship between family variables and disease activity, no partial correlations were significant. As with the knowledge measure, the index of disease activity suffered from a skewed distribution of scores.

Exploratory Analyses

Although not the major focus of the study, analyses were performed to test for the relationships between the children's instruments created for this study (the FACES III-K and the Family Satisfaction-K) and the standard versions of the same measures. Pearson product-moment correlations and subsequent Fisher's (1921) r to z transformations indicated that neither the DFC scores obtained from the FACES III-K designed for this study nor the adolescent scores on the FACES III designed by Olson were related to parent DFC scores, $r(6) = -.05, p > .05$; and $r(14) = .35, p > .05$, respectively. The difference in these two correlations was also not significant, $z = .775, p > .05$.

The Family Satisfaction-K questionnaire was more highly related to the mother's Family Satisfaction scores, $r(6) = .89, p < .01$, than were the adolescent scores from the original Family Satisfaction Questionnaire, $r(14) = .20, p > .05$, and this difference was statistically significant, $z = 2.64, p < .05$. Child version scores of family satisfaction created for this study were also more highly correlated with father scores, $r(6) = .40, p > .05$, than were adolescent satisfaction scores on the original questionnaire, $r(14) = .21, p > .05$, but this difference was not statistically significant, $z = .40, p > .05$.

Thus the FACES III-K created for this study was at least as closely related to parent DFC scores as those scores obtained by adolescents on the standard version. In addition, the correlations between children's scores on the Family Satisfaction-K were significantly more highly related to the mothers' satisfaction scores than were the adolescent's satisfaction scores on the standard version. Child and adolescent scores were equally related in the patient–father correlations for family satisfaction.

Correlations were also performed to test for the relationships among the various compliance estimates. Parent–child comparisons yielded nonsignificant results, suggesting that there was little agreement among family members on global estimates of medication compliance. Primary estimates of global compliance (i.e., those from the person responsible for administered medication) also demonstrated a nonsignificant relationship with medication diary compliance, $r(18) = .27, p > .05$.

The final series of validation analyses focused on the relationships between parent, child, and physician global ratings of disease severity and the relationships among these global estimates and the objective disease activity rating. In contrast to the compliance estimates, all correlations among the physician, parent, and child global estimates of disease activity were signifi-

Table III. Correlations Among Global Estimates of Disease Activity and Objective Ratings of Disease Activity

Global rating	Father global	Mother global	Child global	Objective disease
Physician	.87[c]	.89[c]	.83[c]	.64[a]
Father		.82[c]	.64[c]	.68[b]
Mother			.81[c]	.62[a]
Child				.47

[a] $p < .001$.
[b] $p < .002$.
[c] $p < .0001$.

cant, ranging from $r = .64$ to $r = .89$ (Table III). These results indicated that there was high agreement on the global estimate of disease severity among parent, child, and physician ratings. The correlations between the global estimates of disease severity and the objective disease activity measure also resulted in significant relationships for all but the children's estimates (Table III).

DISCUSSION

The principal goals of the present study were to examine the associations between family functioning and regimen knowledge, medication compliance, and disease activity in children with juvenile rheumatoid arthritis. Of these three primary areas of investigation, family functioning and medication compliance demonstrated a strong relationship across several different measures. The relationship between the FACES III scores and compliance suggested that more extreme levels of family functioning were associated with poorer medication compliance. These findings provide support for the circumplex model of family relations (Olson et al., 1979) in that families experiencing optimal levels of cohesion and adaptability (i.e., those closer to the center of the circumplex) were more closely associated with more adaptive functioning (i.e., better medication compliance).

Other measures of family functioning also demonstrated significant relationships with the diary measure of medication compliance. Family life events evidenced a significant relationship with medication compliance. The results suggest that as the number of family stressors (as reported by the parents) increases, compliance decreases. Similarly, mothers' coping behaviors were significantly related to compliance, indicating that families in which mothers reported a greater number of coping behaviors had children who demonstrated higher levels of medication compliance. Also of importance, fathers' levels of family satisfaction were strongly related to scores on the medication diary. This underscores the importance of including fathers (as well as other family members) when establishing family estimates on any dimension of family functioning.

Because of the small sample and subsequent limited power of analysis, the significant relationships between the cohesion and adaptability dimensions and medication compliance could be considered quite robust. Further, all of the findings were in the predicted directions. A measure such as the compliance diary may be more sensitive to fluctuations in the behavior of its members than would a more abstract rating of compliance. Thus, the current findings support the notion that family relations play an integral role in influencing behavior at an individual level.

An alternative explanation may be that the relationships observed were due to the shared variance in the method of measurement (i.e., self-report) rather than to actual associations between the family and compliance dimensions measured. In essence, subjects willing to endorse family problem areas simply may have been more willing to report problems in other areas (i.e., medication compliance), and subjects reporting "socially desirable" responses likewise did so across the board. However, such an explanation would not clarify why there were no relationships found between the global self-report measure of compliance and family variables, but there were strong relationships between the self-monitoring measure of compliance and family factors.

In addition, self-reported family functioning exhibited no relationship to self-reported regimen knowledge or disease activity. Perhaps no such relationships exist. Alternatively, the inadequate sensitivity of both the knowledge and disease activity measures may have resulted in the restricted range of scores and subsequent lack of significant relationships. In contrast to previous research revealing a direct relationship between life stress and metabolic control in diabetes (Hanson et al., 1987a, 1987b), which utilized reports of life events provided by the adolescent subjects themselves, the present study relied only on parents' perceptions of life events and child's physical disease. Perhaps if children's perceptions of life stress had been evaluated, they might have demonstrated a stronger relationship with physiological indices of disease activity. Future research in this area should focus on developing more adequate measures of regimen knowledge and disease activity. Patients' perceptions of family stress should also be utilized.

Exploratory Analyses

FACES III-K. The secondary goals of the present study were to assess the validity of utilizing the child versions of the FACES III (FACES III-K) and Family Satisfaction (Family Satisfaction-K) questionnaires with younger children. The younger children's scores on the FACES III-K demonstrated a relationship to the adult scores that was similar to those obtained by adolescents on the standard version. This suggests that the FACES III-K may be of practical use with younger children. However, given the small sample, it is suggested that the FACES III-K be evaluated with larger samples and in a variety of settings before considering it a valid measure of family functioning.

Family Satisfaction-K. The relationship of the Family Satisfaction-K measure and the standard version also suggested the validity of the measure, and even suggested a stronger relationship to parental satisfaction than the standard adolescent measure. Child and adolescent scores exhibited similar relationships to father's ratings of family satisfaction, but an even stronger relationship was observed between younger children's and mothers' ratings of family satisfaction, perhaps because younger children spend more time with their mothers and share more similar perceptions with them than do adolescents. Further research of a longitudinal nature is required to investigate the possibility that children's perceptions of family satisfaction do indeed become more independent of their parents' perceptions over time.

Compliance and Disease Activity. The third major set of investigations in the present study attempted to evaluate the relationships among (a) the various compliance measures and (b) the multiple measures of disease activity. Little agreement was observed between parent and child estimates of medication compliance or between the global estimates of compliance and self-monitoring compliance. This emphasizes the importance of utilizing multiple measures for the assessment of compliance and, not surprisingly, suggests that global estimates of compliance may not serve as adequate indicators of actual compliance. In contrast to the compliance data, the findings regarding global estimates of disease activity suggest that parents and children are able to estimate generally the severity of the child's disease (as measured by the physician in the clinic) with a high degree of accuracy. This was further illustrated by the high level of agreement between parent estimates and objective ratings provided by the physician's physical examination. Children's ratings, however, were not associated with the objective physician rating and may suggest that more subjective factors constitute the child's perception of disease activity.

In summary, the present study provides support for considering family functioning as a critical area of investigation with chronically ill populations and suggests that the circumplex model of marital and family systems (Olson et al., 1979) is a useful model in such research. It also emphasizes the need for more precise measurement of disease activity in juvenile rheumatoid arthritis. The most significant limitation of the present study is the small sample and subsequent restricted power of analysis. However, even with these limitations, the present study does provide several methodological suggestions for the study of families of chronically ill children, namely, the importance of assessing multiple respondents across multiple measures and utilizing a theory-driven conceptualization to investigate the relationship of family relations and chronic illness.

REFERENCES

Anderson, K. O., Bradley, L. A., Young, L. D., McDaniel, L. K., & Wise, C. M. (1985). Rheumatoid arthritis: Review of psychological factors related to etiology, effects, and treatment. *Psychological Bulletin, 98,* 358-387.

Anderson, B. J., Miller, J. P., Auslander, W. F., & Santiago, J. V. (1981). Family characteristics of diabetic adolescents: Relationship to metabolic control. *Diabetes Care, 4,* 586-594.

Blechman, W. F., & Zane, S. (1976). Fenoprofen calcium in steriod treated rheumatoid arthritis: Efficacy, safety, and steroid-sparing effect. *Journal of Rheumatology, 2,* 38-42.
Brewer, E. J., Bass, J., Baum, J., Cassidy, J. T., Fink, C., Jacobs, J., Hanson, V., Levinson, J. E., Schaller, J., & Stillman, J. S. (1977). Current proposed revision of JRA criteria. *Arthritis and Rheumatism, 20,* 195-199.
Brewer, E. J., & Giannini, E. H. (1982). Standard methodology and segment I, II, and III Pediatric Rheumatology Collaborative Study Group studies: I. Design. *Journal of Rheumatology, 9,* 109-113.
Deyo, R. A. (1982). Compliance with therapeutic regimens in arthritis: Issues, current status, and a future agenda. *Seminars in Arthritis and Rheumatism, 12,* 233-244.
Fehrenback, A. B., & Peterson, L. (1989). Parental problem solving, stress, and dietary compliance in PKU children. *Journal of Consulting and Clinical Psychology, 57,* 237-241.
Feinstein, A. R. (1979). Compliance bias and the interpretation of therapeutic trials. In R. B. Haynes, D. W. Taylor, & D. L. Sackett (Eds.), *Compliance in health care* (pp. 309-322). Baltimore: Johns Hopkins Press.
Fisher, R. A. (1921). On the probable error of a coefficient of correlation deduced from a small sample. *Metron, 1,* 3-32.
Foster, M., & Berger, M. (1985). Research with families with handicapped children: A multilevel systemic perspective. In L. L'Abate (Ed.), *The handbook of family psychology and therapy* (pp. 741-780). Homewood, IL: Dorsey.
Hanson, C. L., Henggeler, S. W., & Burghen, G. A. (1987a). Model of association between psychological variables and health outcome measures of adolescents with IDDM. *Diabetes Care, 10,* 752-758.
Hanson, C. L., Henggeler, S. W., & Burghen, G. A. (1987b). Social competence and parental support as mediators of the link between stress and metabolic control in adolescents with insulin dependent diabetes mellitus. *Journal of Consulting and Clinical Psychology, 55,* 529-533.
Hanson, C. L., Henggeler, S. W., Burghen, G. A., & Moore, M. (in press). Family systems variables and the health status of adolescents with IDDM. *Health Psychology.*
Harter, H. (1982). The perceived competence scale for children. *Child Development, 53,* 87-97.
Hollingshead, A. B., & Redlich, F. C. (1958). *Social class and mental illness* (pp. 398-407). New York: Wiley.
Hunder, G. G., & Bunch, T. W. (1982). Treatment of rheumatoid arthritis. *Bulletin on the Rheumatic Diseases, 32,* 1-6.
Korsch, B., Fine, R., & Negrete, V. (1978). Noncompliance in children with renal transplants. *Pediatrics, 61,* 872-876.
Koski, M. L., & Kumento, A. (1977). The interrelationship between diabetic control and family life. *Pediatric and Adolescent Endocrinology, 3,* 41-45.
Litt, I. F., & Cuskey, W. R. (1981). Compliance with salicylate therapy in adolescents with juvenile rheumatoid arthritis. *American Journal of Disease of Children, 135,* 434-436.
Litt, I. F., Cuskey, W. R., & Rosenberg, A. (1982). Role of self-esteem and autonomy in determining medication compliance among adolescents with juvenile rheumatoid arthritis. *Pediatrics, 69,* 15-17.
McCubbin, H. I., Larsen, A., & Olson, D. H. (1985). F-COPES: Family crises oriented personal evaluation scales. In D. H. Olson, H. I. McCubbin, H. Barnes, A. Larsen, M. Muxen, & M. Wilson, (Eds.), *Family inventories: Inventories used in a national survey of families across the family life cycle* (pp. 143-159). St. Paul: Family Social Science, University of Minnesota.
McCubbin, H. I., Patterson, J. M., & Wilson, L. R. (1985). FILE: Family inventory of life events and changes. In D. H. Olson, H. I. McCubbin, H. Barnes, A. Larsen, M. Muxen, & M. Wilson, (Eds.), *Family inventories: Inventories used in a national survey of families across the family life cycle* (pp. 105-127). St. Paul: Family Social Science, University of Minnesota.
Minuchin, S., Rosman, B. L., & Baker, L. (1978). *Psychosomatic families: Anorexia nervosa in context.* Cambridge: Harvard University Press.

Neter, J., Wasserman, W., & Kutner, M. H. (1983). *Applied linear regression models.* Homewood, IL: Irwin.
Olson, D. H. (1986). Circumplex model VII: Validation studies and FACES III. *Family Process, 25,* 337-351.
Olson, D. H., McCubbin, H. I., Barnes, H. L., Larsen, A. S., Muxen, M. J., & Wilson, M. A. (1983). *Families: What makes them work.* Beverly Hills: Sage.
Olson, D. H., Portner, J., & Lavee, Y. (1985). FACES III: Family adaptability and cohesion evaluation scales. In D. H. Olson, H. I. McCubbin, H. Barnes, A. Larsen, M. Muxen, & M. Wilson, (Eds.), *Family inventories: Inventories used in a national survey of families across the family life cycle* (pp. 18-42). St. Paul: Family Social Science, University of Minnesota.
Olson, D. H., Sprenkle, D., & Russell, C. (1979). Circumplex model of marital and family systems: I. Cohesion and adaptability dimensions, family types, and clinical application. *Family Process, 18,* 3-28.
Olson, D. H., & Wilson, M. (1985). Family satisfaction. In D. H. Olson, H. I. McCubbin, H. Barnes, A. Larsen, M. Muxen, & M. Wilson (Eds.), *Family inventories: Inventories used in a national survey of families across the family life cycle* (pp. 43-50). St. Paul: Family Social Science, University of Minnesota.
Phillips, P. E. (1981, January). The optimistic outlook for juvenile rheumatoid arthritis. *Drug Therapy,* pp. 71-83.
Podell, R. N. (1975). *Physician's guide to compliance in hypertension.* West Point, PA: Merck.
Rapoff, M. A., Lindsley, C. B., & Christophersen, E. R. (1984). Improving compliance with medical regimens: Case study with juvenile rheumatoid arthritis. *Archives of Physical Medicine and Rehabilitation, 65,* 267-269.
Rapoff, M. A., Purviance, M. R., & Lindsley, C. B. (1988). Educational and behavioral strategies for improving medication compliance in juvenile rheumatoid arthritis. *Archives of Physical Medicine and Rehabilitation, 69,* 439-441.
Rennebohm, R., & Correll, J. K. (1984). Comprehensive management of juvenile rheumatoid arthritis. *Nursing Clinics of North America, 19,* 647-662.
Singsen, B. H., Johnson, M. A., & Bernstein, B. A. (1979). Psychodynamics of juvenile rheumatoid arthritis. In J. J. Miller (Ed.), *Juvenile rheumatoid arthritis* (pp. 249-265). Littleton, MA: PSG Publishing.
Sullivan, D. B. (1982). The pediatric rheumatology clinic. In J. T. Cassidy (Ed.), *Textbook of pediatric rheumatology* (pp. 615-629). New York: Wiley.
Wedgwood, R. J., & Schaller, J. G. (1977, June). The pediatric arthritides. *Hospital Practice,* pp. 83-97.

II

NONCATEGORICAL DISORDERS

8

Family Resources as Resistance Factors for Psychological Maladjustment in Chronically Ill and Handicapped Children[1]

Jan L. Wallander
Sparks Center and Department of Psychology, University of Alabama at Birmingham

James W. Varni
Orthopaedic Hospital and University of Southern California

Lina Babani, Heather Tweddle Banis, and Karen Thompson Wilcox
University of Southern California

The hypothesis that their psychological adjustment is related in part to resources present in their families was investigated in 153 children, age 4–16, who had one of five chronic physical disorders: juvenile diabetes, juvenile rheumatoid arthritis, chronic obesity, spina bifida, or cerebral palsy. Their mothers completed standardized psychometric instruments to measure specific dimensions of family psychological and utilitarian resources and of child adjustment. Variation in children's psychological adjustment was related both to their psychological and utilitarian family resources. Psychological family resources contributed uniquely to the prediction of adjustment beyond that provided by utilitarian family resources. These results are discussed as having implications for the identification of chronically ill and handicapped children at risk for adjustment difficulties.

[1]This research was supported in part by grants from The Crippled Children's Guild through the Behavioral Pediatrics Program at Orthopaedic Hospital, Los Angeles; University of Southern California Faculty Research and Innovation Fund; the Biomedical Research Support Grant program; and National Institute of Child Health and Human Development (grant #HD24322).

About 10% of children experience a serious chronic physical illness (e.g., Pless, 1968; Pless & Douglas, 1971) and they constitute 50% of pediatric practice (Magrab & Calcagno, 1978). Children with chronic physical illness or handicap are at risk for psychological adjustment problems, though there is wide variation in individual functioning (e.g., Breslau, 1985; Rutter, Tizard, & Whitmore, 1970). Wallander, Varni, Babani, Banis, and Wilcox (1988), for example, found 270 children with one of six chronic physical disorders to be reported by their mothers as evidencing on the average more behavioral and social competence problems than expected based on norms for children in general. However, only a small proportion could be considered clinically maladjusted. The majority rather was reported with no problems.

The noted increased risk for, but wide variation in, psychological adjustment among individual children in this population indicates a need to identify factors associated with their adjustment. Varni and Wallander (1988, 1989; Varni, 1987; Wallander, 1987, 1988) have proposed a conceptual model to account for the differential psychosocial adjustment in chronically ill and handicapped children in terms of risk and resistance factors. This model is presented in Figure 1 (see p. 143). Disease or disability parameters, functional independence, and psychosocial stress are major risk factors in this model. A variety of resistance factors are also hypothesized to be important.

Research completed thus far has largely shown a nonsignificant direct relationship between disease or disability parameters and adjustment. For example, there were very few significant differences in the adjustment of children with markedly different chronic physical disorders (Wallander et al., 1988). Different measures of the severity of the child's physical disorder, furthermore, have not been found to be related to behavioral adjustment (Varni, Rubenfeld, Talbot, & Setoguchi, in press-a; Wallander, Feldman, & Varni, 1989; Wallander, Varni, Babani, Banis, et al., 1989), though they are moderately predictive of the children's social adjustment. It remains to be investigated whether disease parameters have an indirect effect on adjustment, for example, by causing increased psychosocial stress (cf. Wallander, Pitt, & Mellins, in press).

However, in continuing to investigate this model attention has begun to be focused on hypothesized resistance factors. Generally subsumed under the rubric of coping resources, three broad types of resistance factors have been distinguished (Wallander, 1987): stable person factors (e.g., temperament, perceived competence), stress processing (e.g., cognitive appraisal, coping behaviors), and social-ecological factors (e.g., family resources, social support). Our approach in this research has been to focus on limited sets of rather specific factors initially to identify those that should be included in subsequent more comprehensive multivariate investigations. A good deal of attention has been paid to social-ecological factors in understanding adaptation to physical disorders (e.g., Gentry & Kobasa, 1984; Moos & Schaeffer,

1984). Building on this led us to focus on characteristics of children's social environment first.

Among social-ecological factors, there is a vast amount of literature indicating the importance of the family for most children's development (cf. Heatherington & Martin, 1979). Several investigators have emphasized family resources as influencing children's adaptation to chronic strain (Garmezy, 1983; Rutter, Cox, Tupling, Berger, & Yule, 1975; Rutter, Yule, et al., 1975). Family resources refer to the broad range of reserves and aids characterizing the family which are potentially available in times of need (McCubbin et al., 1980). Different specific family resources have been distinguished (cf. George, 1980), but of these, psychological family resources have received most attention vis-à-vis chronically ill or handicapped children's adjustment (McCubbin & Patterson, 1981). Psychological resources are defined as the family's characteristic mode of perceiving and interacting with the social world, including within and external to the family (Reiss, 1982).

Research on psychological family resources and chronically ill or handicapped children's adjustment has shown, for example, that higher family cohesion is related to better adjustment among children with sickle cell anemia (Moise, 1980). Diabetic children have been found to have higher self-perceived competence in families high in independence, achievement, activity, and organization (Hauser, Jacobson, Wertlieb, Brink, & Wentworth, 1985). Lower family conflict and higher organization were found to predict greater self-esteem in children with congenital/acquired limb deficiencies (Varni, Rubenfeld, Talbot, & Setoguchi, in press-b). Family psychological characteristics also interacted with child temperament to predict these children's adaptation (Varni, Rubenfeld, Talbot, & Setoguchi, in press-c). Steinhausen, Schindler, and Stephan (1983) found differences in the relationship between psychological family resources and child adjustment in children with different disorders, with a stronger relationship existing in the typically less severe condition of asthma and no relationship in the life-threatening condition of cystic fibrosis. None of the three psychosocial family resource dimensions investigated by Daniels, Moos, Billings, and Miller (1987) were associated with the adjustment of children with juvenile rheumatic disease. In contrast to these studies which have addressed discrete disorders, Pless, Roghmann, and Haggerty (1972) found a general index of family psychological resources to be related to the adjustment of children with a mixture of chronic physical disorders of varying severity. Thus varying findings have been reported, indicating a need to continue to investigate the relationship between family psychological resources and adjustment in children with chronic illness or handicap.

Another family resource implicated in chronically ill or handicapped children's adjustment is the practical resources available to deal with acute and chronic problems and issues. A chronic physical disorder can be characterized as bringing forth a series of problems needing attention as well as a chronic level of strain inherent in the care of such a child (Varni & Wallander, 1988; Wallander & Marullo, 1989). In light of this, utilitarian resources may play a role in the smooth functioning of the family and consequently the adaptation of a chronically ill or handicapped child. For example, financial resources can be used to buy services helpful for the care of such a child or the household more generally. The educational level of parents may contribute to cognitive ability related to appropriate parenting or care of an ill or handicapped child and resolution of problems thereto related.

Both psychological and utilitarian family resources are therefore hypothesized as resistance factors within our heuristic conceptual model. It would be useful to compare the differential and joint relationships existing between these types of family resources and chronically ill or handicapped children's adaptation. In the present study, it was hypothesized that psychological as well as utilitarian family resources would be significantly associated with both behavioral and social adjustment in chronically physically ill or handicapped children. It was also hypothesized that these two family resources would contribute in part independently to the prediction of child adjustment, but that the psychological family resources would add significantly to the prediction of adjustment beyond that contributed by the utilitarian family resources. It is felt these are independent family resources, both worthy of attention.

METHOD

Subjects

To obtain a sufficiently large sample to study psychosocial aspects in children with chronic physical disorders with satisfactory power for multivariate procedures, diagnostic groups were combined. Although each chronic physical disorder has a low incidence, the total prevalence of all is estimated at over 10% (Pless, 1968; Pless & Douglas, 1971). However, little is lost by combining apparently distinct physical disorders because there is great commonality in their psychosocial implications (Pless & Perrin, 1985; Pless & Pinkerton, 1975; Varni & Wallander, 1989). Much research has supported a noncategorical approach to the study of psychosocial aspects of chronic physical disorders (e.g., Stein & Jessop, 1982), including our whole research program, as reviewed in the introduction.

Chronically ill and handicapped children were recruited from the ambulatory care clinics of three teaching hospitals affiliated with a major metropolitan medical school (Orthopaedic Hospital, Children's Hospital of

Los Angeles, The Pediatric Pavilion at the Los Angeles County–University of Southern California Medical Center). These clinics specialized in the multidisciplinary care of children with juvenile diabetes, spina bifida, juvenile rheumatoid arthritis, or cerebral palsy. In addition, children with chronic obesity, defined as 25% over median population weight for the child's age, sex, and height for a minimum duration of 2 years, were recruited from a general pediatrics clinic. This condition was included because it has most of the physical and psychosocial implications of other chronic physical disorders such as chronicity, physical complications (e.g., cardiovascular disease, diabetes), therapeutic adherence problems, and social stigma (Varni & Banis, 1985; Wallander et al., 1988). Clinic master lists were reviewed and mothers of children in the age range of 4 to 16 were contacted either through the mail, over the phone, or when she appeared with her child for a regularly scheduled clinic appointment. Of those approached, 81% agreed to participate. The most commonly cited reason for declining was time constraints.

This resulted in a sample of 153 children between the ages of 4 and 16, with 68 (44%) boys and 85 (56%) girls.[3] The distributions of the children across age intervals and the five chronic physical disorders are presented in Table I, as are the distributions of the educational level of the mothers and their family income. The average child in this sample was 10.4 years old. His/her mother had completed slightly less than 12 years of education and the family had an income of about $24,000 the previous year. The average family in this sample consequently had a socioeconomic status (SES) quite similar to that of the average family in the U.S. population in 1985, when these data were collected.

Procedure

The procedure of this study was completed by the mother either during a regularly scheduled clinic appointment or during a specially scheduled time. It was administered by a psychology graduate student research assistant. Following the signing of the informed consent form, the mother completed a series of instruments specific to the particular data collection in which

[3]This sample made up 57% of that reported on in Wallander et al. (1988). This latter study reported detailed descriptive results on the adjustment of 270 children with one of six chronic physical disorders (including beyond those studied herein children with hemophilia and additional children with spina bifida and cerebral palsy). Both studies were conducted on samples constituted by combining subjects from several separate and distinct data collections on discrete disorders or conditions. All children for whom adjustment and family data were available from these separate data collections were included in the current study. This is a necessary strategy when studying children with low-incidence disorders of the type included herein. It also explains the uneven distribution of the current sample across chronic disorders.

Table I. Subject Characteristics (N = 153)

Characteristic	n	% of sample
Chronic physical disorder		
Juvenile diabetes	74	48
Juvenile rheumatoid arthritis	23	15
Chronic obesity	22	14
Spina bifida	17	11
Cerebral palsy	17	11
Child's age		
4-5	4	3
6-7	29	19
8-9	33	22
10-11	36	24
12-13	17	11
14-15	23	15
16	11	7
Mother's education		
Junior high school or less	41	27
Some high school	26	17
High school diploma	26	17
Community college	41	27
College degree	12	8
Graduate education	7	4
Family income		
State aid only	14	9
≤ $10,000	22	14
$10–20,000	43	28
$20–30,000	26	17
$30–40,000	16	11
≥ $40,000	32	21

she participated, though of relevance to the current study are only the three described below. The research assistant subsequently checked that the instruments were filled out completely and appropriately, or discrepancies were resolved.

Measures

Adjustment was defined in reference to norms for age-appropriate behavior, in particular as it pertains to behaviors associated with maladjustment. Adjustment of these children was assessed using three scales of the 138-item Child Behavior Checklist (CBCL; Achenbach & Edelbrock, 1983). Normative data, stratified for three age groups (4–5, 6–11, 12–16) and each sex, are available for 1,300 nonclinic-referred community children and 2,300 mental health clinic-referred children between the ages of 4 and 16, fairly representing the U.S. population on several dimensions, including race and

SES. Extensive analyses have yielded principal component solutions for the 118 behavior problem items that are different for the two sexes and three age groups. However, the two second-order principal components of Internalizing Behavior Problems and Externalizing Behavior Problems, which exist for all sexes and age groups, serve as summary scales of behavior problems for all children. In addition, there is a summary scale of Social Competence, constituted by 20 items measuring the child's activities, peer relations, and school performance, which is invariant for sex and age groups. Child adjustment was therefore assessed in this study using these three summary scales. Extensive psychometric analyses (Achenbach & Edelbrock, 1983) and subsequent frequent research use have shown these CBCL scales to have excellent test–retest reliability, interparent agreement, and construct validity when completed by parents. Using available norms (Achenbach & Edelbrock, 1983), scores on the three summary scales are computed as normalized *T* scores.

Family psychological resources were defined in terms of the nature and quality of the relationships and system ties existing in the child's nuclear family as a unit. Following much previous research in this field (see introduction), it was measured by administering the 45 items of the Family Environment Scale (FES; Moos & Moos, 1981) pertaining to the subscales of Cohesion, Expressiveness, Conflict, Organization, and Control. The remaining five subscales of the FES, addressing family interests and goals, were deemed less relevant psychological resources for purposes of this study and were not administered. The Cohesion scale is intended to assess the degree of commitment, help, and support members provide for one another; the Expressiveness scale, the extent to which members are encouraged to act openly and express feelings directly; the Conflict scale, the amount of openly expressed anger, aggression, and conflict among members; the Organization scale, the degree of importance ascribed by the family to clear organization and structure in planning family activities and responsibilities; and the Control scale, the extent to which set rules and procedures are used to run family life. All scales were developed on a theoretical–rational basis. The internal consistency (alpha $\geq$ .67) and 2-month test–retest reliability ($r \geq .73$) are adequate for these five scales. Numerous studies provide support for the validity of this instrument for its stated purpose (cf. Moos & Moos, 1981). Subscale scores are reported as *T* scores calculated based on extensive normative data.

Family utilitarian resources was defined in terms of two salient socioeconomic characteristics of a child's family, the family income and maternal education level. These have been found to be highly predictive of children's psychosocial development (Rutter, Cox, et al., 1975; Rutter, Yule, et al., 1975). Family income was measured using a nine-item checklist and maternal educational level using a seven-item category checklist.

RESULTS

Child Psychological Adjustment

This sample of chronically ill or handicapped children obtained a mean *T* score of 57 (SD = 10) on the Internalizing Behavior Problems, 54 (SD = 11) on the Externalizing Behavior Problems, and 41 (SD = 12) on the Social Competence scales of the CBCL. The distribution for each scale around its mean was essentially normal and not markedly influenced by extreme scores (kurtosis = − 0.34– + 0.44; skewness = −0.19– + 0.14). Though not a central feature of this study, comparisons were nonetheless made between this sample and the normative sample of nonclinic-referred community children for the CBCL (Achenbach & Edelbrock, 1983) to provide some information about the relative adjustment of children with chronic physical disorders. *Z* tests indicated that these chronically ill and handicapped children were described as displaying significantly more behavior problems and a poorer social competence than children in the nonclinic community normative sample (all $|Zs| \geq 5.82$, all $ps < .001$). As has been reported upon in detail elsewhere (Wallander et al., 1988), there were very few differences in the psychological adjustment of children with different disorders. Based on one-way ANOVAs and post hoc analyses using the Newman-Keuls procedure, the only significant differences were the juvenile rheumatoid arthritis group's lower Externalizing Behavior Problem scale and the cerebral palsy group's lower Social Competence scale mean scores compared to the other diagnostic groups.

It would be logical to expect somatic complaints to be more frequent in a sample of chronically ill or handicapped children. However, the Internalizing Behavior Problems scale scores for this sample remained significantly higher than those of the nonclinic community normative sample even when items reflecting somatic complaints were disregarded (modified scale *T*-score $M = 55$, $Z = 7.14$, $p < .001$). Separating the study sample into groups of children from low, medium, and high SES families still resulted in significantly higher Externalizing and Internalizing Behavior Problems scale scores for each SES group compared to the normative sample (all $Zs \geq 4.87$, all $ps < .001$). There were no significant relationships between the children's age and their psychological adjustment, $r(151) \leq .04$. Boys, however, obtained significantly higher scores than girls on the Externalizing Behavior Problems scale, $t(151) = 1.98$, $p < .05$, even though *T* scores are derived based only on same-sex norms. However, the mean difference was only one *T*-score point.

Family Psychological Resources

The mean T scores on the five family psychological resource dimensions were 54 (SD = 14) for Cohesion, 52 (SD = 12) for Expressiveness, 48 (SD = 11) for Conflict, 56 (SD = 11) for Organization, and 57 (SD = 10) for Control. The distribution of scores for each scale around its mean was essentially normal, with an exception for the Cohesion scale. Whereas both kurtosis (range = -0.21–$+0.80$) and skewness (range = -0.49–$+0.67$) were minimal for the four other scales, several families obtained extremely high scores on the Cohesion scale, resulting in its kurtosis = 7.25 and skewness = -1.39. Child's age was significantly positively correlated only with the Expressiveness scale; however, the strength of this relationship was weak, $r(151) = .19$, $p < .001$. There were no significant differences on any of the family psychological resources scales due to sex.

Family Resources and Children's Adjustment

Since the above results indicate there were very few differences associated with diagnosis, age, or sex, subsequent analyses were conducted on the total sample (N = 153). Several analyses were completed to investigate whether there was a relationship between family resources and chronically ill or handicapped children's psychological adjustment. First, Pearson product-moment correlations were computed between all relevant variables (see Table II). Both internalizing and externalizing behavior problems were significantly negatively related to family cohesion and organization and positively to conflict. Social competence was significantly positively related to cohesion and expressiveness. However, at most only 9% of the variance in a psychological adjustment dimension could be accounted for by a single family psychological resource dimension, and vice versa. In terms of family utilitarian resources, maternal education was significantly negatively related to both types of behavior problems and positively to social competence. Family income was significantly positively related only to social competence.

Multiple regression analyses were completed to test hypotheses about the separate contribution of the two types of family resources to chronically ill or handicapped children's psychological adjustment (see Table III). Family psychological resources predicted in combination significant proportion of the variance in all three child psychological adjustment dimensions, though the amount was less than 10% for behavior problems and 20% for social competence. Regression coefficients indicated that none of the family psychological resources contributed independently a significant amount to the

Table II. Pearson Product-Moment Correlations Among All Variables ($N = 153$)

	Child adjustment			Psychological resources					Utilitarian resources
Variable	1	2	3	4	5	6	7	8	9
Child adjustment									
1. Internalizing problems									
2. Externalizing problems	$.67^c$								
3. Social competence	$-.26^c$	$-.30^c$							
Family psychological resources									
4. Cohesion	$-.21^b$	$-.23^b$	$.30^c$						
5. Expressiveness	$-.08$	$-.09$	$.26^c$	$.38^c$					
6. Conflict	$.18^a$	$.27^c$	.05	$-.41^c$	$-.05$				
7. Organization	$-.23^c$	$-.14^a$	.05	$.53^c$	.11	$-.42^c$			
8. Control	.04	.07	$-.09$	$.17^a$	$-.08$	.05	.12		
Family utilitarian resources									
9. Maternal education	$-.21^a$	$-.16^a$	$.35^c$	$.22^b$	$.22^b$	$.25^c$	.02	$-.08$	
10. Family income	$-.12$	$-.10$	$.41^c$	$.19^a$	.02	.04	$-.05$	$-.01$	$.44^c$

$^a p < .05$.
$^b p < .01$.
$^c p < .001$.

Table III. Multiple Regression Analysis of the Contribution of Psychological and Utilitarian Family Resources to Child Psychological Adjustment

	Internalizing problems	Externalizing problems	Social competence
		Psychological resources	
Standardized regression coefficients (β)			
Cohesion	−.09	−.17	.45[b]
Expressiveness	.01	−.01	.21
Conflict	.10	.20[a]	.25[b]
Organization	−.17	.03	−.08
Control	.07	.07	−.16[a]
Multiple R	.29[b]	.31[a]	.45[b]
$F(5, 147)$	2.53[b]	2.92[a]	6.93[b]
		Utilitarian resources	
Standardized regression coefficients (β)			
Maternal education	−.32[b]	−.28[a]	.18[a]
Family income	.00	.04	.20[a]
Multiple R	.27[b]	.22[b]	.49[b]
$F(2, 150)$	8.36[b]	8.99[b]	18.46[b]

[a] $p < .05$.
[b] $p < .01$.

variance in internalizing behavior problems and only family conflict did so in externalizing behavior problems. However, three dimensions contributed significantly and independently to the variance in social competence: family cohesion, conflict, and control, in order of their relative contribution.

All three child psychological adjustment measures were significantly predicted by the combination of the two utilitarian resources of maternal education and family income. Less than 7% of the variance in behavior problems was accounted for by these two utilitarian resources, but 24% was in social competence. Maternal education contributed independently and significantly to all three child adjustment dimensions, as indicated by the regression coefficients, while family income did so only for social competence.

The zero-order relationships observed between the psychological and utilitarian family resources (see Table II) and the results of these multiple regression analyses (see Table III) bring into question whether the two types of family resources are independent predictors of psychological adjustment in these children. Alternatively, the relationship observed between family psychological resources and child psychological adjustment could be explained mainly as an artifact of the influence of utilitarian resources on both of these. Hierarchical multiple regression analyses were completed to test the hypothesis that psychological family resources are independent contributors to adjustment. This analysis involves the specification of the order in which sets of predictors are entered into the regression system, allowing the calculation of added contribution of subsequent predictors once the variance in the out-

Table IV. Hierarchial Multiple Regression Analysis Evaluating the Contribution of Psychological Over That of Utilitarian Resources

Statistic	Internalizing problems	Externalizing problems	Social competence
Standardized regression coefficients (β)			
Maternal education	$-.32^d$	$.28^c$	$.18^c$
Family income	.00	.04	$.20^c$
Cohesion	.04	$-.12$	$.41^d$
Expressiveness	.06	.02	.13
Conflict	.13	$.22^c$	$.22^c$
Organization	$-.28^d$	$-.06$	$-.02$
Control	.11	.10	$-.19^c$
Multiple *R*			
Utilitarian	$.27^d$	$.22^d$	$.49^d$
Utilitarian + psychological	$.42^d$	$.40^d$	$.66^d$
F test			
Utilitarian (2, 150)[a]	8.36^d	8.99^d	18.46^d
Utilitarian + psychological (7, 145)[a]	3.42^d	2.92^d	11.78^d
R^2 change[b]	$.11^d$	$.11^d$	$.19^d$

[a]Degrees of freedom for *F* test.
[b]Significance of change in R^2 evaluated by *F* test for increment.
[c]$p < .05$.
[d]$p < .01$.

come already accounted for by prior predictors has been removed. In this case the two utilitarian resources were entered first, followed by the five psychological resource dimensions in predicting each child adjustment dimension separately. This ordering followed the principle of parsimony, when the theoretically simpler structural variables were entered before more complex psychological ones.

The results presented in Table IV indicate that the combination of both utilitarian and psychological family resources account for significant proportions of the variance in all three child psychological adjustment dimensions (all *F*s ≥ 2.92, all *p*s < .01). Again, these family resources had less shared variance with behavior problems (16–18%) than with social competence (43%). The results regarding the added contribution of the family psychological resources over that provided by the utilitarian resources were similar for the three child psychological adjustment dimensions. Psychological family resources added significantly to the prediction of all three adjustment dimensions (all incremental *F*s[5, 143] ≥ 2.92, all *p*s < .01) beyond the contribution of utilitarian resources. The additional variance accounted for by the psychological resources for both types of behavior problems was 11% and for the social competence 19%.

Two family resources, one psychological and one utilitarian, yielded significant regression coefficients within these combined systems in predicting both types of behavior problems. Maternal education made an independent contribution to both behavior problems dimensions, whereas family organization did so for internalizing behavior problems and family conflict for externalizing behavior problems. Five family resources dimensions contributed independently and significantly to the variance in social competence: family cohesion, conflict, control, and income, as well as maternal education. Family cohesion yielded a particularly significant regression coefficient in this system ($\beta = .41$, $p < .01$), while the contribution of the other predictors was about the same (all $|\beta| = .18–.22$, all $ps < .05$).

DISCUSSION

These chronically ill and handicapped children were found to be at increased risk for psychological adjustment problems, as reported by their mothers. This is consistent with several other studies (e.g., Breslau, 1985; Pless et al., 1972; Rutter et al., 1970). Although this is a disturbing outcome, it must be noted that only a portion of these children experience adjustment problems, raising the question of what factors may moderate this differential outcome. The results obtained herein suggest the family resources are significantly related to chronically ill and handicapped children's adjustment. This appears to be more so for their social than behavioral adjustment.

Both psychological and utilitarian family resources appear important components in this relationship. Each type of family resource contributes about equally to the explained variance in child adjustment. It amounts to between 5 and 10% for behavioral adjustment and 20 and 24% for social adjustment. Psychological family resources add significantly to the variance in child adjustment beyond that already accounted by utilitarian family resources. Taken as a whole, these two types of family resources account for about 17% of the variance in the behavioral adjustment and 44% in the social adjustment of chronically ill or handicapped children.

It seems reasonable that social adjustment is more related to family resources than is behavioral adjustment. Admittedly, only a limited range of the social adjustment domain was measured. As defined herein, social adjustment is evidenced largely as involvement in organized clubs, activities, hobbies, and peer interactions and in terms of school performance. Several of these components are dependent on financial resources, for example. Furthermore, all take special effort by parents to maintain in a physically disadvantaged child (e.g., special transportation, adaptive equipment, increased time). Such special efforts are easily disrupted when financial resources are meager, family conflict exists, or the family is disorganized or does not work together, for example. Behavioral adjustment may in comparison be less influenced by such social-environmental factors. Rather, a variety of other factors, such as genetic endowment, temperament, and learning history, are thought to be more important for this outcome. These types of factors are not considered to be family resources in the current definition.

Since there was little consistency in specific types of family resources predicting child adjustment, it appears that the relationship between family resources and child adjustment is rather general. Nonetheless, maternal education appears to be an important factor, as it contributed independently to all dimensions of child adjustment investigated herein. A lower educational level for the mothers was consistently related to poorer social and behavioral child adjustment, even when other family resources were considered. The importance of maternal education may reside in it being a marker for a host of underlying factors, such as maternal intelligence, family size, child-rearing knowledge, and maternal adjustment, which may have causal relationships with child adjustment (cf. Anthony & Cohler, 1987; Farran & McKinney, 1986). Different family psychological resources may be important for different child outcomes, but the strong and unique contribution of family cohesion to the child's social adjustment is noteworthy.

Several potential limitations to this study need to be considered prior to drawing implications. This research was based on a singular perspective, that of the mothers of these children. No independent verification was sought in measuring family resources nor child adjustment. Other unmeasured processes may have biased maternal perceptions, creating the observed relationships, such as maternal depression (Brody & Forehand, 1986). However, since these mothers described their families as appearing less like distressed families (cf. Moos & Moos, 1981) while describing their children as more like distressed children than were normative samples of either type, this concern is lessened somewhat. Response bias should influence reporting of family and child functioning in the same direction.

Another concern is the constitution of this sample. It was uneven on several dimensions and of uncertain representation. Several analyses suggested, however, that diagnosis, age, and sex were essentially unrelated to the outcomes being investigated herein. Furthermore, though this represents a volunteer sample from a population of unknown characteristics, descriptive data suggest it is demographically quite similar to the general population. Finally, it must be acknowledged that this was a cross-sectional correlational study. Concurrently observed relationships cannot be interpreted to suggest causal directions. Obviously, observed relationships can reflect the effect child adjustment may have on family resources just as well as the opposite, at least for the psychological if not the utilitarian resources. Longitudinal studies should follow to investigate causal priority among these variables, now that it has been established relationships do exist between family resources and adjustment in these children. Additionally, it may be fruitful to study how these family factors interact with other factors, such as disease or disability parameters or child temperament (Varni et al., in press-c) to affect child adjustment.

Nonetheless, the obtained results may be used, with potential benefit, to identify from family resources those chronically ill or handicapped children who are at risk for experiencing adjustment problems. For example, children of mothers with little education and/or poorly organized families may be at risk for experiencing internalizing problems. Similarly, families with poor cohesion are at higher risk to have children with a lower social integration. However, a complete explanation of the differential psychosocial outcome in this population needs to include several other factors in addition to family resources. More comprehensive models must be investigated, consequently, including other social-ecological as well as intrapersonal, process, and physical variables (e.g., Wallander, Feldman, & Varni, 1989; Wallander, Hubert, & Varni, 1988; Wallander, Varni, Babani, DeHaan, et al., in press), as suggested by our conceptual model (see Figure 1).

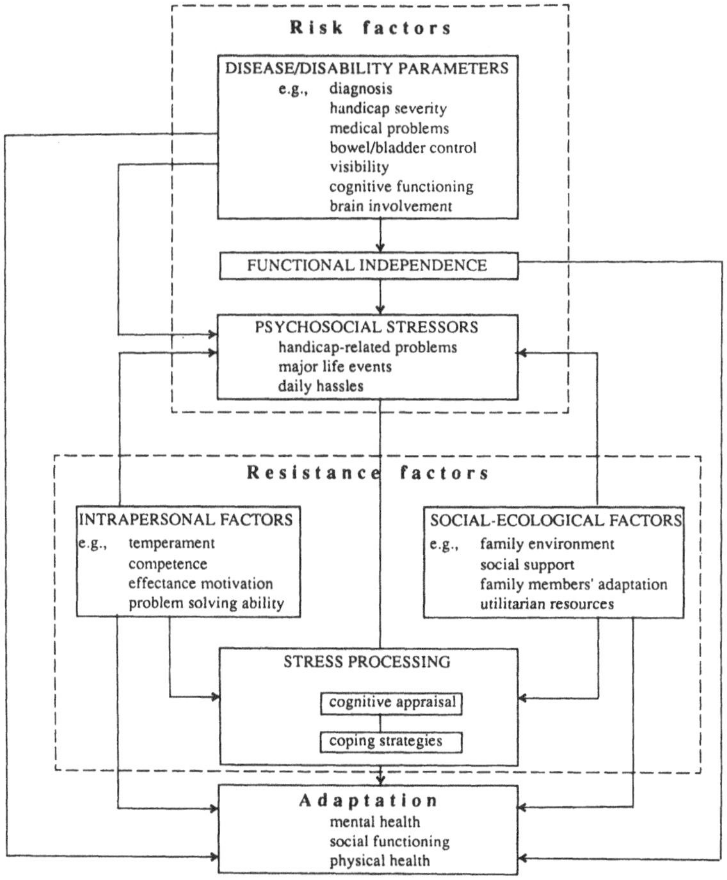

Fig. 1. Risk and resistance factors and the differential psychosocial adjustment of chronically ill and handicapped children.

REFERENCES

Achenbach, T. M., & Edelbrock, C. (1983). *Manual for the Child Behavior Checklist and Revised Behavior Profile.* Burlington: University of Vermont.

Anthony, G. J., & Cohler, B. J. (Eds.). (1987). *The invulnerable child.* New York: Guilford.

Breslau, N. (1985). Psychiatric disorder in children with physical disability. *Journal of the American Academy of Child Psychiatry, 24,* 87-94.

Brody, G. H., & Forehand, R. (1986). Maternal perceptions of child maladjustment as a function of the combined influences of child behavior and maternal depression. *Journal of Consulting and Clinical Psychology, 54,* 237-240.

Daniels, D., Moos, R. H., Billings, A. G., & Miller, J. J. (1987). Psychosocial risks and resistance factors among children with chronic illness, healthy siblings, and healthy controls. *Journal of Abnormal Child Psychology, 15,* 295-308.

Farran, D. C., & McKinney, J. D. (Eds.). (1986). *Risk in intellectual and psychosocial development.* New York: Academic Press.

Garmezy, N. (1983). Stressors of childhood. In N. Garmezy & M. Rutter (Eds.), *Stress, coping and development in children* (pp. 43-84). New York: McGraw-Hill.

Gentry, W. D., & Kobasa, S. C. (1984). Social and psychological resources mediating the stress-illness relationships in humans. In W. D. Gentry (Ed.), *Handbook of behavioral medicine* (pp. 87-115). New York: Guilford.

George, L. (1980). *Role transitions in later life.* Belmont, CA: Brooks/Cole.

Hauser, S. T., Jacobson, A. M., Wertlieb, D., Brink, S., & Wentworth, S. (1985). The contribution of family environment to perceived competence and illness adjustment in diabetic and acutely ill adolescents. *Family Relations, 34,* 99-108.

Heatherington, E. M., & Martin, B. (1979). Family interaction. In H. C. Quay & J. S. Werry (Eds.), *Psychopathological disorders of childhood* (2nd ed., pp. 247-302). New York: Wiley.

Magrab, P., & Calcagno, P. (1978). Psychological impact of chronic pediatric conditions. In P. R. Magrab (Ed.), *Psychological management of pediatric problems* (pp. 3-14). Baltimore: University Park.

McCubbin, H. I., Joy, C. B., Cauble, A. E., Comeau, J. K., Patterson, J. M., & Needle, R. H. (1980). Family stress and coping: A decade review. *Journal of Marriage and the Family, 42,* 855-871.

McCubbin, H. I., & Patterson, J. M. (1981). *Systematic assessment of family stress, resources, and coping: Tools for research, education, and clinical intervention:* St. Paul: University of Minnesota.

Moise, J. R. (1980). *Psychosocial adjustment of children and adolescents with sickle cell anemia.* Unpublished master's thesis, Case Western Reserve Uniersity.

Moos, R. H., & Moos, B. S. (1981). *Family Environment Scale.* Palo Alto, CA: Consulting Psychologists Press.

Moos, R. H., & Schaeffer, J. A. (1984). The crisis of physical illness: An overview and conceptual approach. In R. H. Moos (Ed.), *Coping with physical illness 2: New perspectives* (pp. 3-26). New York: Plenum Press.

Pless, I. B. (1968). Epidemiology of chronic disease. In M. Green & R. J. Haggerty (Eds.), *Ambulatory pediatrics.* Philadelphia: Saunders.

Pless, I. B., & Douglas, J. W. B. (1971). Chronic illness in childhood: Part 1. Epidemiological and clinical characteristics. *Pediatrics, 47,* 405-414.

Pless, I. B., & Perrin, J. M. (1985). Issues common to a variety of illnesses. In N. Hobbs & J. M. Perrin (Eds.), *Issues in the care of children with chronic illnesses* (pp. 41-60). San Francisco: Jossey-Bass.

Pless, I. B., & Pinkerton, P. (1975). *Chronic childhood disorders: Promoting patterns of adjustment.* Chicago: Year Book Medical.

Pless, I. B., Roghmann, K. J., & Haggerty, R J. (1972). Chronic illness, family functioning, and psychological adjustment: A model for the allocation of preventive marital health services. *International Journal of Epidemiology, 1,*271-278.

Reiss, D. (1982). *The family's construction of reality.* Cambridge, MA: Harvard University Press.

Rutter, M., Cox, A., Tupling, C., Berger, M., & Yule, W. (1975). Attainment and adjustment in two geographical areas: I. The prevalence of psychiatric disorder. *British Journal of Psychiatry, 126,* 493-509.

Rutter, M., Tizard, J., & Whitmore, K. (Eds.). (1970). *Education, health, and behavior.* London: Longman.

Rutter, M., Yule, B., Quinton, D., Rowlands, O., Yule, W., & Berger, M. (1975). Attainment and adjustment in two geographical areas: III. Some factors accounting for area differences. *British Journal of Psychiatry, 126,* 520-533.

Stein, R. E. K., & Jessop, D. J. (1982). A noncategorical approach to chronic childhood illness. *Public Health Report, 97,* 354-362.

Steinhausen, H., Schindler, H., & Stephan, H. (1983). Correlates of psychopathology in sick children. *Journal of the American Academy of Child Psychiatry, 22,* 559-564.

Varni, J. W. (1987, August). *Stress, moderator variables, and adaptation in pediatric chronic disorders.* Invited address presented at the Annual Convention of the American Psychological Association, New York.

Varni, J. W., & Banis, H. T. (1985). Behavior therapy techniques applied to eating, exercise, and diet modification in childhood obesity. *Journal of Developmental ad Behavioral Pediatrics, 6,* 367-372.

Varni, J. W., Rubenfeld, L. A., Talbot, D., & Setoguchi, Y. (in press-a). Stress, social support, and depressive symptomatology in children with congenital/acquired limb deficiencies. *Journal of Pediatric Psychology.*

Varni, J. W., Rubenfeld, L. A., Talbot, D., & Setoguichi, Y. (in press-b). Determinants of self-esteem in children with congenital/acquired limb deficiencies. *Journal of Developmental and Behavioral Pediatrics.*

Varni, J. W., Rubenfeld, L. A., Talbot, D., & Setoguchi, Y. (in press-c). Family functioning, temperament, and psychological adaptation in children with congenital/acquired limb deficiencies. *Pediatrics.*

Varni, J. W., & Wallander, J. L. (1988). Pediatric chronic disabilities. Hemophilia and spina bifida as examples. In D. K. Routh (Ed.), *Handbook of pediatric psychology* (pp. 190-221). New York: Guilford.

Varni, J. W., & Wallander, J. L. (1989). *Psychological adjustment of chronically ill and handicapped children: A multivariate model.* Manuscript in progress, Orthopaedic Hospital, Los Angeles.

Wallander, J. L. (1987). *Competence, stress, and disabled children's adjustment* (National Institute of Child Health and Human Development grant HD24322). Birmingham: Sparks Center, University of Alabama at Birmingham.

Wallander, J. L. (1988). *Mentally retarded adolescents' stress and coping.* Unpublished manuscript, Sparks Center, University of Alabama at Birmingham.

Wallander, J. L., Feldman, W., & Varni, J. W. (1989). Disease parameters and psychosocial adjustment in children with spina bifida. *Journal of Pediatric Psychology, 14,* 89-102.

Wallander, J.L., Hubert, N. C., & Varni, J. W. (1988). Child and maternal temperament characteristics, goodness of fit, and adjustment in physically handicapped children. *Journal of Clinical Child Psychology, 17,* 336-344.

Wallander, J. L., & Marullo, D. S. (1989). *Development and evaluation of an inventory to measure mothers' stress related to child's handicap.* Manuscript submitted for publication.

Wallander, J. L., Pitt, L. C., & Mellins, C. A. (in press). Risk factors for maladaptation in mothers of physically or sensory handicapped children: Disability status, functional independence, and psychosocial stress. *Journal of Consulting and Clinical Psychology.*

Wallander, J. L., Varni, J. W., Babani, L., Banis, H. T., DeHaan, C. B., & Wilcox, K. T. (1989). Disability parameters, chronic strain, and adaptation of physical handicapped children and their mothers. *Journal of Pediatric Psychology, 14,* 23-42.

Wallander, J. L., Varni, J. W., Babani, L., Banis, H. T., & Wilcox, K. T. (1988). Children with chronic physical disorders: Maternal reports of their psychological adjustment. *Journal of Pediatric Psychology, 13,* 197-212.

Wallander, J. L., Varni, J. W., Babani, L., DeHaan, C. B., Wilcox, K. T., & Banis, H. T. (in press). The social environment and the adaptation of mothers of physically handicapped children. *Journal of Pediatric Psychology.*

9

The Social Environment and the Adaptation of Mothers of Physically Handicapped Children[1]

Jan L. Wallander
Sparks Center and Department of Psychology, University of Alabama at Birmingham

James W. Varni
Orthopaedic Hospital and University of Southern California

Lina Babani, Christine B. DeHaan, Karen Thompson Wilcox, and Heather Tweddle Banis
University of Southern California

Evaluated relationships between social environmental characteristics and adaptation in 50 mothers of congenitally physically handicapped 6- to 11-year-old children. Mothers reported on utilitarian resources, child adjustment, psychosocial family resources, service utilization, and three dimensions of adaptation. Analyses of the concurrent correlational design indicated significant proportions of the variance in mental and social functioning were explained by features of the social environment. Mother's physical health could not be significantly predicted. Consistently strong contri-

[1]This research was supported in part by grants to J. L. Wallander from the National Institute of Child Health and Human Development (#HD24322), the University of Southern California Faculty Research and Innovation Fund, and Biomedical Research Support Grant Program, and to J. W. Varni from the Crippled Children's Guild through the Behavioral Pediatrics Program at Orthopaedic Hospital, Los Angeles. Appreciation is expressed to Timothy Saar and John Yzaguirre for their help in conducting this research, to all families who participated in it, and to an anonymous reviewer of an earlier version of this manuscript. This study was presented at the Florida Child Health Psychology Conference in Gainesville, 1988.

butions were made by psychosocial family resources in all adaptation domains.

A pediatric chronic physical disorder rarely affects only the child. Numerous studies suggest that these children's families experience adverse effects (Burton, 1975; Haggerty, Roghmann, & Pless, 1975; Ireys, 1981). Because the majority of the burden for the daily care of chronically ill and handicapped children is typically carried by mothers (e.g., Carey, 1982; Wilkin, 1979), particular concern is raised for their adaptation (e.g., Cummings, Bayley, & Rie, 1966; Tew & Laurence, 1973). Mothers of handicapped children experience, on the average, increased psychological distress compared to mothers of healthy children (cf. Blacher, 1984; Byrne & Cunningham, 1985; Gallagher, Beckman, & Cross, 1983). However, there is considerable variation in the observed adaptation of mothers of children with chronic physical disorders and few experience clinical maladjustment. These findings indicate that these mothers' adaptation cannot be explained entirely by the presence of a handicapped child. Rather, more specific features of having a chronically ill or handicapped child must serve to increase their risk for maladaptation, otherwise all would be affected the same. For purposes of prevention and intervention, it becomes important to identify such risk factors as well as those factors that help mothers resist this increased risk.

We have proposed a conceptual model to account for the differential adaptation of parents of chronically ill and handicapped children. It adapts notions put forth by Pless and Pinkerton (1975), Moos and Schaefer (1984), and Lazarus and Folkman (1984) to identify as major risk factors parameters of the child's physical disease or disability, the strain of caring for such a child in activities of daily living, termed functional care strain, and psychosocial stress. The impact of these risk factors on adaptation is, however, hypothesized to be moderated by social-ecological factors, intrapersonal factors, and coping. These are thought to constitute a set of resistance factors. Furthermore, these factors are hypothesized to be related to adaptation in both direct and indirect ways. Disability/disease parameters, in addition to their direct effect on adaptation, are also hypothesized to have indirect effects by increasing functional care strain and psychosocial stress. The relationship between psychosocial stress and adaptation is hypothesized to be moderated by the use of certain coping strategies. Intrapersonal and social-ecological factors have direct effects on adjustment, as well as indirect effects by affecting both the occurrence of psychosocial stress and the quality and type of coping. This conceptual model is depicted in Figure 1.

Because the size of most available samples of chronically ill or handicapped children precludes an evaluation of the complete model, we have be-

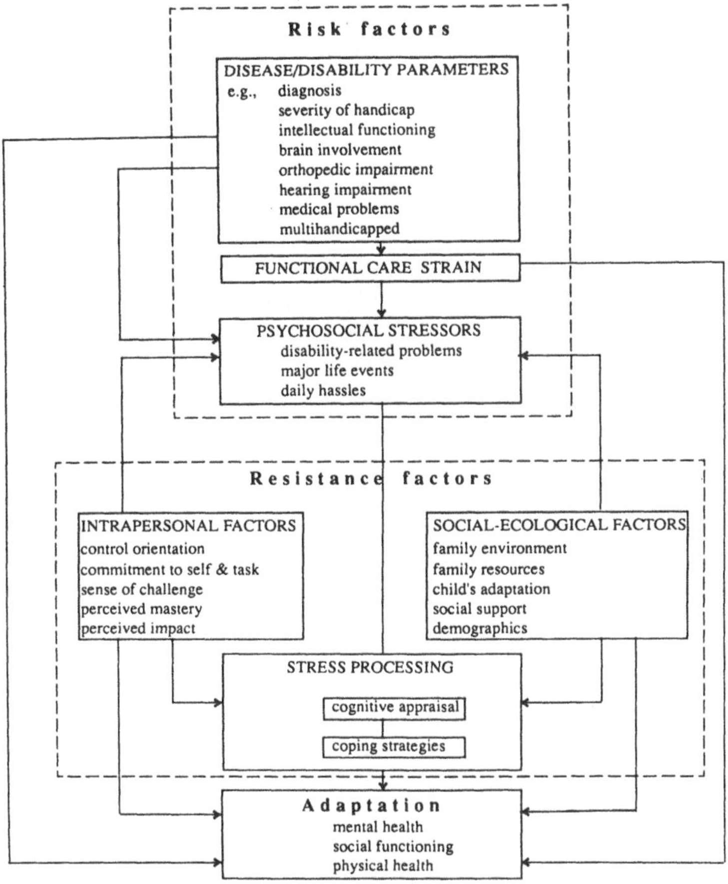

Fig. 1. Conceptual model for research on mothers of physically handicapped children

gun a research program to assess specific components of it. In light of the emphasis placed within traditional medical literature on the direct relationship possibly existing between parameters of the child's physical disorder and maternal adaptation, we focused on them first. Previous studies had reported equivocal findings whether certain physical conditions in the child are associated with poor maternal adaptation (e.g., Breslau, Staruch, & Mortimer, 1982; Chetwynd, 1985; Holroyd & McArthur, 1976; Kazak & Clark, 1986; McKinney & Peterson, 1987; Tavormina, Boll, Dunn, Luscomb, & Taylor, 1981). However, in the two separate studies we have conducted, no relationship was found between the child's physical condition and the mother's adaptation. Multiple dimensions of adaptation, disability status, and functional independence were considered in these two studies. In one study, the adaptation of mothers of congenitally physically handicapped children, ages 6–11, was not significantly related to the children's type of degree of disability nor their functional independence (Wallander et al., 1989). Identical findings were obtained in a second study of a larger sample of mothers with children, ages 2–18, with more varied physically handicapping conditions (Wallander, Pitt, & Mellins, in press). This latter study rather found that psychosocial stress explained a significant proportion of the variance in the mother's mental health. However, a proportion of the association between psychosocial stress and mental health was represented as an indirect effect of child disability status on psychosocial stress. An integration of these risk factors accounted for 57% of the variance in these mothers' mental health but less than 21% in their physical health and social functioning.

In this study we explore the role of another set of factors identified in the conceptual model. Given our previous findings of the stronger relationship existing between psychosocial factors, compared to physical factors, and mental health, we focus herein on the social environment. Much research into adaptation in the general population suggest social-ecological factors have important direct and indirect influences on psychosocial adaptation (see reviews by Gentry & Kobasa, 1984; Moos & Billings, 1982; Turner, 1983). Social-ecological factors refer to attributes of the individual's social environment. Based on research both on adaptation in general and of parents of chronically ill or handicapped children, specific social-ecological factors identified in our model include the utilitarian or practical resources available to the family, the chronically ill or handicapped child's adjustment, psychosocial family resources, and the services available and used for the care of the chronically ill or handicapped child.

The current study thus represents an initial attempt at investigating relationships between the social environment and adaptation of mothers of physically handicapped children, using a conceptually driven multivariate approach. Though the conceptual model is thought to be applicable to any pediatric physical disorder, the current study focuses on mothers of children who have one of two congenital physically handicapping conditions involving central nervous system lesions, namely, cerebral palsy or spina bifida. These are the two most common disorders of this type.

METHOD

Subjects[3]

Children age 6–11 with either spina bifida or cerebral palsy were identified from rosters of ambulatory clinics at Orthopaedic Hospital, Los

[3]This sample is identical to the one reported on in Wallander et al. (1989). A large number of variables were measured in this sample, following our conceptual model (see Figure 1). Differ-

Angeles. Their mothers were sent a letter introducing a research project pertaining to the adjustment of physically handicapped children. A phone call was then made to each mother to answer any questions and request her and her child's participation. Of the 78 mothers who were contacted, 50 consented to participate in the research. Mean age was 35.1 (SD = 7.3) for the mothers and 8.0 (SD = 1.7) for the physically handicapped children. Forty-six percent of the children were diagnosed with spina bifida, 54% were boys, 61% were independently ambulatory (though often with braces or crutches), and 66% were in some type of special education program. High school had been completed by 47% of the mothers and 52% reported a yearly family income at or above $20,000 in 1985, when these data were collected. This indicates that the sample was generally representative of the population in this geographic region at that time. Further descriptive sample statistics are reported in the Results section.

Procedure

This study was completed in the context of a larger data collection pertaining to handicapped children. Written informed consent and assent was first obtained from the mother and child, respectively. They were then separated and a research assistant administered the procedure to each independently. The mother was first interviewed in a semistructured fashion for approximately 30 minutes to obtain information about the child's disability, daily life, and family situation. A number of instruments were then administered in a fixed order to the mother, with those of relevance to this study described below. Of the several procedures administered to the child, relevant to this study are only those used to estimate his/her intellectual functioning. They are described below. With the mother's consent, the child's primary teacher was sent a request to complete several instruments. Relevant to this study is only the form described below requesting the scores from any intellectual assessment completed in the school within the past 2 years. The mother and child were paid $20 plus travel expenses for their participation.

Measures

Child Disability Status

Two parameters of the child's disability were measured. An assistant completed the 5-point Severity of Physical Handicap (Rutter, Tizard, &

---

ent hypotheses relating to different sets of variables were addressed in these two studies. Consequently, none of the main analyses have been duplicated.

Whitmore, 1970) rating scale based on information obtained in the interview with the mother and an hour interaction with the child. This scale describes the degree of the child's physical handicap (0 = none, 4 = total) in objectively defined terms. It was used to measure the child's *handicap severity*. The child's intellectual functioning was estimated using four data sources: the results from the WISC-R Block Design, WISC-R Picture Arrangement, The Peabody Picture Vocabulary Test—Revised (Form L-M), which were administered to the child by an assistant; in addition, the results of any school-administered intelligence tests were requested from the child's teacher and considered. However, standardized administration procedures could not always be followed with these physically handicapped children. Furthermore, handicapped children show more variablility than healthy children in performance across specific intellectual abilities. Consequently, a child's *intellectual functioning range* was estimated by considering all relevant test data and the child's physical ability to meet the task demands of the tests, in a manner typically done in clinical evaluations with physically handicapped children (Sattler, 1988).

Utilitarian Resources

Utilitarian resources are defined as structural characteristics of the family which may aid it in dealing with acute and chronic problems related to the child's handicap. Specific characteristics often discussed in this vein (e.g., Blacher, 1984; Johnson, 1985; Rutter et al., 1975; Whitt, 1984) include family income, mother's education, family size, presence of a child older than the handicapped child, duration of marriage, and mother's age. A standard checklist was administered to the mother to obtain this information.

Child Adjustment

Child adjustment was defined in terms of behaviors displayed which are associated with maladjustment in reference to age norms. As such, child adjustment was assessed by administering the 138-item Child Behavior Checklist (CBCL; Achenbach & Edelbrock, 1983) to the mother. The mother reports to which extent 118 behavior problems described the child, using a 3-point scale. A Total Behavior Problems score is calculated as the sum of all item ratings. In addition, the CBCL contains a Social Competence scale, constituted by another 20 items measuring the child's activities, peer relations, and school performance. These items are answered with differing content-specific answer scales. Extensive psychometric analyses and subsequent frequent research use have shown these two scales to have excellent test–retest reliability, interparent agreement, and construct validity when completed by parents (cf. Achenbach & Brown, 1988). Child adjustment was therefore measured in this study using the total scores from these scales.

Psychosocial Family Resources

Psychosocial family resources are defined as the family's characteristic mode of receiving and interacting with the social world, including within and external to the family (Reiss, 1982). Different specific psychosocial family resources can be distinguished (cf. George, 1980), of which three were considered herein. All were measured from the mother's perspective since her adaptation was the focus of this study.

Family support was defined in terms of the nature and quality of the relationships and system ties existing in the mother's nuclear family. Following much previous research in this field, it was measured with the 27 true–false items of the Family Environment Scale (Moos & Moos, 1981) pertaining to the subscales Cohesion, Expressiveness, and Conflict. The Cohesion Scale is intended to assess the degree of commitment, help, and support members provide one another; the Expressiveness Scale the extent to which members are encouraged to act openly and express feelings directly; and the Conflict Scale the amount of openly expressed anger, aggression, and conflict among members. These are commonly combined, after the direction of scoring on the Conflict subscale is reversed to form a summary score. Because this index has high internal consistency and good construct validity for measuring family support (e.g., Holahan & Moos, 1985, 1986), it was used to define family support.

Marital satisfaction was measured with the Dyadic Adjustment Scale (Spanier, 1976). This is a 32-item questionnaire addressing marital satisfaction, cohesion, consensus, and affective expression. Different answer scales are used as appropriate to the item content. The most widely used scale of its type, it has high reliability and criterion-related and construct validity (e.g., Margolin, Michelli, & Jacobson, 1988). The total score was used to measure marital satisfaction.

Social support network was defined as the number of people who would be available to provide support to the mother when problems are encountered. This type of global structural support (Cohen & Wills, 1985) was measured with the Social Support Questionnaire (Sarason, Levine, Bashom, & Sarason, 1983). This instrument presents 27 problems, for each of which the respondent lists who would be supportive. A score reflecting the mean across problems is calculated. It has very high reliability and good construct validity (cf. Heitzman & Kaplan, 1988; House & Khan, 1985), supporting its use in this study as a measure of social support network.

Service Utilization

A checklist was constructed specifically for this study which lists 20 primary services potentially used by physically handicapped children and their families. They include, among others, The Crippled Children's Service program, physical therapy, counseling, Supplemental Security Income, and special education. The mother indicates which of these services had been used during the child's lifetime. Service utilization was measured as the total number of services used.

Maternal Adaptation

Maternal Adaptation was defined, following prevailing conceptualizations of adult functioning (cf. Ware, Davies-Avery, & Brook, 1980; World Health Organization, 1948), broadly to include three domains: physical, mental, and social adaptation. Two instruments were used to measure these domains: The Malaise Inventory (Rutter et al., 1970) is a 24-item self-report checklist of emotional distress and physical health symptoms on which the mother indicated which have applied to her recently. It was used in this study because of its previous use in research on mothers of exceptional children and in other relevant epidemiological research (e.g., The Isle of Wight Study, Rutter et al., 1970). It has shown good construct validity and test–retest reliability in this context. Two subscales were formed on a content-rational basis from these items to measure two of the adaptation domains. *Mental health* was measured negatively with the 12 items tapping emotional complaints (e.g., "often worried about things," "easily upset or irritated," "frightened of going out alone or of meeting people"). *Physical health* was measured negatively with the other 12 items tapping physical complaints (e.g., "backache," "indigestion," "rheumatism or fibrositis"). Scores on both of these scales were reversed to yield a positive measure of each health domain.

Mother's *social functioning* was assessed using an instrument constructed for this research, the Social and Activities Questionnaire. This 19-item questionnaire elicits objective self-reports of average frequency of engagement of social-recreational activities (e.g., organizations, hobbies) and social contacts of different types with various people (e.g., neighbor, friend, extended family member) over the last year. Social activities and contacts are the two most important aspects of social functioning (e.g., Lazarus & Folkman, 1984; Ware et al., 1980). Involvement in general social activities was assessed with 10 items and frequency of social contacts with nine. A global social function score was calculated from the sum of the standard score from these two subscales.

RESULTS

Sample Characteristics

Descriptive statistics are reported for all social-ecological, child disability status, and maternal adaptation variables in Table I. A broad distribution was obtained for all social-ecological variables.

Child Disability. The ratings of the degree of the child's physical disability indicate that 30% of the children had "slight," 32% "moderate," 27% "severe," and 16% "total" disability. Based on the clinical estimation of children's intellectual functioning, 52% were considered to function in the average or above average, 18% in the borderline, 8% in the mildly retarded, 6% in the moderately or severely retarded, and 16% in the profoundly retarded range of intellectual ability.

Maternal Adaptation. The mothers of these physically handicapped children reported a mean of 2.84 (SD = 2.42) mental and 2.66 (SD = 2.08)

Table I. Descriptive Statistics for All Variables

	M	*SD*	Median[a]
Child disability status			
Handicap severity			Moderate
Intellectual functioning			Average
Utilitarian resources			
Family income			$20–30,000
Maternal education			Some high school
Family size	4.30	2.12	
Older child			No
Years married	8.22	3.56	
Maternal age	35.13	7.28	
Child adjustment			
Behavior problems	59.79	9.14	
Social competence	30.23	12.16	
Psychosocial family resources			
Family support	18.40	3.70	
Marital statisfaction	41.40	29.71	
Social support network	2.16	1.52	
Service utilization	4.98	3.74	
Maternal adaptation			
Mental health	2.84	2.42	
Physical health	2.66	2.08	
Social functioning[b]	0.11	1.22	

[a]Median reported for variables measured with categorical scales.
[b]Score is sum of two standard scores.

physical symptoms complaints on the Malaise Inventory, measures of mental and physical health, respectively. A combined total score was also calculated for these mothers to allow for comparison with the scores from the same questionnaire administered to the mothers in the Isle of Wight epidemiological study (Rutter et al., 1970). These mothers of physically handicapped children reported significantly more total health complaints on the average than mothers in general ($Z = 3.29$, $p < .001$), and an amount indistinguishable from that reported by mothers of psychiatrically disturbed children ($Z = -0.66$, $p =$ ns) on the Isle of Wight (mothers of physically handicapped children, $M = 5.7$; mothers in general, $M = 3.6$; mothers of psychiatrically disturbed children, $M = 6.1$). Because the social functioning measure was developed for this research, no comparisons with normative data were possible.

Preliminary Analyses

Classification Variables. Three series of t tests were first completed to determine whether the sample could be combined for subsequent analyses. One compared groups formed by the child's diagnosis, spina bifida or cerebral palsy; the second series compared groups formed by the child's sex; and the third series compared groups formed by the child's age, 6–8 or 9–11. Group means were compared in each series for the three maternal adaptation measures (mental health, physical health, social functioning). None of these nine comparisons yielded significant classification differences. Furthermore, t tests were completed to compare the children with spina bifida and cerebral palsy in terms of age, sex, ethnic status, family size, presence of older sibling, family income, maternal age, maternal education, and maternal marital status. There were no significant differences between the two diagnostic groups. All subsequent analyses, consequently, were conducted on the full sample without concern for these classification variables.

Utilitarian Resources Composite. Principal component analyses were conducted on the six utilitarian resources variable to attempt to empirically reduce these to a fewer number of nonredundant variables.[4] Results indicated that three components accounted for 73% of the total variance in the utilitarian resource variables. Based on the pattern of the varimax rotated component loading matrix, composite scores were computed by adding the standardized scores of these variables as follows: (a) maternal education, family income, and maternal age (negative) constituted SES-age composite and (b) the presence of an older sibling to the handicapped child and family

[4]Detailed description of the results of these analyses are available from the first author.

size constituted a family structure composite. The (c) duration of marriage did not load on either of these two components and thus remained a variable itself. Subsequent analyses of utilitarian resources were completed on these three variables.

Child Disability Status as a Covariate. The association between child disability status and maternal adaptation needed to be tested. If significant, the former would have to be controlled for in analyses of relationships between the social environment and maternal adaptation. Neither child handicap severity nor intellectual functioning correlated significantly with any of the maternal adaptation dimensions (rs $\leq$ .22) They did not jointly account for a significant proportion of the variance in any of the maternal adaptation dimensions either (R^2s $\leq$ .08). Thus there was no need to enter child disability as a covariate in subsequent analyses.

Social Environment and Adaptation

The zero-order relationships between specific social-ecological variables and adaptation dimensions are presented in Table II. Hierarchical multiple regression analyses were completed to evaluate the contribution of the social environment to the different dimensions of maternal adaptation. The utilitarian resources composite, child adjustment, psychosocial family resources, and service utilization variables were entered as sets of indepen-

Table II. Zero-Order Correlations Between Social-Ecological Variables and Adaptation

	Maternal adaptation		
	Mental	Physical	Social
Utilitarian resources			
SES-age	−.19	.00	.32[a]
Family structure	.17	.14	−.13
Duration of marriage	.23	−.01	−.29[a]
Child adjustment			
Behavior problems	−.08	−.25[a]	.10
Social competence	−.13	−.14	.21
Psychosocial family resources			
Family support	.43[c]	.39[b]	.06
Marital satisfaction	.54[c]	.36[b]	.23
Social support network	.30[a]	.01	.52[c]
Service utilization	.12	.05	.25[a]

[a] $p < .05$.
[b] $p < .01$.
[c] $p < .001$.

dent variables on separate steps in these regression analyses. Theoretical considerations dictated the particular order. Utilitarian resources were entered first since they addressed theoretically simple structural characteristics of the family environment. The remaining social-ecological factors were entered as determined by their proximity to the mother, starting with the handicapped child's adjustment, then the more general psychosocial family resources, and finally the use of community services. This analysis was repeated with each of the three adaptation dimensions being the dependent variable.

To control for and balance Type I and Type II errors in the regression analyses, two strategies recommended by Cohen and Cohen (1983, pp. 166-176) were employed: First, since the three dependent variables were not independent of one another, Bonferroni tests were employed to determine the significance of the *F*s for each hierarchically entered set as well as the final *F*, setting $p < .017$ (.05/3). Moreover, Fisher's Protected *t* tests were employed to evaluate the significance of the contribution of individual independent variables within the hierarchically entered sets. That is, a regression coefficient would not be tested unless the *F* test on the increment in the variance accounted for by the set to which that variable belongs reached significance at $p < .017$. If this criterion were met, the regression coefficients for variables in that set were tested at $p < .05$. The results from these analyses are presented in Table III.

The social environment was significantly ($p < .017$) associated with maternal mental health, $R^2 = .57$, $F(9, 40) = 5.89$, and social functioning, $R^2 = .68$, $F(9, 40) = 9.44$, but not physical health. Psychosocial family resources accounted for a significant increment in the variance in all three adaptation dimensions, beyond that accounted for by utilitarian resources and child adjustment. Between 22 and 34% of the variance in maternal adaptation was jointly explained by psychosocial family resources. More specifically, family support and social support network contributed uniquely to the variance in physical health, marital satisfaction to mental health, and all three specific family psychosocial resources to social functioning, based on their standardized regression coefficients reported in Table III.

Variance in maternal social functioning was significantly explained also by other social-ecological factors. Utilitarian resources accounted by itself for 32% of the variance in this adaptation dimension. Significant unique contributions were made by family structure and duration of marriage. Service utilization, even when added last in the regression system, accounted for a significant additional 11% of the variance beyond that attributable to utilitarian resources, child adjustment, and family psychosocial resources. Aside from psychosocial family resources, no social-ecological factors accounted for a significant proportion of the variance in mental or physical health.

Table III. Hierarchical Multiple Regression Analysis

				Maternal adaptation		
Step	Factor/variable	k^a	Statistic	Mental	Physical	Social
1	Utilitarian resources	3	R^2	.16	.03	.32[c]
2	Child adjustment	2	R^2 change	.03	.03	.03
3	Psychosocial family resources	3	R^2 change	.34[c]	.26[c]	.22[c]
4	Service utilization	1	R^2 change	.04	.02	.11[c]
			Final R^2	.57[c]	.38	.68[c]
	Utilitarian resources					
	SES-Age		β	—[b]	—	.23
	Family structure		β	—	—	−.30[c]
	Duration of marriage		β	—	—	−.28[c]
	Psychosocial family resources					
	Family support		β	.19	.34[c]	−.36[c]
	Marital satisfaction		β	.52[c]	.14	.46[c]
	Social support network		β	.16	.39[c]	.52[c]
	Service utilization		β	—	—	.42[c]

[a] k = number of variables entered on this step.

[b] Indicates this variable was not tested since the R^2-change for its set did not reach significance.

[c] $p < .017$ for R^2 change; $p < .05$ for β.

DISCUSSION

This was an investigation of the relationship between the social environment and the adaptation of mothers with elementary school aged congenitally physically handicapped children. Being guided by a conceptual model, these relationships were investigated for a broad set of social-ecological factors. Furthermore, adaptation was defined broadly to include functioning in the physical, mental, and social domains. Though restricted to mothers of children with one of two physically handicapping conditions, the sample represented a broad set of child, maternal, and family characteristics.

The results indicate that the social environment is strongly related to the mental and social functioning of these mothers. Social-ecological factors in combination accounted for between 57 and 68% of the variance in these adaptation domains. However, these mothers' physical health was not significantly associated with characteristics of their social environment. Children's disability status was not significantly associated with maternal adaptation either. At a general level then, these results support the notion that psychosocial outcomes in mothers of handicapped children are probably better predicted by psychosocial factors than by aspects of the children's physical condition.

Several social-ecological factors were considered herein. Utilitarian resources accounted for significant proportions of the variance in mothers' social functioning. A longer marriage is not a resource, as one might expect, but rather a risk factor as it predicted fewer social activities and contacts for the mothers. Similarly, having a larger family and a child older than the handicapped child were predictive of poorer social functioning. Thus, a younger marriage and smaller family may facilitate a more active social life for mothers of physically handicapped children.

The physically handicapped child's adjustment, as reported by the mothers, contributed no significant incremental variance in the mothers' adaptation. Behavior problems in children are directly associated with poorer physical health in the mothers; however, this association is not strong or independent.

Even though psychosocial family resources were considered in our hierarchical model only after utilitarian resources and child adjustment had been entered, they accounted for significant and sizable increments in the variance in all dimensions of adaptation. This suggests psychosocial characteristics of the mother's immediate social environment are potentially important resistance factors. As expected, better marital satisfaction reported by the mother was associated with better mental health. Better family support and a larger social support group was related to better physical health. Finally, better marital satisfaction, a larger support group, but less family support predicted better social functioning. The final social-ecological factor considered herein, service utilization, was important only for mothers' social adaptation.

To our knowledge there has been no previous report of relationships between this broad set of social-ecological factors and maternal adaptation to raising a handicapped child. This makes it difficult to place these results in a larger context. However, there is much research on the importance of the social support network for the adaptation of parents of chronically ill or handicapped children (e.g., Kazak, 1987; Kazak, Reber, & Snitzer, 1988). The importance of different family variables, furthermore, has been demonstrated in a variety of studies in general, though less so directly for mothers of handicapped children (cf. Johnson, 1985; Seligman, 1983). It is hoped this comparison of various social-ecological factors will facilitate further exploration of this important area. It appears that much of the variation in maternal psychosocial adaptation can be predicted, and possibly better understood, when considering the social environment. At the same time, more research is clearly needed to replicate these findings and extend them to other populations.

Future research would do well to improve upon some of the limitations present in this research. First, this research relied exclusively on maternal reports of all variables. It is felt that the mother's perspective of the child's adjustment and presence of family resources is important to understand her reporting of her adaptation. That is, her perceptions of these aspects of her environment may influence her perceptions of her functioning. At the same time, it is important to determine whether more objective reports of these social-ecological dimensions relate to maternal perceptions as well as more objective determinations of maternal mental and social functioning. Another limitation is of course the concurrent and correlation design of this study. Correlational results cannot be interpreted to indicate causation. It can be fairly easily argued, as a matter of fact, that the mother's adaptation can influence her reporting of her social environment as well as the actual status of this environment. A prospective longitudinal design would be a logical next step to enhance our understanding of causal priority between social-ecological factors and adaptation. The mother's physical health, as measured herein, was not well predicted from social-ecological factors. Possibly more comprehensive measurement procedures of physical health need to be used, rather than the simple symptom checklist employed in this study.

At the same time, research into maternal adaptation to raising a chronically ill or handicapped child would do well to consider other types of factors in addition to the social environment investigated herein. Intrapersonal characteristics of these mothers must also be considered, as identified in our conceptual model (see Figure 1). We have hypothesized that such specific intrapersonal characteristics as hardiness (Keith & Wallander, 1988a, 1989b), temperament (Wallander, Hubert, & Varni, 1988), causal attributional style, sense of mastery, and perceived impact of the handicapped child may be important. Future research should also attempt to compare environmental and intrapersonal factors and investigate their potentially moderating effect in the risk factor–adaptation relationship specified in our model.

REFERENCES

Achenbach, T. M., & Brown, J. S. (1988). *Bibliography of published studies using the Child Behavior Checklist and related material.* Burlington, VT: University Associated in Psychiatry.

Achenbach, T. M., & Edelbrock, C. (1983). *Manual for the Child Behavior Checklist and Revised Behavior Profile.* Burlington, VT: University Associates in Psychiatry.

Blacher, J. (1984). A dynamic perspective on the impact of a severely handicapped child on the family. In J. Blacher (Ed.), *Severely handicapped young children and their families: Research in review* (pp. 3-50). New York: Academic Press.

Breslau, N., Staruch, K. S., & Mortimer, F. A. (1982). Psychological distress in mothers of disabled children. *American Journal of Disease in Children, 136,* 682-686.

Byrne, E. A., & Cunningham, C. C. (1985). The effects of mentally handicapped children on families—a conceptual review. *Journal of Child Psychology and Psychiatry, 28,* 847-864.

Burton, L. (1975). *The family life of sick children: A study of family coping with chronic childhood disease.* London: Routledge & Kegan Paul.
Carey, G. E. (1982). Community care—care by whom? Mentally handicapped children living at home. *Public Health, 96,* 269-278.
Chetwynd, J. (1985). Factors contributing to stress on mothers caring for an intellectually handicapped child. *British Journal of Social Work, 15,* 295-304.
Cohen, J., & Cohen, P. (1983). *Applied multiple regression/correlation analysis for the behavioral sciences* (2nd ed.). Hillsdale, NJ: Erlbaum.
Cohen, S., & Wills, T. A. (1985). Stress, social support, and the buffering hypothesis. *Psychological Bulletin, 98,* 310-357.
Cummings, S. T., Bayley, C., & Rie, H. E. (1966). Effects of the child deficiency on the mother: A study of mothers of mentally retarded, chronically ill, and neurotic children. *American Journal of Orthopsychiatry, 36,* 595-608.
Gallager, J., Beckman, P., & Cross, A. (1983). Families of handicapped children: Sources of stress and its amelioration. *Exceptional Children, 50,* 10-19.
Gentry, W. D., & Kobasa, S. C. (1984). Social and psychological resources mediating the stress-illness relationships in humans. In W. D. Gentry (Ed.), *Handbook of behavioral medicine* (pp. 87-115). New York: Guilford.
George, L. (1980). *Role transitions in later life.* Belmont, CA: Brooks/Cole.
Haggerty, R. J., Roghmann, K. J., & Pless, I. B. (1975). *Child health in the community.* New York: Wiley.
Heitzmann, C. A., & Kaplan, R. M. (1988). Assessment methods for measuring social support. *Health Psychology, 7,* 75-109.
Holahan, C. J., & Moos, R. H. (1985). Life stress and health: Personality, coping, and family support in stress resistance. *Journal of Personality and Social Psychology, 49,* 739-747.
Holahan, C. J., & Moos, R. H. (1986). Personality, coping, and family resources in stress resistance: A longitudinal analysis. *Journal of Personality and Social Psychology, 51,* 389-395.
Holroyd, J., & McArthur, D. (1976). Mental retardation and stress on parents: A contrast between Down's Syndrome and childhood autism. *American Journal of Mental Deficiency, 80,* 431-436.
House, J. S., & Kahn, R. L. (1985). Measures and concepts of social support. In S. Cohen & S. L. Syme (Eds.), *Social support and health* (pp. 83-108). New York: Academic Press.
Ireys, H. T. (1981). Health care for chronically disabled children and their families. In *Better health for our children: A national strategy* (Vol. 4, pp. 321-353, DHHS Publication No. 70-55071). Washington, DC: U.S. Government Printing Office.
Johnson, S. B. (1985). The family and the child with chronic illness. In D. C. Turk & R. D. Kerns (Eds.), *Health, illness, and families: A life-span perspective* (pp. 220-254). New York: Wiley.
Kazak, A. (1987). Families with disabled children: Stress and social networks in three samples. *Journal of Abnormal Child Psychology, 15,* 137-146.
Kazak, A. E., & Clark, M. W. (1986). Stress in families of children with mylomeningocele. *Developmental Medicine and Child Neurology, 28,* 220-227.
Kazak, A. E., Reber, M., & Snitzer, L. (1988). Childhood chronic disease and family functioning: A study of phenylketonuria. *Pediatrics, 81,* 224-230.
Keith, B. R., & Wallander, J. L. (1988a, April). *Hardiness as a stress-resistance factor in mothers of physically handicapped children.* Paper presented at the Florida Conference on Child Health Psychology, Gainesville.
Keith, B. R., & Wallander, J. L. (1988b, August). *Longitudinal study of stress and hardiness in a clinical population.* Paper presented at the meeting of the American Psychological Association, Atlanta.
Lazarus, R. S., & Folkman, S. (1984). *Stress, appraisal, and coping.* New York: Springer.
Margolin, G., Michelli, J., & Jacobson, N. S. (1988). Assessment of marital interactions. In A. S. Bellack & M. Hersen (Eds.), *Behavioral Assessment: A practical handbook* (3rd ed., pp. 441-489). New York: Pergamon.

McKinney, B., & Peterson, R. A. (1987). Predictors of stress in parents of developmentally disabled children. *Journal of Pediatric Psychology, 12,* 133-150.
Moos, R. H., & Billings, A. G. (1982). Conceptualizing and measuring coping resources and processes. In L. Goldberger & S. Breznitz (Eds.). *Handbook of stress: Theoretical and clinical aspects* (pp. 212-230). New York: Free Press.
Moos, R. H., & Moos, B. S. (1981). *Family Environment Scale.* Palo Alto, CA: Consulting Psychologists Press.
Moos, R. H., & Schaefer, J. A. (1984). The crisis of physical illness: An overview and conceptual approach. In R. H. Moos (Ed.), *Coping with physical illness 2: New perspectives* (pp. 3-25). New York: Plenum Press.
Pless, I. B., & Pinkerton, P. (1975). *Chronic childhood disorders: Promoting patterns of adjustment.* Chicago: Year Book Medical.
Reiss, O. (1982). *The family's construction of reality.* Cambridge, MA: Harvard University Press.
Rutter, M., Tizard, J., & Whitmore, K. (Eds.). (1970). *Education, health, and behavior.* London: Longman.
Rutter, M., Yule, B., Quinton, D., Rowlands, O., Yule, W., & Berger, M. (1975). Attainment and adjustment in two geographical areas: III. Some factors accounting for area differences. *British Journal of Psychiatry, 126,* 520-533.
Sattler, J. M. (1988). *Assessment of children's intelligence and special abilities* (3rd ed.). San Diego: Author.
Sarason, I. G., Levine, H. M., Basham, R. B., & Sarason, B. R. (1983). Assessing social support: The Social Support Questionnaire. *Journal of Personality and Social Psychology, 44,* 127-139.
Seligman, M. (Ed.). (1983). *The family with a handicapped child: Understanding and treatment.* New York: Grume & Stratton.
Spanier, G. B. (1976). Measuring dyadic adjustment: New scales for assessing the quality of marriage and similar dyads. *Journal of Marriage and the Family, 38,* 15-28.
Tavormina, J., Boll, R., Dunn, N., Luscomb, R., & Taylor, J. (1981). Psychosocial effects on parents of raising a physically handicapped child. *Journal of Abnormal Child Psychology, 9,* 121-131.
Tew, B. J., & Laurence, K. M. (1983). Mothers, brothers, and sisters, of patients with spina bifida. *Developmental Medicine and Child Neurology, 15*(Suppl. 29), 69-77.
Turner, R. J. (1983). Direct, indirect, and moderating effects of social support on psychological distress and associated conditions. In H. B. Kaplan (Ed.), *Trends in theory and research* (pp. 105-155). New York: Academic Press.
Wallander, J. L., Hubert, N. C., & Varni, J. W. (1988, April). *Temperament characteristics, goodness of fit, and adaptation in physically handicapped children and their mothers.* Paper presented at the Florida Conference on Child Health Psychology, Gainesville, FL.
Wallander, J. L., Pitt, L. C., & Mellins, C. A. (in press). Risk factors threatening adaptation in mothers of physically or sensorally handicapped children: An integrative model. *Journal of Consulting and Clinical Psychology.*
Wallander, J. L., Varni, J. W., Babani, L., Banis, H. T., DeHaan, C. B., & Wilcox, K. T. (1989). Disability parameters, chronic strain, and adaptation of physically handicapped children and their mothers. *Journal of Pediatric Psychology, 14,* 23-42.
Ware, J. E., Davies-Avery, A., & Brook, R. H. (1980). *Conceptualization and measurement of health for adults in the Health Insurance Study* (Vol. 6, Analysis of relationships among health status measures, R-1987/6-HEW). Washington, DC: U.S. Government Printing Office.
Whitt, J. K. (1984). Children's adaptation to chronic illness and handicapping conditions. In M. G. Eisenberg, L. C. Sutkin, & M. A. Jansen (Ed.), *Chronic illness and disability through the life span: Effects on self and family* (pp. 69-102). New York: Springer.
Wilkin, D. (1979). *Caring for the Mentally handicapped child.* London: Croom Helm.
World Health Organization. (1948). *Basic documents.* Geneva, Switzerland: Author.

10

Adjustment of Siblings of Handicapped Children: A Comparison[1]

Lily L. Dyson
University of Washington

Compared 55 older siblings (ages 7½ to 15 years) of young handicapped children (ages 1–7 years) with 55 matched siblings of nonhandicapped children. Results of standardized children's assessment scales show that siblings of handicapped children are comparable to siblings of nonhandicapped children in self-concept, behavior problems, and social competence. Differences, however, appear along certain psychological dimensions and great variations exist within each group of siblings. Further, demographic and personal attributes are differentially related to measures of adjustment in different groups of siblings. Implications for research and intervention are drawn.

The effect of a child's handicap is not limited to the child. When a family has a handicapped child, all members are affected (Fewell, 1986). As siblings share an intimate and intense relationship (Sutton-Smith & Rosenberg, 1970), a handicapped child will have a special impact on the siblings. A practical concern is the nature of the impact and factors that may influence that impact.

[1]This report is based on the author's doctoral dissertation. I thank my committee members, Drs. Eugene Edgar, Owen White, Keith Crnic, James Morishima, Martha Perry, and Joanne McMillan. I am also grateful for the children, parents, and teachers who have helped the completion of this study. The project was funded by a grant from the Washington Association for Retarded Citizens Research Trust Fund. A portion of this paper was presented at the International Early Childhood Conference on Children with Special Needs, Nashville, Tennessee, November 1988.

Common assumptions exist that handicapped children have a harmful effect on siblings and that siblings of handicapped children experience more adjustment difficulty than children with no handicapped brothers or sisters (San Martino & Newman, 1974). These assumptions are drawn from reasonable considerations, including the residual effects of parental stress due to the care of the handicapped child (Lavigne & Ryan, 1979), increased home responsibility (Breslau, Weitzman, & Messenger, 1981; Farber, 1959) but decreased parental attention and family resources (McAndrew, 1976; McKeever, 1983; Siemon, 1984), and finally, pathological identification with the handicapped child (Featherstone, 1980; Kaplan, 1969).

Research, however, has produced conflicting results on the effect of handicapped children on siblings. Negative effects have been found (Farber, 1959; Ferrari, 1987; Fowle, 1969; Gath, 1973; Harvey & Greenway, 1984; Tew & Lawrence, 1973), as well as the absence of negative effects (Caldwell & Guze, 1960; Ferrari, 1984; Gath, 1972; Gayton, Friedman, Tavormina, & Tucker, 1977; Graliker, Fishler, & Koch, 1962; Schwirian, 1976). Simultaneously positive and negative consequences have also been reported (Cleveland & Miller, 1977; Grossman, 1972).

Professionals are cognizant that the effect of handicapped children on siblings may be influenced by extraneous factors such as the family's socioeconomic status (SES), birth order, sex of the handicapped child and the sibling, type and severity of the handicap. Equal confusion surrounds the effects of these characteristics. SES alone was reported to be influential in some studies (Farber, 1959; Gath, 1972), but was found to interact with sibling sex in other studies (Gath, 1974; Grossman, 1972). Still another study (Schwirian, 1976) discerned no such interaction effects. Disagreement also exists regarding whether older sisters or older brothers are more adversely affected (cf. Breslau, 1982; Cleveland & Miller, 1977; Farber, 1959; Fowle, 1969; Gath, 1974; Grossman, 1972; Lavigne & Ryan, 1979; Schwirian, 1976). Still others detected no difference due to sex (Kowalski, 1980; Tew & Laurence, 1973) or birth order per se (Tew & Laurence, 1973). As with sex of the sibling, disparate reports concern the effect of gender of the handicapped child (cf. Ferrari, 1984; Gath, 1974; Grossman, 1972), type of handicap (cf. Breslau et al., 1981; Lavigne & Ryan, 1979), and severity (cf. Breslau et al., 1981; Grossman, 1972; Kowalski, 1980; Tew & Laurence, 1973).

Conflicting findings are partly attributed to methodological weaknesses. These encompass a lack of a control group (Caldwell & Guze, 1960; Farber, 1959; Fowle, 1969; McAndrew, 1976), the use of nonequivalent comparison groups (e.g., Breslau et al., 1981; Harvey & Greenway, 1984; Lavigne & Ryan, 1979), an indirect measure based on parental interviews (Farber, 1959; Fowle, 1969; Schwirian, 1976), and a reliance on a single measure such as the current psychological state (e.g., Breslau et al., 1981; Lavigne & Ryan, 1979) or self-concept (Gayton et al., 1977; Harvey & Greenway, 1984). Although the pertinence of adequate comparison groups is apparent for a valid evaluation, direct and multiple measures have also been advocated by reviewers for accurately assessing siblings of handicapped children (Simeonsson & McHale, 1981).

Discrepant results, however, continue to surface with improved experimental designs. While siblings of handicapped children were found to be not different from control children in self-concept and behavior adjustment (Ferrari, 1984) and in self-concept alone (Dyson & Fewell, in press; Lobato, Barbour, Hall, & Miller, 1987), siblings of diabetic children were reported (Ferrari, 1987) to have a lower self-concept. Lobato et al. (1987) also found brothers of handicapped children to be more depressed and more aggressive and sisters more aggressive than control children. Similar inconsistencies have arisen among these studies concerning the effects of personal characteristics such as sex (cf. Ferrari, 1984, 1987; Lobato et al., 1987). A common weakness of these studies, however, is a small sample ($N < 30$).

Less disputed but also implicated in studies of siblings of handicapped children are attributes such as family size (Gath, 1974; Kazak & Clark, 1986) and age spacing (Breslau, 1982). Other factors associated with adjustment of siblings may include parents' education and age of the child, for these are common factors affecting a child's development.

Disparate research findings on the effect of a handicapped child on siblings are of little utility both for understanding and for intervention for families of handicapped children. Further clarification is needed. This is important as medical advances and the emphasis on mainstreaming will result in more severely handicapped children being cared for at home. If the presence of a handicapped child at home would harm the development of siblings, family intervention is urgently required. The identification of personal factors that may influence the effect of a handicapped child on siblings would particularly aid intervention.

This study examined the adjustment of siblings of handicapped children and identified its personal and demographic correlates, as compared with children with nonhandicapped siblings. Adjustment was measured by self-concept, behavior problems, and social competence. Two hypotheses were tested: (a) There would be differences between siblings of handicapped children and siblings of nonhandicapped children in self-concept, behavior problems, and social competence, and (b) there would be personal and demographic characteristics related to self-concept, behavior problems, and social competence in siblings of handicapped children.

METHOD

Subjects

The subjects were 110 older siblings of children under 7 years of age. They were equally divided into two groups: the handicapped group consisting of siblings of children with a diagnosed handicap and the nonhandicapped group comprising siblings of children with no known handicap. The ages of the subjects ranged from 7½ to 14½, most (89%) were between 8 and 12 years. Sixty subjects resided in a major city and vicinity in the west coast of Canada and 50 in a Northwest metropolitan area of the United States. The two groups were matched by the age and sex, their younger sibling's age range (under 7 years of age), family structure (single vs. two-parent family), geographical region (Canada vs. U.S.), and socioeconomic class.

Based on the Hollingshead (1975) scale, most (81%) of the families were of the middle SES. The handicapped and the nonhandicapped groups did not differ in the total socioeconomic rating ($p > .05$). Further, the overwhelming majority (91%) of the families in each group were two-parent families and only six families had only one adult living in the house. Mothers of the nonhandicapped group had significantly more formal education than mothers of the handicapped group ($p < .04$), whereas no difference appeared in the fathers. Major subject characteristics are presented in Table I.

The primary diagnoses of the handicapped children included (a) mental retardation ($n = 18$), (b) physical and sensory handicaps ($n = 22$), (c) speech disorders ($n = 8$), (d) learning and behavior disorders ($n = 3$), and (e) developmental delays ($n = 4$). Different degrees of severity were reported by parents: 16 were mildly, 26 moderately, 8 severely, and 5 profoundly handicapped.

All of the handicapped children were enrolled in a special program, whereas all nonhandicapped younger siblings were attending a regular preschool, day care, or kindergarten program. All older siblings, those of handicapped and of nonhandicapped children, were enrolled in regular schools.

Instrumentation

The subjects and their parents completed a set of questionnaires which included a demographic form for parents' completion and child and family assessment scales.

The Piers-Harris Children's Self-Concept Scale (CSCS). The CSCS (Piers & Harris, 1969), completed by the subject, is a self-report and self-referenced instrument designed for children Grades 4 to 12, or younger. The

Table I. Selected Subject Characteristics

Characteristics	Handicapped group	Nonhandicapped group
Age of subjects (years)		
Range	7½–14½	7½–14½
M	9.6	9.8
SD	1.7	2.0
Sex of subjects (*n*)		
Male	35	35
Female	20	20
Age of younger sibling (years)		
Range	1–6	1–6
M	4.1	4.3
SD	1.4	1.7
Sex of younger sibling (*n*)		
Male	30	27
Female	25	28
Region[a]		
Canada	30	30
U.S.	25	25
Family structure[b]		
2-parent	50 (91)	50 (91)
1-parent	5 (10)	5 (10)
SES[b]		
Lower	14 (26)	4 (7)
Lower-middle	8 (15)	19 (35)
Middle-middle	31 (56)	24 (46)
Upper-middle	2 (3)	7 (13)

[a]Number of subjects in each group.
[b]Number of subjects in each group. Percentages shown in parentheses.

scale consists of 80 first-person declarative statements such as, "I am smart," requiring the child to respond with "Yes" or "No." The CSCS, standardized on 1,183 children, has an internal consistency of between .78 to .93 and the test–retest reliability of from .71 to .77. In addition to a total scale score, the CSCS yields 6 cluster scores: Factor 1: Behavior; Factor 2: Intellectual and School Status; Factor 3; Physical Appearance and Attributes; Factor 4: Anxiety; Factor 5: Popularity; and Factor 6; Happiness and Satisfaction. The higher a score is, the higher the self-concept is.

The Child Behavior Checklist (CBCL). The CBCL (Achenbach, 1981) assesses the behavior problems and social competence of children, ages 4 to 16 years, as reported by parents and others who know the child well (Achenbach & Edelbrock, 1983). The scale consists of two main parts: the Behavior Problems and Social Competence Scales. There are 118 items related to behavior problems, each scored on a 3-point scale from *not true* (0), *somewhat true* (1), to *very true* (2). The social competence items record the amount and quality of the child's competence in sports, organization, and chores and in academic skills and peer interaction.

Normed on both referred and nonreferred children (N = 1,300), the CBCL scale is psychometrically sound with adequate reliability and validity (Freeman, 1985; Kelley, 1985). The Behavior Problems Scale contains eight or nine factors depending on the age and sex of the child, and two broad bands labeled Internalizing and Externalizing. The CBCL produces a total behavior problem score and a social competence score in addition to factor and subscale scores. The higher a behavior problem score is, the more negative the behavior is. However, a high social competence score indicates more social competence. Parents rated the older participating sibling. The Social Competence Scale has three subscales: Activities, Social, and School.

Procedure

Families of handicapped children were recruited from a total of nine programs and agencies serving handicapped children or their families in Canada and the United States. These programs and agencies included early intervention programs, special education programs, associations for retarded citizens, and public health clinics. The selection criteria for the handicapped group were families with a child under the age of 7 years with a diagnosed developmental handicap and an older child between the age of 7½ to 15 years. The diagnosis was based on the assessment and diagnosis made by the child's intervention or special education program. To avoid overrepresentation by some families, only one older sibling from each family was included.

Families of nonhandicapped children were recruited from regular preschool, day care, and kindergarten programs in Canada and the United States. A total of 22 programs assisted in the recruitment. In Canada, the programs were drawn from a government list. Regular preschools and day care centers in the same region as the special programs for the handicapped children were contacted by phone. Those centers with families meeting the selection criteria assisted in recruiting families. Only one day care center refused. In the United States, child care facilities came from a list supplied by a community college preschool teacher training program and from individual preschool teachers. Thus, the families and children were representative of the population in each region. The same selection criteria for the handicapped children were applied to the nonhandicapped group. Additionally, the families had to match families of handicapped children in the personal and demographic characteristics described earlier.

Qualified families were identified by their respected programs and, upon informed consent, received the questionnaires and child and family assessment scales, described earlier, to be completed at home. Only one family completed the scales with the investigator reading the items.

RESULTS

A total of 207 packets of questionnaires and scales were distributed with 144 (70%) returned. The return rate was higher for the nonhandicapped group (74%) than the handicapped group (64%). However, only 110 sets of questionnaires and scales were included in the final analyses due to one incompleted scale and a lack of matched subject attributes.

Differences Between Groups on Self-Concept, Behavior Problems, and Social Competence

Descriptive statistics (means, standard deviations, ranges, and medians) on self-concept, behavior problems, and social competence for the handicapped group are shown in Table II. A one-way multivariate analysis of variance (MANOVA) was performed on the three dependent variables: self-concept, behavior problems, and social competence, to test for a significant difference between the two groups. The multivariate test was not significant, $F(3, 100) = 1.98$, $p < .31$, indicating that the two groups did not differ from each other on the combined variables. Examination of the univariate tests also revealed no significant differences at the .05 level.

Separate MANOVAs comparing the two groups were further applied to the 6-factor scores of the CSCS, to the 8 subscales of the Behavior Problems scale, and to 3 subscales of the Social Competence scale of the CBCL. No significant differences between the groups were found on the subscales of the CSCS ($p < .10$). On the CBCL, however, a significant difference between groups was found on the subscales of the Social Competence scale, $F(3, 100) = 4.89$, $p < .01$. The univariate tests showed that on this scale the two groups differed only on the Activities subscale. Siblings of handicapped children were rated less active in sports and nonsports activities than siblings of nonhandicapped children, $F(1, 102) = 8.63$, $p < .01$.

As the Behavior Problems scale of the CBCL has designated different subscales and broad bands for different age ranges and sexes (Achenbach

Table II. Descriptive Statistics on Self-Concept, Behavior Problems, and Social Competence for the Handicapped and the Nonhandicapped Group

	Handicapped group				Nonhandicapped group			
	M	*SD*	Range	Median	*M*	*SD*	Range	Median
Self-concept	64.75	8.26	43–78	64.0	64.43	11.01	35–79	65.0
Behavior problems	20.95	13.61	1–58	20.0	25.07	16.42	3–81	21.0
Social competence	20.26	3.59	7–27	20.6	20.63	3.09	13–28	21.3

& Edelbrock, 1983), comparisons were made along the four sex-by-age groups: (a) girls ages 7 to 11, (b) girls ages 12 to 15, (c) boys ages 7 to 11, and (d) boys ages 12 to 15. This classification, however, resulted in greatly unequal number of subjects in each category (from 4 to 37) due to fewer children over 12 years of age. As meaningful MANOVAs could not be performed under the circumstances, *t* tests were applied to examine any differences between the handicapped and the nonhandicapped group. None of the *t* tests discriminated the two groups among the girls of any age range. For boys, significant differences appeared on ages 7 to 11 on the Schizoid subscale, $t(40) = -2.32$, $p < .03$, and ages 12 to 15 on the Aggression factor, $t(11) = -2.38$, $p < .04$. Marginal differences also appeared on the Withdrawal factor, $t(54) = -1.86$, $p = .07$ for ages 7 to 11, and on the Externalizing, $t(11) = -2.01$, $p = .07$, and Hyperactivity factor, $t(11) = -1.93$, $p = .08$, for ages 12 to 15. In all of these differences, the nonhandicapped group scored higher, indicating more behavior problems.

Within-Group Variations in Response

Table II also shows the ranges and medians of scores for self-concept, behavior problems, and social competence for the handicapped and the nonhandicapped group. As seen, a wide range of scores emerged for each measure for each group. For example, a range as wide as 35 points appeared in self-concept scores in the handicapped group. On the same measure, a greater discrepancy of 44 points was observed in the nonhandicapped group. Greater variations were seen in the behavior problems scale for both groups.

Demographic and Personal Characteristics Related to Adjustment

To explore the relationship between demographic and personal characteristics and adjustment, a MANOVA was performed with a $2 \times 2 \times 2$ (SES $\times$ Sex $\times$ Group) factorial design. No main or interaction effects were found. Similarly, while a $2 \times 2 \times 2$ MANOVA with younger child's sex, older sibling's sex, and group found a significant interaction effect, $F(3, 100) = 3.81$, $p < .05$, subsequent ANOVA showed no difference due to any gender. For a further analysis, age specing was categorized into four categories. A MANOVA with $2 \times 4 \times 2$ design (Gender $\times$ Age Spacing $\times$ Group) detected no effects as well.

The effect of severity and type of handicap was assessed with analysis of variance (ANOVA). The SES categories were condensed from 4 to 3 with the upper-middle class being included in the middle-middle class and types of handicap were reduced from 5 to 3 with speech disorders, developmental delay, and learning and behavior disorders being combined. Likewise, severity of handicap was compressed from 4 to 3, the profound being combined with the severe degree.

ANOVA showed no effect of severity of handicap on any measure of adjustment. The type of handicap, however, discriminated the groups, the most prominent effect was on behavior problems, $F(2, 52) = 5.82$, $p < .01$, followed by self-concept $F(92, 52) = 3.17$, $p < .05$. Post hoc multiple comparisons with the Scheffé test showed that siblings of mentally retarded children ($M = 12.7$) had significantly fewer behavior problems than siblings of children with physical or sensory handicaps ($M = 25.6$), or siblings of the combined group of children with speech disorders, learning and behavior disorders, and developmental delays ($M = 24.0$). Likewise, post hoc t tests showed that siblings of mentally retarded children had significantly higher self-concept ($M = 68.6$) than siblings of children with physical or sensory handicaps ($M = 62.9$, $p < .05$) or siblings of children with other handicaps (speech disorders, developmental delays, or learning and behavior disorders) ($M = 62.8$, $p < .05$).

In social competence, the ANOVA showed the effect of type of handicap to be only short of statistical significance ($p > .06$). Post hoc t tests, however, showed that siblings of mentally retarded children had significantly higher social competence ($M = 21.8$) than siblings of children with physical or sensory handicaps ($M = 19.8$, $p < .05$) or siblings of children with speech disorders, learning and behavior disorders, or developmental delays ($M = 19.0$, $p < .05$). These results were based on children who shared only such common characteristics as having a handicapped younger sibling with the same age range and being within the same range themselves.

The Pearson correlation procedure was applied to continuous demographic variables, resulting in the following significant correlations: Age of the handicapped child ($r = .26$, $p < .05$) and age spacing ($r = -.27$, $p < .05$) correlated with behavior problems, while family size ($r = .24$, $p < .05$) and mother's education ($r = .27$, $p < .05$) correlated with social competence. For the nonhandicapped group, age of the younger sibling ($r = -.24$, $p < .05$) and mother's education ($r = -.38$, $p < .01$) correlated with behavior problems. Mean scores for adjustment measures and correlated demographic attributes are summarized in Table III for the handicapped and the nonhandicapped group, with age, age spacing, number of children (family size), and number of years of education of the parents categorized.

Comparison of Regional Samples

No difference in any adjustment measure appeared between the Canadian and the American sample either on the regional basis (handicapped and

Table III. Mean Scores for Adjustment Measures and Correlated Demographic and Personal Attributes for the Handicapped and the Nonhandicapped Group

Demographic and personal attributes	Adjustment measure		
Handicapped group			
	Behavior problems		
	M	*SD*	*n*
Age of handicapped child[a]			
1-2	12.00	10.11	6
3-4	19.04	12.27	23
4-7	24.69	14.49	26
Total	20.94	13.61	55
Age spacing[b]			
2-3	25.37	15.23	16
4-5	21.52	12.20	17
6-7	19.90	14.35	10
9-10	11.75	8.95	4
Total	21.65	13.67	47
	Social competence		
No. of children			
1-2	20.13	4.42	16
3-4	19.92	3.15	34
5-7	22.96	2.84	5
Total	20.26	3.58	55
Mother's education (years)			
9 or less	19.00	2.23	4
12	19.07	3.95	21
14	21.30	2.90	19
16 and more	21.19	3.85	11
Total	20.26	3.58	55
Nonhandicapped group			
	Behavior problems		
	M	*SD*	*n*
Age of younger sibling[a]			
1-2	29.00	1.00	3
3-4	29.35	18.70	28
5-7	19.43	13.16	23
Total	25.11	16.57	54
Mother's education (years)			
12	31.95	19.49	20
14	25.64	13.27	14
16 or more	18.14	12.43	21
Total	25.07	16.42	55

[a]The range of age in years.
[b]Spacing in years.

nonhandicapped groups combined) or within each group (handicapped and nonhandicapped group separately). As well, no group differences (handicapped vs. nonhandicapped) emerged within the Canadian or American sample.

DISCUSSION

The first hypothesis that siblings of handicapped children would differ in adjustment from siblings of nonhandicapped children is not supported. Overall, siblings of handicapped children display the same level of self-concept, behavior problems, and social competence as matched siblings of nonhandicapped children.

The results concur with other reports that siblings of handicapped children do not display a lower self-concept (Dyson & Fewell, in press; Ferrari, 1984; Gayton et al., 1979; Kazak & Clark, 1986; Lobato et al., 1987). This study, nonetheless, contrasts with other reports in that siblings of handicapped children hold a low self-concept (Ferrari, 1987; Harvey & Greenway, 1984). The results also support other studies reporting no higher rates of psychopathological behavior (Breslau et al., 1981; Ferrari, 1984; Gath, 1972; Lavigne & Ryan, 1979) but more social competence in siblings of handicapped children than siblings of healthy children (Ferrari, 1984). Further support for the finding is the report that siblings of mentally retarded children live a normal social life (Graliker et al., 1962).

There are, however, indications that siblings of handicapped children differ from other siblings on some psychological dimensions. Siblings of handicapped children in general were less active in extracurricular activities than other siblings. Further, although sisters of handicapped children did not differ from sisters of nonhandicapped children on any psychological dimension, there were differences among the brothers. Between the ages of 7 and 11, brothers of handicapped children showed fewer fantasizing, deviant, and isolated behaviors than brothers of nonhandicapped children. For the age range of 12 to 15, brothers of handicapped children were less aggressive and hyperactive and tended to have fewer externalizing behavior problems than brothers of nonhandicapped children.

Of special interest is the variability in adjustment that appeared in both groups of siblings. In all siblings, some displayed an exceptionally high self-concept and social competence but few behavior problems, while others showed just the opposite. The variability suggests the presence of individual differences in adjustment among children whether they have a handicapped sibling or not. Most children are well adjusted but others experience difficulties.

The second hypothesis that there would be personal attributes related to adjustment in siblings of handicapped children is confirmed. A significant attribute was the type of handicap. Siblings of mentally handicapped children in general showed better behavior adjustment, a higher self-concept, and more social competence than siblings of children with physical or sensory handicaps or siblings of children with milder handicapping conditions. Little adjustment difference was found between children whose siblings have a physical or sensory handicap and children whose siblings have other handicaps (speech disorders, learning and behavior disorders, or developmental delay). The discrepancy between siblings of mentally retarded children and siblings of other types of handicapped children may be explained by the differential social consequences. Mental retardation may in general evoke earlier and more social and family acceptance than other disabilities such as sensory and physical handicaps, developmental delays, speech disorders, and learning disabilities. Some of these handicaps (e.g., developmental delay) may not be well defined and some may involve an apparent handicap (e.g., physical or sensory) despite the absence of intellectual deficit. These conditions could produce uncertainty or frustration in the family to harm the sibling's self-concept and behavior adjustment.

Further association existed between behavior problems and the age of the handicapped child and age spacing between the handicapped child and her sibling. The older a handicapped child, the more behavior problems were reported of the sibling. This finding coincides with the observation that families of handicapped children experience increasing isolation as these children become older (Suelzle & Keenan, 1981). Moreover, the larger the age gap, the better the sibling's behavior adjustment was. Again, this confirms the report that closer age spacing in younger brothers is linked to poor psychological functioning and aggressive behavior (Breslau, 1982). Family size and mother's education were also related to the siblings' adjustment. The larger the family and the higher the mother's education, the more social competence a sibling showed. The effect of family size supports the finding that siblings of handicapped children from larger families have a higher self-concept in the aspects of popularity and physical appearance than do siblings from two-child families (Kazak & Clark, 1986). Cautious interpretations of these results, however, are required because of the generally weak though significant correlations between measures.

For siblings of nonhandicapped children, the influence of demographic characteristics was limited to only the behavior problems. This measure was related to the mother's education and the age of the younger sibling. Mothers with higher education reported fewer behavior problems in the older siblings. Further, contrary to the handicapped group, the older a nonhandicapped child was, the fewer behavior problems the sibling had.

This study fails to confirm the reported effects of SES, gender, and severity of handicap. Instead, the study finds adjustment of siblings of handicapped children is related to the type of handicap, age of the handicapped child, age spacing between the handicapped child and the sibling, family size, and mother's education. Different demographic and personal characteristics, however, are differentially related to siblings of nonhandicapped children.

CONCLUSION

Clearly, a handicap alone in a sibling is not a sufficient factor affecting a child's adjustment. More salient factors appear to be characteristics present in the handicapped sibling, the child him/herself, and the family—a similar conclusion reached by Ferrari (1984) and others (Lobato, 1983, Simeonsson & McHale, 1981).

Other potential resources affecting reaction to a handicapped sibling may be psychological attributes as indicated by preliminary studies (Ferrari, 1984; Gath & Gumley, 1987; Grossman, 1972). Future study should explore psychological mediators of adjustment. Research must also clarify the potential of type of handicap in affecting a sibling's adjustment.

Most important, the findings suggest that programs and intervention should focus on these children currently experiencing adjustment difficulty, perhaps due to the presence of a handicapped brother or sister. Intervention should consider the personal and family characteristics that may affect the adjustment of the siblings. Equal attention is urged for children with no handicapped siblings but nonetheless with social and emotional difficulties.

REFERENCES

Achenbach, T. M. (1981). *Child Behavior Checklist.* Burlington: University of Vermont.

Achenbach, T. M., & Edelbrock, C. (1983). *Manual for the Child Behavior Checklist and Revised Child Behavior Profile.* Burlington: University of Vermont.

Breslau, N. (1982). Siblings of disabled children: Birth order and age-spacing effects. *Journal of Abnormal Child Psychology, 10,* 85-96.

Breslau, N., Weitzman, M., & Messenger, K. (1981). Psychologic functioning of siblings of disable children. *Pediatrics, 67,* 344-353.

Caldwell, B., & Guze, S. E. (1960). A study of the adjustment of parents and siblings of institutionalized and noninstitutionalized retarded children. *American Journal of Mental Deficiency, 64,* 845-861.

Cleveland, D. S., & Miller, N. B. (1977). Attitudes and life commitments of older siblings of mentally retarded adults: An exploratory study. *Mental Retardation, 15,* 38-41.

Dyson, L., & Fewell, R. R. (in press). A comparison of the self-concept of siblings of handicapped children and sinblings of nonhandicapped children. *Journal of the Division for Early Childhood.*

Farber, B. (1959). Effects of a severely retarded child on family integration. *Monographs of the Society for Research in Child Development, 24*(2, Serial No. 71).
Featherstone, H. (1980). *A difference in the family: Life with a disabled child.* New York: Basic Books.
Ferrari, M. (1984). Chronic illness: Psychosocial effects on siblings—I. Chronically ill boys. *Journal of Child Psychology and Psychiatry, 25,* 459-476.
Ferrari, M. (1987). The diabetic child and well sibling: Risks to the well child's self-concept. *Children's Health Care, 15*(3), 141-147.
Fewell, R. R. (1986). A handicapped child in the family. In R. R. Fewell & P. F. Vadasy (Eds.), *Families of handicapped children: Needs and supports across the life span* (pp. 3-34). Austin: Pro-Ed.
Fowle, C. M. (1969). The effects of the severely mentally retarded child on his family. *American Journal of Mental Deficiency, 73,* 468-473.
Freeman, B. J. (1985). Review of Child Behavior Checklist. In J. V. Mitchell, Jr. (Ed.), *The ninth mental measurements yearbook* (pp. 300-301). Lincoln: The Buros Institute of Mental Measurements, University of Nebraska.
Gath, A. (1972). The mental health of siblings of congenitally abnormal children. *Journal of Child Psychology and Psychiatry, 13,* 211-218.
Gath, A. (1973). The school-aged siblings of mongol children. *British Journal of Psychiatry, 123,* 161-167.
Gath, A. (1974). Sibling reactions to mental handicap: A comparison of the brothers and sisters of Mongol children. *Journal of Child Psychology and Psychiatry, 15,* 187-198.
Gath, A., & Gumley, D. (1987). Retarded children and their siblings. *Journal of Child Psychology and Psychiatry, 28,* 715-730.
Gayton, W. F., Friedman, S. B., Tavormina, J. F., & Tucker, P. (1977). Children with cystic fibrosis: I. Psychological test finding of patients, siblings and parents. *Pediatrics, 59,* 888-894.
Graliker, B. V., Fishler, K., & Koch, R. (1962). Teenage reaction to a mentally retarded sibling. *American Journal of Mental Deficiency, 66,* 838-843.
Grossman, F. K. (1972). *Brothers and sisters of retarded children: An exploratory study.* Syracuse, NY: Syracuse University Press.
Harvey, D. H., & Greenway, A. P. (1984). The self-concept of physically handicapped children and their nonhandicapped siblings: An empirical investigation. *Journal of Child Psychology and Psychiatry, 25,* 273-284.
Hollingshead, A. B. (1975). *Four factor index of social status.* Unpublished manuscript, Yale University.
Kaplan, F. (1969). Siblings of the retarded. In S. B. Sarason & J. Doris (Eds.), *Psychological problems in mental deficiency* (4th ed., pp. 186-208). New York: Harper & Row.
Kazak, A. E., & Clark, M. W. (1986). Stress in families of children with myelomeningocele. *Developmental Medicine & Child Neurology, 28,* 220-228.
Kelley, M. L. (1985). Review of Child Behavior Checklist. In J. V. Mitchell Jr. (Ed.), *The ninth mental measurements yearbook* (pp. 301-303). Lincoln, NE: The Buros Institute of Mental Measurements, University of Nebraska.
Kowalski, J. L. (1980). The attitudes and self-concept of adolescent siblings of handicapped children. *Dissertation Abstracts International, 41,* 03A, 1020.
Lavigne, J., & Ryan, M. (1979). Psychologic adjustment of siblings of children with chronic illness. *Pediatrics, 63,* 616-626.
Lobato, D., Barbour, L., Hall, L. J., & Miller, C. T. (1987). Psychosocial characteristics of preschool siblings of handicapped and nonhandicapped children. *Journal of Abnormal Child Psychology, 15,* 329-338.
McAndrew, I. (1976). Children with a handicap and their families. *Child Care, Health and Development, 2,* 213-327.
McKeever, P. (1983). Siblings of chronically ill children: A literature review with implications for research and practice. *American Journal of Orthopsychiatry, 53,* 209-218.
Piers, E. V., & Harris, D. B. (1969). *The Piers-Harris Children's Self-concept Scale (The way I feel about myself).* Nashville: Counselor Recordings and Tests.

San Martino, M., & Newman, M. B. (1974). Siblings of the retarded: A population at risk. *Child Psychiatry and Human Development, 4,* 168-177.
Schwirian, P. M., (1976). Effects of the presence of a hearing impaired preschool child in the family on behavior patterns of older "normal" siblings. *American Annals of the Deaf, 121,* 373-380.
Siemon, M. (1984). Siblings of the chronically ill or disabled child: Meeting their needs. *Nursing Clinics of North America, 19*(2), 295-307.
Simeonsson, R. J., & McHale, S. M. (1981). Reviews: Research on handicapped children: Sibling relationships. *Child Care, Health, and Development, 7,* 153-171.
Suelzle, M., & Keenan, V. (1981). Changes in family support networks over the life cycle of mentally retarded persons. *American Journal of Mental Deficiency, 86,* 267-274.
Sutton-Smith, B., & Rosenberg, B. C. (1970). *The sibling.* New York: Holt, Rinehart & Winston.
Tew, B., & Laurence, K. M. (1973). Mothers, brothers, and sisters of patients with spina bifida. *Developmental Medicine and Child Neurology, 15*(Suppl. 6), 69-76.

11

The Role of Maternal Employment and Depression in the Psychological Adjustment of Chronically Ill, Mentally Retarded, and Well Children[1]

Lynn S. Walker
Vanderbilt University School of Medicine

Juan Antonio Ortiz-Valdes and J. R. Newbrough
George Peabody College of Vanderbilt University

Used path analysis to test a conceptual model of the relationship among maternal employment status, maternal depression, and reported child behavior problems. Ss were 95 mothers of children in 4 conditions: cystic fibrosis, diabetes, mental retardation, and well. Regardless of child chronic condition or family SES, mothers not employed outside the home had higher levels of depression than employed mothers. Maternal depression, in turn, was associated with higher levels of reported child behavior problems. Controlling for SES and maternal depression, mental retardation was associated with more child behavior problems, but chronic illness (cystic fibrosis and diabetes) was not associated with more behavior problems. The findings underscore the need to examine the adjustment of children with chronic disorders

[1]This research was supported by grants from NICHD (HD 6351) and from NIDDK (AM 20593). The authors gratefully acknowledge the cooperation of the Metropolitan Nashville Public Schools, the Cystic Fibrosis Foundation, and the Diabetes Research and Training Center and Cystic Fibrosis Clinic of Vanderbilt University Medical Center. Thanks to Naomi Breslau for comments on a draft of the manuscript, and to Michael Swafford for consultation regarding data analysis. Ortiz-Valdes is now at the Department of Psychology, Instituto Tecnico y Estudios Superiores, Guadalajara, Mexico.

in the context of their mothers' well-being, particularly when mothers are the principal informants regarding child adjustment.

Early studies of children with chronic illness or handicap suggested that these disorders were generally associated with psychological disturbance. More recent investigations indicate that maladjustment is less prevalent than originally thought and by no means inevitable for children with chronic disorders (for reviews, see Drotar & Bush, 1985; Johnson, 1985). As a result, the current challenge for research in this area is to identify factors that intervene in the relationship between chronic disorder and child psychological adjustment.

The role of the family is frequently the focus of investigations seeking to understand the development of child psychopathology (e.g., Garmezy & Tellegen, 1984; Holahan & Moos, 1987). Maternal depression, for example, has been linked to child behavior problems (Billings & Moos, 1983; Pound, Cox, Puckering, & Mills, 1985). Several explanations have been offered for this finding. For example, there is evidence that depressed mothers have parenting styles that may contribute to child adjustment difficulties (Forehand, Lautenschlager, Faust, & Graziano, 1986; Kochanska, Kuczynski, Radke-Yarrow, & Welsh, 1987). Also, it appears that depression affects mothers' perceptions or tolerance of their children's behavior such that they are more likely to label their children as disordered and refer them for treatment (Breslau, Davis, & Prabuki, 1988; Brody & Forehand, 1986; Griest, Forehand, Wells, & McMahon, 1980). These findings are of particular relevance in the study of families of children with chronic disorders because a high rate of maternal depression is reported in these families (Breslau, Staruch, & Mortimer, 1982). Thus, it is possible that maternal depression is a significant factor contributing to the reported incidence of behavior problems in children with chronic disorders.

The relatively high incidence of depression in mothers of children with chronic disorders is not surprising, given the special demands they face. In a recent analysis of women's family roles, Baruch, Biener, and Barnett (1987) argued that women are particularly vulnerable to stress because their family roles often combine a high level of psychological demands with a low level of control. Certainly this describes the situation of mothers who are responsible for the well-being of children with disorders that have unpredictable and often uncontrollable effects on the child.

Baruch et al. (1987) proposed that for some women, the balance of psychological demands and control is more favorable in the workplace than at home. In this case, employment may serve as a buffer against stress arising in family roles. Several studies indicate higher levels of emotional and physical well-being among women who occupy the three roles of wife, mother, and employee compared with women who occupy fewer roles (Pietromonaco, Manis, & Frohardt-Lane, 1986; Stewart & Salt, 1981; Thoits, 1983; Verbrugge, 1982). For women with multiple roles, frustration in any single role may be offset by the rewards of other roles that provide alternate sources of stimulation, self-esteem, and social status. In the case of mothers of children with chronic conditions, employment may provide both temporary relief from caretaking concerns and the opportunity for self-expression and achievement in another realm. The resulting benefits to the mother's mental health would indirectly benefit the child.

In this study we examined the effects of employment status and child chronic disorder on depression in mothers of children in several diagnostic groups. In addition to mothers of well children who served as a comparison group, we selected mothers of children in three chronic conditions characterized by different features (cf. Rolland, 1984): (a) cystic fibrosis, which is a life-threatening chronic illness, (b) juvenile diabetes, which is not usually fatal during childhood, and (c) mental retardation without physical handicap or illness. We hypothesized that the presence of a child with any of these disorders would be associated with higher maternal depression than in families of well children (see Fig 1). Further, cystic fibrosis was expected to have the strongest link to maternal depression because of the potentially greater sense of powerlessness associated with this life-threatening illness in comparison to the other disorders. Regardless of the child's diagnostic condi-

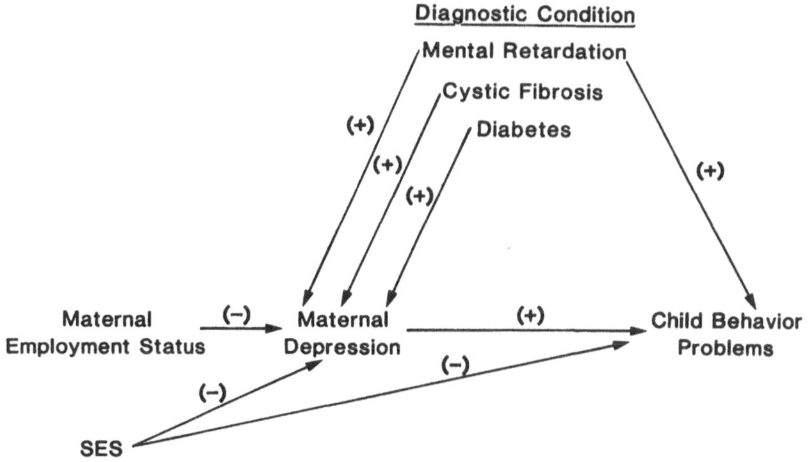

Fig. 1. Conceptual model showing direction of expected relationships.

tion, maternal employment outside the home was predicted to be associated with lower maternal depression.

Maternal depression, in turn, was expected to have a direct effect on reported child behavior problems, with depressed mothers reporting more behavior problems. We also considered the effect of type of child disorder on behavior problems. There is evidence that the psychosocial impact on the child may be similar for many chronic disorders (Wallander, Varni, Babani, Banis, & Wilcox, 1988). However, when intellectual impairment is associated with chronic disorder, it represents a special risk factor for increased psychopathology (Breslau, 1985; Breslau & Marshall, 1985; Rutter, Graham, & Yule, 1970). Thus, we considered the effects of mental retardation and the two chronic illnesses separately, and predicted that only mental retardation would have a direct effect on child behavior problems.

The model was tested using path analysis. We controlled for socioeconomic status (SES) because lower social class has been linked to depression (Hollingshead & Redlich, 1958) and to higher rates of diagnosed child psychopathology and parent-reported child behavior problems (Achenbach & Edelbrock, 1983).

METHOD

Sample

Subjects were 95 mothers of children in four diagnostic groups: diabetes, cystic fibrosis, mental retardation, and well. For each of the four diagnostic groups, mothers of children in three age groups were recruited: middle childhood (8–10 years of age), early adolescence (11–14 years of age), and late adolescence (15–19 years of age). There were 8 subjects in each age group for each condition, with the exception of the oldest age group in the cystic fibrosis condition which was missing a subject (this was due to the high mortality rate for cystic fibrosis and thus lower availability of mothers of older adolescents with cystic fibrosis). Subjects were recruited in order to obtain 4 mothers of boys and 4 mothers of girls within each age group for each diagnostic condition. This was achieved except in the case of the older age groups for cystic fibrosis which had more boys than girls (among early adolescents, 6 boys and 2 girls; among late adolescents, 5 boys and 2 girls). Children with intellectual deficits, evidenced by placement in a special class, were excluded from the diabetes, cystic fibrosis, and well groups in order not to confound physical and mental disorder.

All target children were living at home with their families and attending public schools. The mean number of children in the family was 3.33,

2.12, 2.43, and 3.29 for the mental retardation, diabetes, cystic fibrosis, and well groups, respectively. The percentage of single-parent mothers was 29% each for the mental retardation and diabetes groups, 13% for the cystic fibrosis group, and 12% for the well group. Additional characteristics and sources of subjects for each group are described below.

Diabetes. Mothers of 24 children with diabetes were recruited from the Diabetes Research and Training Center of a university medical center and from the private practices of local physicians. All children were insulin-dependent and had been diagnosed with diabetes for at least a year. Mothers of children currently hospitalized were excluded.

Cystic Fibrosis. Mothers of 23 children with cystic fibrosis were recruited from the Cystic Fibrosis Clinic of the same university medical center, private practices of physicians in the region, and the local Cystic Fibrosis Foundation. Mothers of children who were currently hospitalized or in the terminal phase of the disease were excluded. All children had received the diagnosis of cystic fibrosis within the first 2 years of life.

Mental Retardation. This group of 24 children was recruited through special education classes in local schools. Only classrooms for children classified in the moderate range of mental retardation were used.

Well. Mothers of 24 children with no known mental or physical disorder were recruited from the records of general pediatrics clinics of the same university medical center. Mothers were eligible for the study if their children had recently been seen at the clinic for a routine examination or acute minor illness, provided the child had no current physical complaint, chronic disorder, or intellectual impairment (defined by placement in a special education class for all or part of the school day). Families in which any member had a serious illness or disability were excluded from this group.

Procedure

All instruments were verbally administered in a personal interview with the mother. The majority of interviews were conducted in the mothers' homes. Some interviews were conducted in other locations (e.g., the clinic, mother's workplace) according to the mothers' preferences and convenience.

Measures

Maternal Depression. The Center for Epidemiological Studies Depression (CES-D) Scale (Radloff, 1977) was used to measure maternal depression. This 20-item scale was originally developed to measure depressive symptomatology in the general population. Item responses are scored from 0 to 3 on a scale of frequency of occurrence of the symptom within the past week. Higher scores are associated with increased symptomatology. The instrument has high internal consistency (.85 in the general population) and moderate test–retest reliability (ranging from .32 to .67 depending on the time interval between test administrations and whether life event stressors occurred during the intervening time period). Validity has been established by correlation with clinical ratings of depression (Radloff, 1977). The usual cutoff score for "significant symptomatology" is 16.

Child Adjustment. The Child Behavior Checklist (CBCL; Achenbach & Edelbrock, 1983) provides a standardized description of children's problem behaviors as reported by their parents. It consists of 118 behavior problem items each scored on a 3-point scale. The social competence scale was not used in this study. For the purposes of data analysis, each child's raw scores for Total Behavior Problems were converted to *T* scores according to the appropriate age and sex group norms for the Revised Child Behavior Checklist Profile.[3]

Maternal Employment Status. Gainful employment outside the home was treated as a dichotomous variable. Mothers who reported full- or part-time employment were considered employed.

Family Socioeconomic Status. Family SES, as measured by the Hollingshead Four-Factor Index of Social Status (Hollingshead, 1975), was used as a control variable. Scores on the measure range from 8 (lowest SES) to 66 (highest SES).

RESULTS

The four diagnostic groups were first compared with respect to family SES and proportion of employed mothers. Results of an analysis of variance revealed no significant difference in family SES among the groups, $F(3, 90) = 0.18$, ns. The majority of families in each group were in the middle class. Chi-square analysis indicated no significant difference in the proportion of employed mothers across the four groups, χ^2 (3) = 4.44, ns. One half to two thirds of the mothers in each group were employed.

Bivariate relationships between predictor variables and dependent variables were examined prior to testing the conceptual model. Table I pre-

[3]The Total Behavior Problems score was used because it includes behavior items that have low factor loadings on the CBCL Internalizing and Externalizing scales and are not included in those subscales (cf. Achenbach & Edelbrock, 1983). These behavior items tend to be rare in the normal population but were frequently endorsed by mothers of mentally retarded children in the present study. Thus, the Total Behavior Problems score gives the most complete picture of the target children in the study.

Table I. Means and Standard Deviations for Child Behavior Problems and Maternal Depression for the Diagnostic Groups and for Employed Versus Nonemployed Mothers

		Child behavior problems		Maternal depression	
	n	*M*	*SD*	*M*	*SD*
Diagnostic group					
Mental retardation	24	63.63	8.59	9.67	9.75
Diabetes	24	56.63	9.45	8.29	7.60
Cystic Fibrosis	23	55.48	8.18	11.26	10.38
Well	24	58.58	10.23	10.12	10.08
Maternal employment status					
Employed	62	56.85	9.48	7.64	7.33
Not employed	33	61.91	8.88	13.91	11.47

sents the means and standard deviations for CBCL Total Behavior Problems t scores and for maternal depression on the CES-D for the four diagnostic groups and for employed versus nonemployed mothers. One-way analysis of variance indicated a significant effect for child condition on behavior problems, $F(3, 91) = 3.67$, $p < .01$. Mothers of mentally retarded children reported significantly more behavior problems than mothers of children with cystic fibrosis or diabetes. Contrary to expectations, the level of self-reported depression was not significantly higher for mothers of children in the chronic condition groups than for mothers of well children, $F(3, 91) = 0.39$, ns. The relationship of maternal employment status to child behavior problems and to maternal depression was examined with t tests. Employed mothers, in comparison to nonemployed mothers, reported significantly lower levels of both child behavior problems, $t(93) = 2.53$, $p < .01$, and depression, $t(93) = 3.24$, $p < .01$.

The data were also examined for possible effects of child sex and age group on the dependent variables. *T* tests indicated no significant difference between mothers of girls versus boys with respect to child behavior problems, $t(93) = 1.15$, ns, and maternal depression, $t(93) = 1.27$, ns. Analysis of variance yielded no significant difference among the child age groups for behavior problems, $F(2, 92) = 0.64$, ns, and maternal depression, $F(2, 92) = 1.08$, ns. Thus, child sex and age group were excluded from further analyses.

Path analysis was used to test the conceptual model (for a discussion of path analysis, see Pedhazur, 1982). First, the relationship between the hypothesized predictor variables and maternal depression was examined. Child diagnostic condition was dummy coded (i.e., subjects were assigned a dichotomous code for the presence or absence of each of the three chronic conditions). Maternal employment status was represented as a dichotomous variable. Child diagnostic condition, maternal employment status, and family SES were entered simultaneously into a regression equation predicting maternal depression. The resulting equation was significant, $F(5, 88) = 3.67$, $p < .01$ $R^2 = .17$. Examination of regression coefficients indicated that both SES and maternal employment status were significant predictors of maternal depression (see Figure 2). Controlling for the child's diagnostic condition, higher SES and maternal employment outside the home were associated with less depression ($p < .01$ and .05, respectively). Controlling for the effects of SES and maternal employment, there was no significant association between child condition and maternal depression. Interaction terms were constructed representing the interaction of maternal employment and child condition. These were entered into the regression equation but did not yield significant regression coefficients and failed to explain additional variance in maternal depression, indicating that the effect of maternal employment on depression did not vary across child conditions.

Next, maternal depression, child diagnostic condition, and family SES were entered simultaneously into a regression equation predicting child behavior problems. The resulting equation was significant, $F(5, 88) = 7.52$, $p < .0001$, $R^2 = .30$. Significant regression coefficients were obtained for maternal depression ($p < .001$), family SES ($p < .05$). and for the mental retardation condition ($p < .05$). Controlling for other variables in the equation, maternal depression was associated with the judgment of more child behavior problems. Lower social class and child mental retardation were also associated with more reported behavior problems.

Our conceptual model did not include a path from maternal employment status to child behavior problems. In order to test our assumption that maternal employment does not directly influence reported child behavior problems, we added maternal employment status to the equation predicting child behavior problems. Controlling for the other predictor variables already in the equation, maternal employment did not have a significant regression coefficient and did not explain additional variance. This finding supports the conceptual model, suggesting that maternal employment status does not have a direct effect on child behavior problems but rather exercises an effect indirectly, through maternal depression.

DISCUSSION

Results of this study indicate that maternal depression may play an important role in the adjustment of children with chronic disorders. Mothers who were more depressed reported more behavior problems in their children. Although this is not evidence of a causal relationship, the association

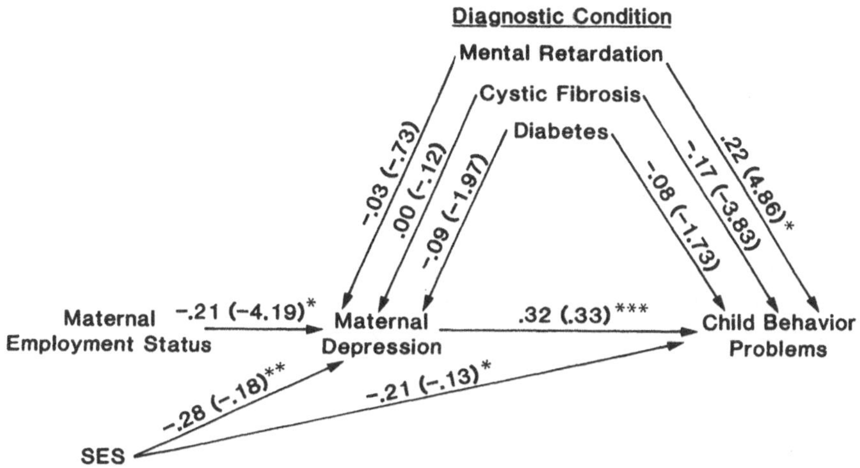

Fig. 2. Results of path analysis showing standardized (unstandardized) regression coefficients. $N = 95$. $^{*}p < .05$; $^{**}p < .01$; $^{***}p < .001$. By using dummy coding in multiple regression, one obtains coefficients that give the effect on the dependent variable of having a child in a given group (e.g., mental retardation, cystic fibrosis, or diabetes) as opposed to having a child in the control group of well children, holding other variables in the equation constant (i.e., SES, maternal employment status). So, for example, the unstandardized regression coefficient of .73 represents the effect of child mental retardation on maternal depression and can be interpreted as follows: controlling on maternal employment and SES, having a child with mental retardation *rather than a child in the control group* lowers the maternal depression score by 0.73 points. Since maternal depression scores on the CES-D may range from 0 to 60, this is neither statistically nor substantively significant. In the case of dummy variables such as diagnostic condition in the example just cited, unstandardized regression coefficients are easier to interpret than standardized coefficients. As an example of the interpretation of standardized regression coefficients, consider the coefficient of .32 leading from maternal depression to child behavior problems. As maternal depression goes up 1 standard deviation, the child behavior problem score goes up by approximately ⅓ standard deviation, controlling on SES and child diagnostic condition.

between maternal depression and reported child behavior problems is noteworthy for two reasons. First, much of the literature on the adjustment of children with chronic disorders is based on maternal reports. If these investigations had controlled for maternal depression, it is likely that they would have yielded lower rates of child maladjustment. Thus, to the extent that current assumptions are based on reports of mothers whose perceptions may have been distorted by depression, they probably overestimate the risk of psychopathology in children with chronic disorders.

Second, the link between maternal depression and reported child behavior problems has clinical implications. Parent perceptions of the child are the determining factor in clinic referral (Lobitz & Johnson, 1975; Rickard, Forehand, Wells, Griest, & McMahon, 1981). Consequently, maternal depression may be an important variable in the clinic referral process for children with chronic disorders. This underscores the need to include an evaluation of parent adjustment when assessing clinic-referred children. In some cases, treatment may need to focus on the parent in addition to the child.

There is evidence elsewhere in the literature suggesting that maternal report bias is not the only factor responsible for a link between maternal depression and CBCL scores. Others have demonstrated that maternal depression does not diminish the validity of the Child Behavior Checklist (Friedlander, Weiss, & Traylor, 1986). Furthermore, studies using both mothers' and independent observers' judgments of child behavior show that mothers' reports are influenced not only by their own mood but also by actual child behavior (Brody & Forehand, 1986; Griest et al., 1980; Schaughency & Lahey, 1985). Thus, while acknowledging the potential role of bias in depressed mothers' reports of child behavior, one might speculate about causal mechanisms that also operate; for example, child deviance may contribute to maternal depression, or maternal depression may be associated with parenting behavior that contributes to child adjustment difficulties. Alternatively, both maternal depression and child behavior problems may arise as a consequence of other factors, such as family disruption.

Whatever the causes of depression in mothers of children with chronic disorders, in this study depression was less for mothers employed outside the home. This may be because employment provides respite from the demands of caretaking, access to another social support network, or an alternative arena for accomplishment. Numerous factors contribute to the impact of employment on a mothers' mental health, for example, the type of work, her desire to work, the extent to which she is supported by her husband, and so on (Kessler & McCrae, 1982; Walker & Wallston, 1985). These should be considered in further explorations of the impact of employment on mothers of children with chronic disorders. In addition, there may be circumstances unique to families of children with chronic disorders that moderate the impact of employment on mothers' well-being. It is possible, for example, that under conditions of acute child illness or hospitalization, employed mothers would experience greater role overload and consequently more distress than mothers who are not employed.

The study results suggest that maternal employment has an indirect effect, through maternal depression, on reported child behavior problems. Related findings were reported by Ghodsian, Zajicek, and Wolkind (1984) in a study of mothers of young children. They found evidence that a mother's employment mitigates the relationship between her depression and child behavior problems. Future research might seek to identify additional family variables, such as marital distress, that have direct or indirect effects on the adjustment of children with chronic disorders.

As expected, we found that mental retardation was associated with significantly higher levels of reported behavior problems, even after controlling for SES and maternal depression. Our samples were such that we could separate the effects of mental retardation and chronic physical disorders on child behavior problems. In research using samples of children where physical and intellectual impairment sometimes coexist (e.g., cerebral palsy), the level of retardation should be assessed, as this study and others (Breslau, 1985; Rutter et al., 1970) suggest that cognitive deficits may be the key variable linking chronic disorder and behavior problems.

In contrast to the findings for mental retardation, chronic physical illness was not associated with more child behavior problems. Controlling for SES and maternal depression, neither mothers of children with diabetes nor mothers of children with cystic fibrosis reported more child behavior problems than mothers of well children who had attended the medical center pediatric clinics. Caution must be used in interpreting this finding due to the relatively high CBCL behavior problem scores in the well group (see Table I) in comparison to the CBCL normative sample (cf. Achenbach & Edelbrock, 1983). It is possible that the well group in this study does not reflect a normal population. However, recent studies using the CBCL with community samples have also found higher rates of behavior problems than for the CBCL normative sample (Costello et al., 1988). Thus, the well group in this study may reflect a current trend of increased maternal reports of child behavior problems.

The present findings parallel those of recent empirical investigations (Cowen et al., 1986; Lewis & Khaw, 1982; Walker, Ford, & Donald, 1987) that failed to find the magnitude of dysfunction reported in earlier observations of families with chronically ill children. Differences in the circumstances of data collection may account in part for inconsistencies in the literature. In studies of chronically ill children, research interviews are commonly conducted in hospital clinics when the child is present for medical evaluation. Even if the child is not acutely ill at the time, it is likely that the prospect of an interview and assistance from health care professionals serves to focus the mother's attention on troubling child behaviors that are not ordinarily salient. If the child has recently been ill and restricted from normal activities, behavior problems may be temporarily increased. In addition, concern about the outcome of the medical visit and the inconvenience occasioned by travel to medical centers that are often far from home may heighten the mother's personal distress and result in a research protocol that does not reflect the typical level of well-being for mother or child. Results of the present study, which was conducted in the families' homes during a stable phase of the disorder, may more accurately describe the day-to-day adjustment of these mothers and children.

In summary, results of the study showed a significant relationship between employment status and depression in mothers of children with chronic disorders. Controlling for SES and the type of child condition, lack of employment outside the home was associated with higher maternal depression. Maternal depression, in turn, was associated with significantly higher levels of reported child behavior problems. Regarding the relationship between child chronic disorder and behavior problems, mental retardation was associated with more behavior problems, but chronic illness (diabetes and cystic fibrosis) was not associated with more behavior problems than reported by mothers of well children of similar SES who had attended the pediatric clinic. Taken together, these findings underscore the need to examine the adjustment of children with chronic disorders in the context of their mothers' well-being, particularly when mothers are the principal informants regarding child adjustment.

REFERENCES

Achenbach, T. M., & Edelbrock, C. (1983). *Manual for the Child Behavior Checklist and Revised Child Behavior Profile.* Burlington: University of Vermont.

Baruch, G. K., Biener, L., & Barnett, R. C. (1987). Women and gender in research on work and family stress. *American Psychologist, 42,* 130-136.

Billings, A. G., & Moos, R. H. (1983). Comparisons of children of depressed and nondepressed parents: A social-environmental perspective. *Journal of Abnormal Child Psychology, 11,* 463-486.

Breslau, N. (1985). Psychiatric disorder in children with physical disabilities. *Journal of the American Academy of Child Psychiatry, 24,* 87-94.

Breslau, N., Davis, G. C., & Prabucki, K. (1988). Depressed mothers as informants in family history research—are they accurate? *Psychiatry Research, 24,* 345-359.

Breslau, N., & Marshall, I. A. (1985). Psychological disturbance in children with physical disabilities: Continuity and change in a 5-year follow-up. *Journal of Abnormal Child Psychology, 13,* 199-216.

Breslau, N., Staruch, K. S., & Mortimer, E. A. (1982). Psychological distress in mothers of disabled children. *American Journal of Diseases of Children, 136,* 682-686.

Brody, G. H., & Forehand, R. (1986). Maternal perceptions of child maladjustment as a function of the combined influence of child behavior and maternal depression. *Journal of Consulting and Clinical Psychology, 54,* 237-240.

Costello, E. J., Edelbrock, C., Costello, A. J., Dulcan, M. K., Burns, B. J., & Brent, D. (1988). Psychopathology in pediatric primary care: The new hidden morbidity. *Pediatrics, 82,* 415-424.

Cowen, L., Mok, J., Corey, M., MacMillan, H., Simmons, R., & Levison, H. (1986). Psychologic adjustment of the family with a member who has cystic fibrosis. *Pediatrics, 77,* 745-753.

Drotar, D., & Bush, M. (1985). Mental health issues and services. In N. Hobbs & J. M. Perrin (Eds.), *Issues in the care of children with chronic illness* (pp. 514-550). San Francisco: Jossey-Bass.

Forehand, R., Lautenschlager, G. J., Faust, J., & Graziano, W. G. (1986). Parent perceptions and parent-child interactions in clinic-referred children: A preliminary investigation of the effects of maternal depressive moods. *Behavior Research and Therapy, 24,* 73-75.

Friedlander, S. Weiss, D. S., & Traylor, J. (1986). Assessing the influence of maternal depression on the validity of the Child Behavior Checklist. *Journal of Abnormal Child Psychology, 14,* 123-133.

Garmezy, N., & Tellegen, A. (1984). Studies of stress-resistant children. In F. Morrison, C. Lord, & D. Keating (Eds.), *Advances in applied developmental psychology* (Vol. 1, pp. 231-287). New York: Academic Press.

Ghodsian, M., Zajicek, E., & Wolkind, S. (1984). A longitudinal study of maternal depression and child behavioral problems. *Journal of Child Psychology and Psychiatry, 91,* 91-109.

Griest, D. L., Forehand, R., Wells, K., & McMahon, R. (1980). An examination of differences between nonclinic and behavior problem clinic-referred children and their mothers. *Journal of Abnormal Psychology, 89,* 497-500.

Holahan, C. J., & Moos, R. H. (1987). Risk, resistance, and psychological distress: A longitudinal analysis with adults and children. *Journal of Abnormal Psychology, 96,* 3-13.

Hollingshead, A. B. (1975). *Four-factor index of social status.* Working paper, Department of Sociology, Yale University.

Hollingshead, A. B., & Redlich, F. C. (1958). *Social class and mental illness: A community study.* New York: Wiley.

Johnson, S. B. (1985). The family and the child with chronic illness. In D. C. Turk & R. D. Kerns (Eds.), *Health, illness, and families* (pp. 220-254). New York: Wiley.

Kessler, R. C., & McRae J. A. (1982). The effect of wives' employment on the mental health of married men and women. *American Sociological Review, 47,* 210-227.

Kochanska, G., Kuczynski, L., Radke-Yarrow, M., & Welsh, J. D. (1987). Resolution of control episodes between well and affectively ill mothers and their children. *Journal of Abnormal Child Psychology, 15,* 441-456.

Lewis, B. L., & Khaw, K. T. (1982). Family functioning as a mediating variable affecting psychosocial adjustment of children with cystic fibrosis. *Behavioral Pediatrics, 101,* 636-640.

Lobitz, G. K., & Johnson, S. M. (1975). Normal versus deviant children: A multi-method comparison. *Journal of Abnormal Child Psychology, 3,* 353-374.

Pedhazur, E. J. (1982). *Multiple regression in behavioral research,* New York: Holt, Rinehart and Winston.

Pietromonaco, P. R., Manis, J., & Frohardt-Lane, K. (1986). Psychological consequences of multiple social roles. *Psychology of Women Quarterly, 10,* 373-382.

Pound, A., Cox, A., Puckering, C., & Mills, M. (1985). The impact of maternal depression on young children. In J. E. Stevenson (Ed.), *Recent research in developmental psychopathology* (pp. 3-10). New York: Oxford.

Radloff, L. S. (1977). The CES-D scale: A self report depression scale for research in the general population. *Applied Psychological Measurement, 1,* 385-401.

Rickard, K. M., Forehand, R., Wells, K. C., Griest, D. L., & McMahon, R. J. (1981). Factors in the referral of children for behavioral treatment: A comparison of mothers of clinic-referred deviant, clinic-referred nondeviant, and clinic children. *Behavior Research and Therapy, 19,* 201-205.

Rolland, J. S. (1984). Toward a psychosocial typology of chronic and life-threatening illness. *Family Systems Medicine, 2,* 245-262.

Rutter, M., Graham, P., & Yule, W. (1970). *A neuropsychiatric study in childhood.* London: Lavenham Press.

Schaughency, E. A., & Lahey, B. B. (1985). Mothers' and fathers' perception of child deviance: Roles of child behavior, parental depression, and marital satisfaction. *Journal of Consulting and Clinical Psychology, 53,* 718-723.

Steward, A. S., & Salt, P. (1981). Life stress, lifestyles, depression, and illness in adult women. *Journal of Personality and Social Psychology, 40,* 1063-1069.

Thoits, P. A. (1983). Multiple identities and psychological well-being: A reformulation and test of the isolation hypothesis. *American Sociological Review, 48,* 174-187.

Verbrugge, L. M. (1982). Women's social roles and health. In P. Berman & E. Ramey (Eds.), *Women: A developmental perspective* (Publication No. 82-2298, pp. 49-78). Bethesda, MD: National Institutes of Health.

Walker, L. S., Ford, M. B., & Donald, W. (1987). Cystic fibrosis and family stress: Effects of age and severity of illness. *Pediatrics, 79,* 239-246.

Walker, L. S., & Wallston, B. S. (1985). Social adaptation: A review of dual earner family literature. In L. L'Abate (Ed.), *Handbook of family psychology and family therapy* (pp. 698-740). Homewood, IL: Dow Jones-Irwin.

Wallander, J. L., Varni, J. W., Babani, L., Banis, H. T., & Wilcox, K. T. (1988). Children with chronic physical disorders: Maternal reports of their psychological adjustment. *Journal of Pediatric Psychology, 13,* 197-212.

III

INTERVENTION PROGRAMS AND ISSUES

12

Diabetes in Adolescence: Effects of Multifamily Group Intervention and Parent Simulation of Diabetes[1]

Wendy Satin, Annette M. La Greca, Marjorie A. Zigo, and Jay S. Skyler
University of Miami

Insulin-dependent diabetes mellitus (IDDM) is a complex, chronic disease that is difficult to control during adolescence. This study evaluated the effects of a 6-week, family-oriented, group intervention on adolescents' metabolic control and psychosocial and family functioning. Thirty-two families were randomly assigned to one of three groups: multifamily (MF), multifamily plus parent simulation of diabetes (MF+S), and control (C). Outcome measures included glycosylated hemoglobin (Hb A1); perceptions of diabetes; estimates of youngsters' self-care; and family functioning. Adolescents in the MF+S group displayed significant decrements in Hb A1, and adolescents in both intervention groups reported more positive perceptions of a "teen-ager with diabetes" at posttreatment, relative to controls. Adolescents participating in smaller family groups demonstrated clinically significant improvements in Hb A1 that were maintained at 6-month follow-up. Parent reports suggested that adolescents in the intervention groups improved their diabetes care. Findings support the use of multifamily groups plus parent simulation of diabetes as an intervention strategy for adolescents with IDDM.

Diabetes mellitus is a chronic metabolic disorder, the successful management of which places daily demands on the patient. These include daily insulin

[a]This research was supported in part by grant P01-HL-36588 from the National Institutes of Health, Public Health Service.

injections, adherence to a meal plan, balancing physical activity with food intake and insulin dosage, and monitoring of the metabolic state through frequent blood and/or urine testing (Skyler, 1986). Coping with diabetes is difficult at any age, but problems arise during adolescence that present additional challenges.

Adolescence is a period of marked change in physical, cognitive, and social/emotional development; these normal developmental processes further complicate diabetes management. Establishing a sense of autonomy and independence from the family, for example, is a developmental task that pervades the adolescent period and presents a special challenge for those with diabetes. It often is difficult for families to strike the right balance between showing an interest and allowing the adolescent the freedom to develop into an independent adult. Among adolescents with diabetes, it is common for parents to be involved in some aspects of diabetes management (Etzwiler & Sines, 1962), particularly the meal-related aspects of care (La Greca, 1982). However, parents often have difficulty relinquishing control when their youngster displays less than optimal levels of self-care. In many cases, the combination of diabetes and adolescence creates considerable tension and stress for the patient, parents, and the health care team (Skyler, 1980; Tattersall & Lowe, 1981). Thus, it is not surprising that acceptable levels of metabolic control often are very difficult to achieve for adolescents with this disease (Tattersall, 1987).

The importance of considering the adolescent with diabetes in the context of his or her family is further underscored by recent empirical findings. Research on psychosocial factors in diabetes clearly highlights the significant role of the family in the course and management of diabetes (see reviews by Anderson & Auslander, 1980, and Johnson, 1988). Youngsters with diabetes who come from conflictual or dysfunctional families typically display behavioral or psychosocial adjustment problems (Wertlieb, Hauser, & Jacobson, 1986), as well as difficulties with metabolic control (Anderson, Miller, Auslander, & Santiago, 1981; Minuchin, Rosman, & Baker, 1978). In contrast, positive family variables, such as support, cohesion, and organization, have been associated with youngsters' behavioral adjustment (Hauser, Jacobson, Wertlieb, Brink, & Wentworth, 1985; Wertlieb et al., 1986) and better metabolic status (Anderson et al., 1981). Although these studies were correlational, it is likely that a complex, bidirectional interplay exists between youngsters' family functioning and their diabetes care (La Greca, 1988).

In view of these findings, we reasoned that efforts to increase family support and positive family interactions around diabetes management might lead to improvements in metabolic status and overall psychosocial functioning for adolescents with diabetes. Moreover, since families are not alone in their problems in dealing with diabetes, we specifically examined the utility of multifamily group sessions for facilitating youngsters' adaptation to diabetes and metabolic control. Group interventions have been strongly advocated for the treatment of diabetes (Blum & Galatzer, 1982; Brink, 1982; Citrin, La Greca, & Skyler, 1985; Citrin, Zigo, La Greca, & Skyler, 1982; Marrero et al., 1982; Tattersall, McCulloch, & Aveline, 1985), yet, to date, no controlled evaluations of family groups have been reported. In fact, the virtual absence of outcome studies on family-oriented intervention programs for youngsters with diabetes has been noted (Johnson, 1988).

In addition to assessing the impact of a multifamily group intervention, we also examined the utility of teaching parents to appreciate the complexities of diabetes management by having them simulate diabetes for a 1-week period. We reasoned that parents might better understand the daily demands their youngsters encountered if they themselves had to face those demands, even for a limited time.

To test these views, we asked adolescents with diabetes and their parents to participate in a randomized study, to assess the impact of both multifamily group meetings and parent simulation of diabetes on youngsters' metabolic control as well as their psychosocial and family functioning. We hypothesized that the multifamily group interventions would produce significant improvements in youngsters' metablic status (Hb A1) relative to control adolescents, and that the groups with the additional parent simulation of diabetes would improve more than those receiving family intervention alone. We additionally hypothesized that, relative to controls, positive changes in youngsters' self-perceptions and parents' estimates of their youngsters' self-care would result from the interventions. Although no specific hypotheses were advanced concerning changes in general family functioning and attitudes toward diabetes as a result of the interventions, we monitored adolescents' and parents' perceptions in these areas as well.

METHOD

Subjects

Thirty-two adolescents (12 male and 20 female) with insulin-dependent diabetes mellitus (IDDM) and their parents participated in the study. The mean age (± *SD*) of the adolescents was 14.6 (± 2.6) years. Their mean duration of diabetes was 5.9 (±4.3) years. Families of adolescents with IDDM were recruited from those receiving medical care at the Diabetes/Metabolic Unit, University of Miami Hospitals and Clinics. Criteria for inclusion were families with an adolescent (age 12 to 19 years, inclusive) with IDDM, and willingness of the family to consent to participate in the protocol, including random allocation. We did not attempt to preselect families with particular characteristics, as diabetes management and control are difficult problems for most adolescents with IDDM and their families (Tattersall, 1987; Tattersall & Lowe, 1981).

Recruitment occurred over a 3-month period, and was accomplished by posting a notice in the Diabetes Unit regarding the availability of this research project. The families who participated were primarily from middle-income levels. Most of the adolescents (69%) came from intact, two-parent families, with the remaining youngsters (31%) residing in single-parent households. Although the characteristics of families who did not elect to participate in this project are unknown, it is likely that the selection procedures favored families who were receptive toward behavioral/psychosocial interventions and who were concerned about their youngsters' metabolic functioning. The three experimental groups did not differ on family demographics.

The adolescents who participated in the study represented a range of metabolic status, although the majority of youngsters (84%) displayed fair to poor control. In our laboratory, the range of Hb A1 values for nondiabetic adolescents is 6.0 to 8.5%; Hb A1 values for adolescents in this study ranged from 8.2 to 22.1%. Of the youngsters with IDDM, 16% were considered to have good metabolic control (Hb A1 < 9%); 39% had fair control (Hb A1 between 9 and 14%); and 45% had poor metabolic control (Hb A1 > 14%). These metabolic status levels were distributed equivalently across the three experimental groups.

Families were assigned to groups, as described below. Table I lists the gender, age, diabetes duration, and glycosylated hemoglobin (Hb A1) levels for adolescents assigned to each group. No significant group differences were observed for any of these variables.

Procedure

Group Assignment

All adolescents and their parents gave informed written consent prior to their voluntary participation in the study. Subsequently, families were randomly assigned to one of three groups. All adolescents and parents, regardless of group assignment, received identical psychosocial and family evaluations at the beginning of the study, and again after 6 weeks. In addition, metabolic control was assessed at baseline, and 3 and 6 months after study enrollment.

Families assigned to Group I, a multifamily (MF) group, met together for six weekly sessions of 90 minutes each, to discuss diabetes management

Table I. Subject Characteristics for Adolescent Subjects[a]

	Group I MF (n = 11)	Group II MF + S (n = 12)	Group III C (n = 9)
Gender	4M; 7F	3M; 9F	5M; 4F
Age (years)	15.0(2.4)	14.9(2.8)	13.7(2.7)
Duration of diabetes (years)	6.3(5.1)	5.2(3.8)	6.3(4.3)
Glycosylated hemoglobin	13.4%(1.3)	12.6%(0.9)	12.9%(1.4)

[a]MF = multifamily group; MF + S = multifamily plus parent simulation group; C = wait-list control group. Standard deviations are in parentheses.

and attitudes toward diabetes (described below) and to receive guidance and support from each other and from the group leaders (a psychologic social worker and a nurse practitioner). This group included 11 adolescents, 11 mothers, and 7 fathers.

Families in Group II, a multifamily plus parent simulation (MF + S) group, met together as those in Group I, with the addition that parents were asked to simulate diabetes management for 1 week, as detailed below. This group included 12 adolescents, 10 mothers, and 9 fathers.

For those families assigned to Group III, the control group (C), no specific intervention was provided. These families participated in all phases of assessment, and were offered intervention at the conclusion of the study. This group included 9 adolescents, 8 mothers, and 5 fathers.

In order to keep the multifamily groups at a manageable size (3 to 5 families per group), families were assigned to the experimental and control groups in three cycles. In the first cycle, 14 families were randomly assigned, 5 to Group I, 5 to Group II, and 4 to Group III. However, the resulting large group was felt to inhibit communication. Subsequent groups were limited to 3–4 families to facilitate communication in the group sessions. In the following two cycles, 9 families were randomized in each cycle, with groups of 3 to 4 families for each of the multifamily groups. Thus, the total number of families in each of the three groups was as follows: 11 in Group I, 12 in Group II, and 9 in Group III.

Content of Groups

The content and structure of the two multifamily interventions were identical, with the exception of the additional simulation exercise for the MF + S group. For both interventions, the first 2 weeks were devoted to establishing the group process, using principles of group therapy (Yalom, 1970). (These principles are described in detail, with specific reference to diabetes, in Citrin et al., 1985.) Group leaders stressed that diabetes was a family disease, encouraging family members to work together in diabetes management. Initial discussions focused on the families' feelings about diabetes, and how diabetes affected various family members. After this initial "grieving" about diabetes, the group discussions focused more on diabetes management, and specifically on what the family could do to improve treatment adherence. This theme continued throughout the 6-week intervention.

The two group leaders served primarily as discussion facilitators, and helped the families to process issues that arose regarding diabetes management and feelings about diabetes. The philosophy of the leaders was to promote independent problem solving among the families, rather than to offer specific advice on diabetes management. Given the high degree of patient involvement in diabetes care, the emphasis was on enhancing families' communication about diabetes, and their problem-solving skills, so that they could use these skills as new diabetes management problems arose. Families were encouraged to avoid a perfectionistic "all or nothing" approach to diabetes management, but rather to grow into better management, and to expect occasional lapses in adherence, in the context of a demanding and complex chronic disease.

Group sessions began with a discussion of "old business," or additional thoughts and reactions that group members had about the previous session. Next, the families were encouraged to share specific diabetes-related issues or management problems that arose during the week. This constituted the bulk of the session. The emphasis was on discussing each family member's feelings about the situation, as well as other group members' reactions to similar situations. Family members were encouraged to communicate with each other in an assertive and positive manner (see La Greca & Citrin, 1984, for specific examples of assertive diabetes-related communication). Following this discussion, family members focused on how the situation might be resolved. Suggestions and input were elicited from all group members. Families then role-played adaptive solutions to the problem. Typical issues that arose during these sessions were how to handle the different food preferences and dietary restrictions of various family members; how to encourage adolescents to monitor glucose more frequently; and how to handle siblings' reactions to the youngster with diabetes.

For those in the MF + S group, the parent simulation exercise was introduced during the third session. The adolescents "taught" their parents how to manage their "diabetes" by reviewing the necessary management tasks. Many of the parents seemed impressed with their adolescents' knowledge of diabetes management.

The parent simulation exercise consisted of (a) administration of twice daily measured injections of normal saline, using insulin syringes and according to a dosage scheme calculated as if the parent had IDDM, and altered on the basis of urine glucose determinations and "hypoglycemic" episodes; (b) four times daily measurement of urinary glucose and ketones, using simulated urine (vials of fluid containing variable amounts of glucose and acetone), recording the results in a diabetes-monitoring diary; (c) following a meal plan based on a three-day food record and using exchange lists for meal planning, including three meals and three snacks daily, and omitting concentrated sweets; (d) following an exercise prescription and recording exercise experiences; (e) recording of major and minor episodes of "hypoglycemia," a minor episode defined as a delayed meal or snack, or failure to consume extra food with extra activity, and a major episode defined as a missed meal or snack; and (f) submitting to a blood test for glycosylated hemoglobin. In addition, failure to take insulin was recorded as "ketoacidosis," and failure to comply with the meal plan was recorded as "uncontrolled diabetes." During the simulation exercise, the adolescents served as "coach"for their parents. This simulation exercise is similar to that used by Welborn and Duncan (1980) to sensitize the health care team to diabetes management issues.

During the subsequent group session, the leaders encouraged the families to discuss and process their reactions to the simulation exercise (e.g., "How did you think you were doing?" "What did you find hard?" "What could you have used help with?" "How does this affect the way you view your teenager?"). The group leaders did not provide specific feedback to the parents on their performance of the simulation exercise, but rather encouraged families to evaluate their own performance. The parents typically reported that the management tasks were very difficult.

Measures

Metabolic Status

Youngsters' metabolic control was assessed prior to the study, and again 3 and 6 months later, by determination of total glycosylated hemoglobin (Hb A1), a measure of average glycemic control over the previous 6 to 10 weeks (Bunn, 1981; Goldstein et al., 1982; Jovanovic & Peterson, 1981). The Isolab microcolumn method was used, as previously described (Abraham et al., 1978; Reeves, Seigler, Ryan, & Skyler, 1982). High levels of Hb A1 are indicative of poor glycemic functioning. Decrements of 1–2% are considered clinically significant improvements (Goldstein et al., 1982; Jovanovic & Peterson, 1981).

Attitudes/Perceptions

Semantic differentials (Osgood, Suci, & Tannenbaum, 1957) were used to assess adolescents' and parents' perceptions of a teen-ager with diabetes, parents of a teen-ager with diabetes, the family of a person with diabetes, medical staff caring for people with diabetes, and diabetes. Each semantic differential contained 10 bipolar items scored on a 7-point scale. Total scores could range from 10 to 70, with low scores indicative of positive attitudes. Semantic differentials have been demonstrated to have acceptable reliability and validity (Osgood et al., 1957), and have been used in research with adolescents and adults with IDDM (Seigler, La Greca, Citrin, Reeves, & Skyler, 1982).

Adolescents' ratings of "a teen-ager with diabetes," specifically were used to assess their self-perceptions. Previous research with this instrument (Seigler et al., 1982) obtained very high and significant correlations between this semantic differential and subjects' self-concept scores (*r*s ranged from .56 to .94; mean $r = .80$).

Estimates of Adolescents' Self-Care

Parents additionally were asked to indicate their impressions of their adolescents' level of self-care, both prior and subsequent to treatment. Parents responded to the question, "How would you estimate your child's overall self-care?," using a 5-point scale. The anchors for this scale were (1) *very careful,* (2) *somewhat careful,* (3) *neither careful nor careless,* (4) *somewhat careless,* and (5) *careless.* Thus, lower ratings reflected parents' impressions of greater carefulness in their adolescent's diabetes care.

Family Environment Scale (FES; Moos, 1974)

The FES was administered to all adolescents and parents, at pre- and posttreatment. This measure includes 10 subscales that assess various aspects of family functioning: cohesion, expressiveness, conflict, independence, achievement orientation, intellectual and cultural orientation, active recreational orientation, moral-religious emphasis, organization, and control. There are 90 items (10 per subscale) that are scored either true or false; higher scores reflect the degree to which the subscale describes the family. The FES has been widely used in research on families and diabetes (e.g., Anderson et al., 1981).

Statistical Analysis

Initially, when specific a priori hypotheses were tested (e.g., those regarding Hb A1, adolescents' perceptions of a "teen-ager with diabetes," and parents' estimates of their youngsters' self-care), planned comparison *t* tests (Winer, 1971, pp. 171-175) were conducted on the pre- to posttreatment change scores, to compare each of the intervention groups (MF and MF + S) with the control group (C). For the measure of metabolic control, this procedure was repeated for the pretreatment to follow-up change scores.

Other dependent measures (i.e., semantic differentials, perceptions of family functioning) were analyzed using a two-factor (Group × Time) repeated measures analysis of variance (ANOVA). For these analyses, the alpha level for each ANOVA was adjusted based on the number of tests conducted per measure, to minimize the possibility of Type I error. Thus, the alpha level was set at .01 (.05/5) for the semantic differentials, and at .005 (.05/10) for the FES.

Reported results are based primarily on our analyses for the entire sample. Despite the small number of subjects per treatment group, we also examined pre- to posttreatment changes for families in the later cycles of the study, excluding those in the first (pilot) cycle, as it was our impression that the smaller groups allowed greater communication among the families. These analyses were done only for the variables that tested a priori hypotheses. For the most part, these latter analyses were consistent with the findings for the total sample, and are reported only where discrepant from the main results.

RESULTS

Pretreatment Analyses

Prior to analyzing treatment-related changes for the dependent variables, the experimental groups were compared on all pretreatment measures, as a check on the randomization procedure. No significant group differences were obtained for any of the measures; thus, the groups were considered to be comparable.

Glycosylated Hemoglobin

Six weeks after the intervention period (i.e., 3 months after baseline), Hb A1 values had risen by 0.52% (± 1.36) for the adolescents in the MF group, and by 0.27% (±0.45) for those in the C group. In contrast, values decreased by 1.21% (±0.72) for those in the MF + S group. (Lower scores indicate better metabolic control.) Planned comparison tests revealed that those in the MF + S group demonstrated significant improvements in metabolic control, in comparison to the control subjects ($p < .05$).

This analysis was repeated using the 6-month follow-up measure of Hb A1, to ascertain the longer term impact of the interventions. At that juncture, all three groups displayed a decline in glycosylated hemoglobin; however, these changes from pretreatment levels were not significant. The mean (± *SD*) decrements in Hb A1 from the preintervention values were 0.32% (± 1.32) for the MF group, 1.10% (±0.98) for the MF + S group, and 0.01% (±0.87) for the C group.

Further analyses were performed for subjects randomized in the second and third study cycles (with smaller group size), excluding those in the first cycle. The pretreatment levels of Hb A1 for adolescents in each group were 15.6% (±1.1) for MF; 13.9% (±1.0) for MF + S; and 14.3% (±1.2) for C. These pretreatment levels were not significantly different. Three months later, the planned comparisons again revealed that adolescents in the MF + S group demonstrated significant improvements (i.e., decrements) in glycosylated hemoglobin relative to control subjects ($p < .01$). Also, the two multifamily groups combined showed improvements in metabolic functioning relative to control subjects ($p < .05$). Compared to pretreatment levels, Hb A1 values decreased by 2.56% (±1.88) for those in the MF group, 2.59% (±0.76) in the MF + S group, and rose by 0.66% (±0.70) in the control group.

In these subjects, glycosylated hemoglobin values obtained at 6 months follow-up showed significant improvements, relative to pretreatment levels, for those in the MF ($p < .05$) and MF + S ($p < .01$) groups compared to the control group. Hb A1 values decreased from the preintervention values by 3.06% (±1.54) in the MF group, and by 2.93% (±0.84) in the MF + S group, while values rose by 0.38% (±0.71) from preintervention values for control subjects.

Attitudes and Perceptions

Data for adolescents' and parents' attitudes are shown in Table II, as are the parents' estimates of their youngsters' level of self-care. For the adolescents, improvement was noted in their attitudes toward "a teen-ager with diabetes," for those in the MF ($p < .05$) and MF + S groups ($p < .01$) relative to the controls. Control subjects reported more negative perceptions of a teen-ager with diabetes at posttreatment (see Table II). No other signifi-

Table II. Adolescent and Parent Attitudes and Parent Perception of Child Self-Care[a]

	Group I MF		Group II MF + S		Group III C	
	Pre	Post	Pre	Post	Pre	Post
Adolescents						
Semantic differentials						
Teen-ager	33.64	29.00	32.55	28.09	25.22	29.55
Family	27.45	30.36	27.82	26.36	23.33	29.44
Parent	25.36	26.64	28.18	26.36	24.11	30.44
Med staff	25.64	23.27	25.09	20.36	21.89	20.11
Diabetes	44.00	43.45	43.73	40.09	38.78	31.33
Mothers						
Semantic differentials						
Teen-ager	38.73	32.27	30.30	28.10	26.63	27.50
Family	29.64	28.27	27.90	26.80	25.38	24.63
Parent	30.00	27.19	32.90	28.10	25.75	24.75
Med staff	25.09	20.91	21.70	18.10	19.75	12.13
Diabetes	37.45	42.73	51.70	49.40	39.75	35.88
Perception						
Self-care	2.90	2.20	2.00	1.78	2.38	2.25
Fathers						
Semantic differentials						
Teen-ager	26.43	24.71	32.22	34.00	27.20	27.40
Family	27.71	32.00	30.56	31.44	22.60	24.00
Parent	26.14	32.14	27.44	31.56	23.40	23.60
Med staff	24.14	29.00	22.56	21.00	18.60	23.40
Diabetes	41.29	51.14	43.22	47.78	36.00	37.40
Perception						
Self-care	2.14	1.86	2.22	1.88	2.00	2.25

[a]MF = multifamily group; MF + S = multifamily plus parent simulation group; C = wait-list control group. Lower values reflect more positive perceptions.

cant changes were noted in adolescents' perceptions as a function of intervention. However, over time, there was a tendency for all adolescents to report more positive attitudes toward a "medical staff caring for people with diabetes," $F(1, 31) = 3.22$, $p < .084$, and toward "diabetes," $F(1, 31) = 3.16$, $p < .086$.

No significant treatment-related changes were observed for mothers or fathers on the semantic differentials (alpha = .01). Some interesting trends were observed over time for parents' perceptions, regardless of group membership. Over time, mothers tended to report more positive attitudes toward "medical staff caring for people with diabetes," $F(1, 28) = 4.04$, $p < .055$, and fathers reported more negative perceptions of "a parent with diabetes," $F(1, 20) = 4.46$, $p < .05$.

Estimates of Adolescents' Self-Care

Mothers tended to report that their adolescents were more careful about their diabetes care at posttreatment, relative to pretreatment levels, regardless of group membership, $F(1, 28) = 3.81$, $p < .07$. (See Table II.) However, for those who participated in the second and third study cycles (with smaller groups), only mothers in the MF and MF + S groups reported increased perceptions of their youngsters' overall self-care, whereas mothers in the C group reported a decrement in their youngsters' self-care ($ps < .05$). The pre- and posttreatment means for each of these groups were as follows: MF (3.50 vs. 2.00); MF + S (2.80 vs. 1.20), and C (1.75 vs. 2.25). (Lower scores indicate greater self-care.)

For the fathers, no significant treatment effects were observed for the ratings of their adolescents' self-care; however, the pattern of the means was identical to the mothers' ratings, in that fathers in the MF and MF + S groups reported an improvement in their adolescents' self-care, those in the C group did not. (See Table II.)

Family Environment Scale

For the adolescents and parents, no significant changes on the subscales of the FES were observed (alpha = .005).

DISCUSSION

Effects of Intervention on Metabolic Control

Glycosylated hemoglobin has become the standard of reference for assessment of metabolic control of diabetes, as it reflects integrated glycemia over the previous 6- to 10-week period (Bunn, 1981; Goldstein et al., 1982; Jovanovic & Peterson, 1981). With a single random blood sample, the physician can make a quantitative assessment of overall patient progress. Decrements of glycosylated hemoglobin of the order of 1–2% represent clinically significant improvements in metabolic control (Goldstein et al., 1982; Jovanovic & Peterson, 1981). Improvements in glycemic control among individuals with IDDM have been associated with the prevention, delay, or reversal of some of the negative health outcomes associated with this disease (Skyler, 1987). Moreover, as an independent assessment of metabolic control, glycosylated hemoglobin avoids problems of patients presenting unreliable home monitoring information (Mazze et al., 1984) and may, in fact, help identify psychological problems (Citrin, Ellis, & Skyler, 1980).

Thus, adolescents' levels of glycosylated hemoglobin were used to assess the impact of our family intervention strategies. Adolescents receiving multifamily group intervention plus parent simulation of diabetes (MF + S) displayed statistically and clinically significant improvements in glycosylated hemoglobin levels from pretreatment to posttreatment, relative to controls. This suggests that improvements in diabetic control were apparent for youngsters whose parents participated in the family groups with the diabetes simulation exercise. No changes in glycosylated hemoglobin levels were evident for adolescents in either the multifamily (alone) or the waiting-list control groups, when the entire sample was considered.

However, it was our impression that the family group sessions were more effective, and involved more active family participation, in the second and third cycles of the study than in the first. This may have been a consequence of the smaller family groups (3 to 4 families in the later cycles, 5 families in the first). It also may have been a consequence of the greater experience of the group leaders. Thus, we reexamined the glycosylated hemoglobin data for those families participating in the second and third cycles of the study. These analyses revealed that youngsters in both intervention groups displayed significant improvements in metabolic functioning relative to controls, and the impact of these interventions was sustained when glycosylated hemoglobin levels were reexamined 6 months after intervention. Moreover, the magnitude of these improvements in Hb A1 (2.5–3%) are considered clinically significant by medical standards. No changes in glycosylated hemoglobin were evident for the control adolescents.

These data provide support for the effectiveness of multifamily groups, coupled with a parent simulation exercise, for improving metabolic control among adolescents with IDDM. Multifamily groups per se also appear to have a positive impact on metabolic control, although further replication is desirable as the effect was not observed for the entire sample. This is the first study to provide empirical support for a family-oriented group intervention strategy for adolescents with IDDM. Moreover, given the extreme difficulties of improving diabetic control among youngsters in this age group (Tattersall, 1987; Tattersall & Lowe, 1981), our findings are very encouraging of further attempts to involve families in the treatment of adolescents with diabetes.

Although improvements in metabolic control evidenced by adolescents in the intervention groups were interesting and clinically important, it was not clear from our data what actually was responsible for these improvements. It is possible that the adolescents became more careful with their diabetes management as a result of the intervention, and this, in turn, may have led to better metabolic control. For those in the second and third study cycles, mothers' ratings of their youngsters' self-care were significantly better at posttreatment for those in the MF and MF + S groups, relative to controls.

Fathers' perceptions of their adolescents' self-care followed the same pattern, although the changes were not significant. Given the recent advent of a standardized measure for assessing treatment adherence among youngsters with IDDM (Johnson, Silverstein, Rosenbloom, Carter, & Cunningham, 1986), subsequent studies might target or monitor adolescents' adherence behaviors more specifically, when evaluating the effects of intervention efforts in IDDM.

Although our data did not address this issue directly, some indirect evidence suggests that behavioral changes in diabetes management were apparent for those receiving psychological intervention. We examined the percentage of families within each experimental group that voluntarily participated in various diabetes-related activities after treatment termination. These activities included the adolescent attending a special diabetes camp session for the first time, the youngster agreeing to use a dextrometer to monitor daily blood glucose concentrations, the family agreeing to participate in subsequent diabetes research projects, and requesting special consultation sessions with the staff dietitian for the purpose of improving dietary management. Levels of participation were considerably higher for those in the intervention groups than for controls; 50% of the MF families and 55% of the MF + S families participated in these kinds of activities versus only 22% of the control group families.

These findings suggest that psychological intervention may have precipitated behavioral changes in diabetic management that may have been responsible, at least in part, for the improved glycosylated hemoglobin levels. Further research on this issue is important and desirable.

Perceptions of Diabetes and Family Functioning

Analyses of the semantic differentials revealed positive changes in adolescents' ratings of a "teen-ager with diabetes" for those in the two intervention groups relative to control adolescents, suggesting that adolescents who participated in multifamily interventions viewed themselves more positively as a result. This finding is in concert with our clinical impressions; during the group sessions, several youngsters expressed that they felt very good about their parents' interest in their diabetes and participation in the group sessions. However, parents' diabetes-related perceptions did not change as a function of intervention.

Some interesting trends were observed in adolescents' and parents' perceptions of diabetes over time, regardless of group membership. These trends must be interpreted cautiously, however, as they are not statistically significant. Adolescents and mothers in all three groups tended to give more positive ratings to "medical staff who work with diabetes" at posttreatment. Over time, the adolescents also tended to report more positive attitudes toward "diabetes." We interpret these findings to suggest that involving youngsters and parents in clinical research can affect their perceptions of health care professionals in a positive manner. Perhaps our research interests communicated a personal interest in the care and well-being of our patients and their families.

In contrast with the teen-agers and their mothers, fathers tended to report more *negative* perceptions of "parents with diabetes" over time, across all subject groups. This suggests that fathers may view themselves more negatively after participating in clinical research. This may reflect fathers' greater awareness of difficulties in diabetes management and a more realistic attitude toward their own involvement in diabetes care. Fathers are traditionally less involved in the daily routine of diabetes than are mothers (Etzwiler & Sines, 1962; Johnson, 1988). Perhaps fathers viewed themselves more negatively due to the heightened realization of their limited participation in these daily activities. It would be of interest to reassess fathers' perceptions after a more extended follow-up period, as these negative self-evaluations may have precipitated a more positive involvement in their youngster's diabetic care.

In contrast to the findings for the diabetes-specific semantic differentials, no significant time or intervention effects were observed for adolescents' and parents' perceptions of family functioning on the FES. Although the absence of change in adolescents' and parents' perceptions of family functioning was disappointing, our interventions focused directly and exclusively on family issues surrounding diabetes management and coping with common diabetes-specific problems. It is quite possible that the FES is not sufficiently sensitive to detect changes in how families handle diabetes-related issues on a daily basis. Other investigators have raised similar concerns regarding the sensitivity of global measures of family functioning with diabetic individuals (Johnson, 1988; Schafer, McCaul, & Glasgow, 1986); however, efforts to develop diabetes-specific measures of family functioning that are valid and reliable with adolescents and their families have been very disappointing (Schafer et al., 1986).

In point of fact, the rather negligible changes in family functioning observed in the present study, coupled with positive change in adolescents' metabolic control, are suggestive of behavioral changes in how adolescents and families manage diabetes (as a result of intervention) *without* initiating any major shifts or disruptions in family life. It may be wise for future investigations of family interventions in IDDM to assess general family functioning, in conjunction with diabetes-specific measures, in order to monitor any potential adverse effects that may result from intervention.

Conclusions

The present study is the first to report on the outcome of a family-oriented group intervention for adolescents with IDDM. The findings support the use of a multifamily group intervention, with parent simulation of diabetes, for improving the metabolic status of adolescents with IDDM.

Although the outcome measures did not differentiate between those receiving multifamily intervention alone and those receiving intervention plus parent simulation of diabetes, only the latter group performed consistently better than control subjects. Thus, firm conclusions cannot be drawn regarding the effectiveness of multifamily groups alone for improving the metabolic status of adolescents with diabetes. Further investigation and replication of the family interventions evaluated by this study would be desirable. Moreover, it is recommended that future interventions monitor adolescents' treatment adherence, in addition to levels of glycosylated hemoglobin, in order to determine whether behavioral changes in diabetes management underlie positive metabolic changes. Given the difficulty of achieving acceptable levels of metabolic control in adolescents with IDDM, intervention efforts are critical for improving the long-term health outlook for youngsters affected by this disease.

REFERENCES

Abraham, E. C., Huff, T. A., Cope, N. D., Wilson, J. B., Bransome, E. D., & Huisman, T. (1978). Determination of the glycosylated hemoglobins (Hb A1) with a new microcolumn procedure: Suitability of the technique for assessing the clinical management of diabetes mellitus. *Diabetes, 27,* 931-937.

Anderson, B. J., & Auslander, W. F. (1980). Research on diabetes management and the family: A critique. *Diabetes Care, 3,* 696-702.

Anderson, B. J., Miller, J. P., Auslander, W. F., & Santiago, J. (1981). Family characteristics of diabetic adolescents: Relationship to metabolic control. *Diabetes Care, 4,* 586-594.

Blum, A., & Galatzer, A. (1982). Group counseling for diabetic patients. *Pediatric and Adolescent Endocrinology, 10,* 230-233.

Brink, S. (1982). Youth and parent groups for patients with juvenile onset type 1 diabetes mellitus. *Pediatric and Adolescent Endocrinology, 10,* 234-240.

Bunn, H. F. (1981). Evaluation of glycosylated hemoglobin in diabetic patients. *Diabetes, 30,* 613-617.

Citrin, W., Ellis, G. J., & Skyler, J. S. (1980). Editorial. Glycosylated hemoglobin: A tool in identifying psychological problems? *Diabetes Care, 3,* 563-564.

Citrin, W., La Greca, A. M., & Skyler, J. S. (1985). Group intervention in type 1 diabetes mellitus. In P. I. Ahmed & N. Ahmed (Eds.), *Coping with juvenile diabetes* (pp. 181-204). Springfield, IL: Charles C. Thomas.

Citrin, W., Zigo, M. A., La Greca, A. M., & Skyler, J. S. (1982). Group strategies for diabetes in adolescence. *Pediatric and Adolescent Endocrinology, 10,* 219-223.

Etzwiler, D. D., & Sines, L. K. (1962). Juvenile diabetes and its management: Family, social, and academic implications. *Journal of the American Medical Association, 181,* 304-308.

Goldstein, D. E., Parker, K. M., England, J. D., England, J. D., Jr., Wiedmeyer, H. M., Rawlings, S. S., Hess, R., Little, R. R., Simonds, J. F., & Breyfogle, R. P. (1982). Clinical application of glycosylated hemoglobin measurements. *Diabetes, 31* (Suppl. 3), 70-78.

Hauser, S., Jacobson, A., Wertlieb, D., Brink, S., & Wentworth, S. (1985). The contribution of family environment to perceived competence and illness adjustment in diabetic and acutely ill adolescents. *Family Relations, 34,* 99-108.

Johnson, S. B. (1988). Diabetes mellitus in childhood. In D. K. Routh (Ed.), *Handbook of pediatric psychology* (pp. 9-31). New York: Guilford.

Johnson, S. B., Silverstein, J. H., Rosenbloom, A. L., Carter, R., & Cunningham, W. (1986). Assessing daily management in childhood diabetes. *Health Psychology, 5,* 545-564.

Jovanovic, L., & Peterson, C. M. (1981). The clinical utility of glycosylated hemoglobin. *American Journal of Medicine, 70,* 331-338.

La Greca, A. M. (1982). Behavioral aspects of diabetes management in children and adolescents. *Diabetes, 32* (Suppl.), 47.

La Greca, A. M. (1988). Children with diabetes and their families: Coping and disease management. In T. Field, P. Mc Cabe, N. Schneiderman (Eds.), *Stress and coping across development* (pp. 139-159). Hillsdale, NJ: Erlbaum.

La Greca, A. M., & Citrin, W. (1984). How to talk to your parents. *Diabetes Forecast, 37,* 45, 68.

Marrero, D. G., Meyers, G. L., Golden, M. P., West, D., Kershnar, A., & Lau, N. (1982). Adjustment to misfortune: The use of a social support group for adolescent diabetics. *Pediatric and Adolescent Endocrinology, 10,* 213-218.

Mazze, R. S., Shamoon, H., Pasmantier, R., Lucido, D., Murphy, J., Hartmann, K., Kuykendall, V., & Lopatin, W. (1984). Reliability of blood glucose monitoring by patients with diabetes mellitus. *American Journal of Medicine, 77,* 211-217.

Minuchin, S., Rosman, B., & Baker, L. (1978). *Psychosomatic families.* Cambridge, MA: Harvard University Press.

Moos, R. (1974). *Family Environment Scale.* Palo Alto, CA: Consulting Psychologists Press.

Osgood, C., Suci, G., & Tannenbaum, P. (1957). *The measurement of meaning.* Urbana: University of Illinois Press.

Reeves, M., Seigler, D. E., Ryan, E. A., & Skyler, J. S. (1982). Glycemic control in insulin-dependent diabetes mellitus: Comparison of outpatient intensified conventional therapy with continuous subcutaneous insulin infusion. *American Journal of Medicine, 72,* 673-680.

Schafer, L. C., McCaul, K. D., & Glasgow, R. E. (1986). Supportive and nonsupportive family behaviors: Relationships to adherence and metabolic control in persons with type 1 diabetes. *Diabetes Care, 9,* 179-185.

Seigler, D. E., La Greca, A. M., Citrin, W. S., Reeves, M. L., & Skyler, J. S. (1982). Psychological effects of intensification of diabetic control. *Diabetes Care, 5* (Suppl. 1), 19-23.

Skyler, J. S. (1980). Diabetes in adolescence: The forgotten years. In S. Podolsky (Ed.), *Clinical diabetes mellitus: Modern management* (pp. 463-479). New York: Appleton-Century-Crofts.

Skyler, J. S. (1986). Insulin dependent diabetes mellitus. In P. O. Kohler (Ed.), *Clinical endocrinology* (pp. 491-573). New York: Willey.

Skyler, J. S. (1987). Why control blood glucose? *Pediatric Annals, 16,* 713-724.

Tattersall, R. B. (1987). Psychological aspects of diabetes in childhood and adolescence. *Pediatric Annals, 16,* 728-740.

Tattersall, R. B., & Lowe, J. (1981). Diabetes in adolescence. *Diabetologia, 20,* 517-523.

Tattersall, R. B., McCulloch, D. K., & Aveline, M. (1985). Group therapy in the treatment of diabetes. *Diabetes Care, 8,* 180-188.

Welborn, T. A., & Duncan, N. (1980). Diabetic staff simulation of insulin dependent diabetic life. *Diabetes Care, 3,* 679-681.

Wertlieb, D., Hauser, S. T., & Jacobson, A. M. (1986). Adaptation to diabetes: Behavior symptoms and family context. *Journal of Pediatric Psychology, 11,* 463-479.

Winer, B. J. (1971). *Statistical principles in experimental design.* New York: McGraw-Hill.

Yalom, I. (1970). *The theory and practice of group psychotherapy.* New York: Basic Books.

13

Familial Similarities of Changes in Cognitive, Behavioral, and Physiological Variables in a Cardiovascular Health Promotion Program[1]

Thomas L. Patterson, James F. Sallis, Philip R. Nader, Robert M. Kaplan, and Joan W. Rupp
University of California, San Diego

Catherine J. Atkins and Karen L. Senn
San Diego State University

A number of studies have demonstrated that physiological and behavioral cardiovascular disease (CVD) risk factors aggregate within families. This fact, and the potential mediating role that the family plays in behavior change, have led to the development of family-based CVD risk reduction programs, including the San Diego Family Health Project. The aggregation of behavioral, physiological, and cognitive changes within families was assessed during a 1-year intervention. We found evidence of modest but significant aggregation of change. There was more aggregation of change in behavioral variables than in physiological or cognitive variables. More significant correlations were found among 3-day food record measures than among 24-hour recall dietary measures, suggesting an influence of assessment method. Aggregation of change within families was stronger within generations than across generations. These data point to the importance of involving all age groups in health promotion programs.

[1]This work was supported by NHLBI grant HL-30872 to P. R. Nader.

The role of the family as a mediator of health-related behaviors, such as dietary and physical activity patterns, appears to be important and long-lasting (Baranowski & Nader, 1985; Sallis & Nader, 1988). Dietary habits (Eastwood, Brydon, Smith, & Smith, 1982; Patterson, Rupp, Sallis, Atkins, & Nader, 1988) and physical activity habits (Gottlieb & Chen, 1985; Sallis, Patterson, Buono, Atkins, & Nader, 1988), as well as related physiological variables such as blood pressure (Feinleib, Garrison, & Havlik, 1980; Patterson, Kaplan, Sallis, & Nader, 1987), serum lipoproteins (Karlin et al., 1982; Morrison, Namboodiri, Green, Martin, & Glueck, 1983), and obesity (Charney, Goodman, McBride, Lyon, & Pratt, 1976; Garn & Clark, 1976; Patterson, Sallis, Kaplan, & Nader, in press) aggregate to varying degrees within families. These observations have stimulated the development of health behavior change interventions that target entire families.

Several mechanisms of family influence are available for alteration in family-based interventions. There is evidence that parental control of environmental variables (e.g., availability of foods in the home) (Birch & Marlin, 1982), parental modeling of health behaviors (Gottlieb & Chen, 1985; Harper & Sanders, 1975), and direct parental instructional prompts (Klesges, Malott, Boschee, & Weber, 1986) are effective in altering child health behaviors. These powerful mechanisms may account for the relative success of family-based health behavior change interventions (Farris, Frank, Webber, & Berenson, 1985; Kirks & Hughes, 1986; Nader, Baranowski, Vanderpool, Dworkin, & Dunn, 1983), and weight-loss programs that target children and parents (Brownell, Kelman, & Stunkard, 1983; Epstein, Koeske, Wing, & Valoski, 1986; Epstein, Nudelman, & Wing, 1987; Epstein, Wing, Koeske, Andrasik, & Ossip, 1981; Israel & Saccone, 1979; Israel, Stolmaker, Sharp, Silverman, & Simon, 1984).

In at least one weight-loss program, short-term weight losses were highly correlated between parents and children (Epstein et al., 1981). Long-term (5-year) effects of a family-based obesity treatment were found to generalize to nonparticipating obese children (Epstein et al., 1987). These results indicate that, at least in obesity treatment programs, family members tend to make similar changes. However, health promotion programs target cognitive, behavioral, and physiological changes, and it is important to explore the extent of family aggregation of changes in all these dimensions in response to family-based interventions. Family interventions are based on the belief that families influence one another (Sallis & Nader, 1988), and this should be evidenced by family aggregation of changes. However, this intrafamily influence has rarely been examined. It is hypothesized that families will be similar in their responses to family-based interventions. Findings of familial aggregation of change would support the rationale for continuing to develop family-based health promotion programs. Cognitive, behavioral, and physiological changes during a 1-year intervention were studied in Mexican-American and non-Hispanic white families (referred to as Anglo). Similarities were explored in spouse, mother–child, father–child, and sibling pairs so that the specific patterns of aggregation within families can be described.

METHODS

Subjects

For purposes of this project, family was defined as at least one adult and one child sharing usual household functions. Families of fifth- and sixth-grade children were recruited from elementary schools in the San Diego Unified School District. Census tract data were used to identify schools with large numbers of Mexican-American or Anglo families of lower to middle socioeconomic status (SES). The Hollingshead (1965) two-factor index of social position indicated that the participants ranged from middle class to the lower part of the SES distribution ($M = 2.8$, $SD = 1.2$). Families were excluded from participation if there was evidence of preexisting cardiovascular disease, total cholesterol above the 95th percentile for that age and sex, an indication of high blood pressure (defined in adults as taking blood pressure (BP) medications or, either a mean of three BP determinations of 150 mm Hg systolic or 95 mm Hg diastolic; in children either reading above the 95th percentile for that age and sex), or some chronic illness that would prohibit an individual from participating in the exercise/diet program promoted in the San Diego Family Health Project (Nader et al., 1986). Families who volunteered to participate were very similar on demographic variables and health habits to nonparticipants at the same schools (Atkins et al., 1987).

A total of 206 families (95 Anglo and 111 Mexican-American families) were recruited into the study. Approximately one half ($n = 101$) of the families were assigned randomly to participate in a cardiovascular health intervention described below. The remaining 105 families were assigned to a no-treatment control condition. Since the focus of this paper was on aggregation of change in families exposed to a health behavior change intervention, the control families were excluded from the analyses.

A total of 90 intervention families (42 Anglo and 48 Mexican-American families) were measured at baseline and 1 year, the completion of the intervention (i.e., 89% of the original families). For this analysis we combined data from both ethnic groups. Descriptive data regarding selected subject characteristics are presented in Table I. Additional subject data on the total subject population can be found elsewhere (Nader et al., 1986).

Intervention Program

The San Diego Family Health Project intervention was based on social learning theory (Bandura, 1977) and was designed to assist families in making long-term changes in their physical activity and dietary behaviors (i.e., reduce sodium and saturated fat intake and increase aerobic activity). The 1-year intervention was structured into 12 weeks of intensive intervention followed by six maintenance sessions distributed over a 9-month period. Ethnically homogeneous groups of families attended evening meetings for 90 minutes of training in self-monitoring, setting realistic goals, problem-solving, self-rewarding goal achievement, and supporting family and group members. The intervention groups were structured to maximize cultural, group, and family support for behavioral change, experiential learning, and intrinsic enjoyment of health behaviors. The intervention was conducted in Spanish and was culturally adapted for the Mexican-American families.

Intervention sessions were conducted at area schools and each session consisted of four parts. First, there was an aerobic exercise session with proper warm-up and cool-down. Then separate adult and child education segments provided new information and skills each sesion. Next, during the behavior management segment, families discussed progress and problems, set short-term goals, and adjusted personal behavior change programs. The final segment of each session was a heart-healthy snack that was prepared by a different family each week. The first session was introductory and included training in self-monitoring. Sessions 2 through 4 focused on physical activity; 5 through 7 covered sodium intake; and 8 through 10 concentrated on saturated and total fat intake. Session 11 reviewed and integrated all areas. Session 12 was a heart-healthy potluck dinner celebrating "graduation" from the intensive intervention. Maintenance sessions covered behavior chaining, ordering in restaurants, grocery shopping, resisting peer pressure, and planned and unplanned breaks in exercise and dietary routines.

Each participant maintained a notebook containing instructional materials, self-monitoring forms, and recipes. Additional materials including posters, games, role-playing situations, and slide shows were developed by a team of psychologists, health educators, a dietitian, and an exercise physiologist.

Measurement Procedures

Baseline measures were collected between October 1984 and February 1985. Follow-up measures were completed immediately after the 1 year intervention; between October 1985 and February 1986. Up to four family members were measured by staff who were trained, certified, and periodically monitored to ensure that standardized protocols were followed.

Assessment Procedures

Dietary Behavior

Collection of nutritional intake data was accomplished by three methods: a 24-hour dietary recall interview, a 3-day food diary, and a food frequency questionnaire. Because of the well-known difficulties of assessing nutritional intake, it is preferable to use multiple measurement methods (Block, 1982).

The 24-hour dietary recall interview was conducted using standardized techniques and food models. Nutrition assessors were trained using Nutrition Coordinating Center procedures (Dennis, Ernest, Hjortland, Tillotson, & Granibsch, 1980) plus modifications to improve accuracy of children's reports (Frank, Berenson, Schilling, & Moore, 1977). Results were coded and analyzed for 27 nutrients at the Nutrition Coordinating Center at the University of Minnesota (Dennis et al., 1980). For this analysis, the percentage of calories from total fat (24-hour total fat), total caloric intake (24-hour Kcals), and milligrams of sodium (24-hour sodium) were used. Test–retest reliability, in the present study, with 30 adults and children interviewed the same day by different nutrition assessors yielded a 91% agreement on the description of 438 food items. Dietary intake values for all groups of subjects fell within normal ranges.

Each participant kept a 3-day food diary for 1 weekend day and 2 weekdays prior to each assessment. The food diaries were reviewed for completeness by nutrition assessors and then assigned a Food Record Rating of average fat and cholesterol intake (3-day fat score) using the scoring system developed for the Multiple Risk Factor Intervention Trial (Remmell, Gorder, Hall, & Tillotson, 1980). The average American diet would receive a score above 20. The range of 10–14 represents some fat modifications. A score of 4–9 indicates Phase 1-2 of the American Heart Association Diet and a score less than 3 represents Phase 3. Average milliequivalents of sodium per day were also calculated from the 3-day food diary (3-day sodium) (Jacobson, Liebman, & Moyer, 1983; Pennington & Church, 1980). Reliability of scoring was .91 for fat and .89 for salt scores (n = 20 adults and children) in the present study. Scores below 100 represented achievement of the 3-gram sodium goal for the project.

A 50-item food frequency questionnaire developed for the Special Project in Nutrition (SPIN) at the Gladstone Foundation in San Francisco was shortened to 36 items and modified to be culturally sensitive to our particular population. This questionnaire focused on sodium- and fat-containing foods. A ratio of the frequency of consumption of the 9 low sodium and/or fat foods to the 27 high sodium and/or fat foods (Food Frequency Score) was determined for *each* individual.

Assessment of Physical Activity

The measure used in the current study to assess physical activity is the 7-day Physical Activity Recall (PAR), which has been well described (Blair, 1984; Sallis et al., 1985). It is an interviewer-administered 1-week recall, with modifications to allow separate scoring of work and leisure activity. Interviewers accounted for only the portion of the day in which subjects engaged in moderate, hard, and very hard intensity activities. Same-day reliability using different assessors was 0.78 ($n = 43$) in the present study. For the purposes of this analysis we used the overall summary score, kilocalories per kilogram of body weight per day (KKD). The procedure has been validated in adults (Taylor et al., 1984) and in children (Wallace, McKenzie, & Nader, 1985).

Assessment of Physiological Indicators

Blood Pressure. The mean of three consecutive BP readings taken after a 5-minute rest period was used for this analysis. The measurement and staff certification procedures developed in the Hypertension Detection and Follow-Up Program (Curb, Labarthe, Cooper, Cutter, & Hawkins, 1983) were used for adults. For children, the cuff selection and fourth phase determination procedures suggested by Berenson (1980) and H. S. Kahn (personal communication, 1983) were utilized. In order to reduce observer bias, random-zero sphygmomanometers (DeGaudemaris, Folsom, Prineas, & Luepker, 1985) were used for all readings. Fourth-phase BP, recorded at the point at which the Korotkoff sounds became muffled, was used as the diastolic BP for children, while fifth phase was used as the diastolic BP for adults. Same-day reliability across different assessors for first-phase blood pressure was 0.87 for adults ($n = 53$) and children ($n = 47$). For fifth phase, BP in adults reliability was 0.79 ($n = 53$) and for children reliability for fourth-phase blood pressure was 0.57 ($n = 47$). All measurements were taken between the hours of 7:00 and 9:30 a.m. in the fasting state.

Body Mass Index. Weight was measured without shoes or heavy objects in pockets. Height was obtained using a secured height anthropometer. The Quetelet index (kg/m^2) was used as a measure of body mass index.

Assessment of Cognitive Change

Knowledge. An adult and a child scale were developed to measure knowledge of health behaviors related to cardiovascular diseases. The scales assess knowledge of dietary sodium, dietary fat, and exercise among both adults and children. These scales focus on "behavioral capability" rather than the link between behavior and disease. It is believed that the type of information measured in these scales is more closely related to behavior changes sought in contemporary CVD prevention trials (cf. Parcel & Baranowski, 1981). The psychometric characteristics of the scales have been reported previously (Vega et al., 1987), and they have been shown to have adequate reliability.

Self-Efficacy. Self-efficacy was measured by having subjects rate the confidence in their ability to change specific dietary and exercise behaviors. There were four questions on reducing fat intake (e.g., confidence that they can "use unsaturated vegetable oil instead of lard or shortening in cooking") and two questions concerning confidence in ability to reduce salt intake (e.g., confidence that they can "reduce salt you add both in cooking and at the table by half or more"). Two questions on exercise (e.g., confidence that they can do vigorous activity such as jogging, running, and swimming laps for 20 minutes three or more times a week) have been shown to predict actual exercise changes (Sallis et al., 1986). For the purposes of the present study, we have analyzed subjects' total confidence scores.

Analysis

SPSS-X programs were used for all analyses. One-year change scores were computed for each variable by subtracting baseline from 1-year values. Change scores were correlated between each of six family pairs: spouses, fathers and younger children, fathers and older children, mothers and younger children, mothers and older children, and siblings. Younger children were fifth- or sixth-grade subjects whereas older children were older siblings who participated in the intervention. All families had at least one fifth- or sixth-grade child. No children younger than the fifth- or sixth-grade cohort were measured.

To assess the impact of random associations, mothers, fathers, and children were randomly assigned to different families. The correlational analyses were then repeated on the randomly assigned pairs.

RESULTS

Descriptive statistics for each of the measures are presented in Table I. As can be seen, there were moderate changes in the expected direction in dietary behaviors and blood pressure but not in exercise. In general, mothers made the largest and most consistent changes across measures.

Aggregation of Behavioral Indicators

Dietary Behaviors. All family pairs except fathers and older children were significantly correlated on change in fat consumed as measured by the 3-day diet record (see Table II). In contrast, only sibling pairs were significantly correlated for change in milligrams of fat consumed as measured by the 24-hour diet recall. For salt/sodium intake, when the 3-day salt score was examined, spouses, siblings, and mother–older child pair correlations were all significant. Dietary sodium changes as assessed by the 24-hour recall were significantly but negatively correlated for father–younger child pairs only. Changes in the food frequency index were not significantly related for any family dyad.

Physical Activity. All pairs except young children and their parents were significantly correlated on change in physical activity as measured by the physical activity recall. Siblings and spouses showed the strongest concordance in KKD change.

Physiologic Indicators. Siblings' blood pressure changes were significantly correlated for both systolic and diastolic blood pressures. Spouses' changes in diastolic blood pressures were correlated but not their change in systolic blood pressure. Fathers' and their younger children's changes in body mass index were significantly negatively correlated. No other family pair's changes in body mass index were significantly related.

Cognitive Variables. The correlations between the knowledge gain of family pairs was significant for spouse and sibling pairs. No significant relationships were found between parents and children. Changes in self-efficacy were nonsignificantly correlated for all pairs except the mother–younger child pair.

Aggregation Within Randomly Constituted "Families"

Comparisons of randomly paired nonrelated "family" dyads are presented in Table III. Only one of the targeted behavior change correlations

Table I. Means (and Standard Deviations), for All Measures by Family Status for Families Who Participated in a Family Health Promotion Intervention

	Father (n = 52)		Mother (n = 98)		Younger child (n = 100)		Older child (n = 54)	
	Baseline	1 year	Baseline	1 year	Baseline	1 year	Baseline	1 year
Age (years)	37.9 (6.9)		35.4 (6.0)		11.6 (0.9)		12.5 (2.2)	
3-day fat score[a]	27.8 (10.2)	21.5 (6.7)	20.3 (8.1)	16.4 (6.6)	22.1 (6.5)	19.3 (7.4)	23.7 (8.3)	19.6 (7.9)
24-hour total fat[b]	0.40 (0.09)	0.38 (0.09)	0.40 (0.10)	0.35 (0.10)	0.37 (0.07)	0.36 (0.08)	0.35 (0.08)	0.36 (0.08)
3-day sodium (mg)	115.2 (42.5)	103.3 (47.3)	98.6 (43.4)	71.7 (34.7)	107.0 (46.1)	91.8 (38.8)	113.2 (43.6)	87.7 (34.7)
24-hour sodium (mg)	3,378 (1,813)	3,458 (2,078)	2,597 (1,319)	2,259 (1,444)	2,918 (1,262)	3,036 (1,843)	2,678 (1,070)	2,746 (1,460)
Food frequency[c]	0.39 (0.28)	0.60 (0.30)	0.44 (0.31)	0.73 (0.56)	0.42 (0.30)	0.51 (0.37)	0.44 (0.34)	0.62 (0.45)
Exercise kilocalories per kilogram per day	39.8 (8.9)	36.2 (2.7)	36.8 (3.4)	35.5 (5.2)	38.5 (4.1)	35.1 (4.8)	37.9 (4.2)	35.2 (3.2)
Systolic BP	120.5 (13.6)	114.6 (14.5)	111.1 (12.2)	108.3 (12.0)	101.3 (9.0)	100.9 (9.2)	99.3 (10.8)	100.7 (11.0)
Diastolic BP	78.7 (11.4)	75.6 (11.4)	72.0 (9.7)	71.5 (10.0)	68.0 (8.7)	64.4 (14.0)	64.8 (10.8)	55.3 (26.9)
Body mass index (kg/m^2)	26.6 (4.8)	26.5 (5.1)	26.5 (7.1)	26.6 (6.1)	19.1 (3.7)	20.0 (4.2)	19.3 (4.2)	20.1 (4.1)
Knowledge	9.8 (3.7)	12.0 (3.5)	9.6 (4.4)	11.8 (3.4)	3.9 (1.9)	5.9 (2.2)	3.9 (2.3)	5.5 (2.3)
Self-efficacy	33.4 (7.2)	33.8 (7.3)	33.4 (5.6)	33.0 (7.5)	28.6 (7.5)	29.4 (8.4)	28.9 (6.1)	29.8 (8.2)

[a]See Dietary Behavior assessment for description.
[b]Percent of calories from all fats calculated from 24-hour diet recall.
[c]Ratio of low sodium, low fat food to high sodium, high fat food items endorsed.

Table II. Correlations in One-Year Changes Observed Between Family Pairs Who Had Participated in Health Behavior Change Program

Observed change	Spouses	Father–younger child	Father–older child	Mother–younger child	Mother–older child	Siblings
Targeted behavior						
3-day fat scores	.51[b]	.20	.34	.10	.62[b]	.35[b]
3-day salt scores	.38[b]	.49[b]	.20	.44[b]	.49[b]	.46[b]
24-hour total fat	.23	–.05	.15	.18	.09	.36[a]
24-hour total sodium (mgs)	.12	–.48[b]	–.17	–.31	–.03	.11
Food frequency index	.01	.05	.04	.14	.11	.12
Kilocalories expended during exercise	.43[b]	.07	.36[a]	.11	.31[b]	.49[b]
Physiologic indicators						
Systolic BP	.09	–.06	.26	.05	.14	.36[b]
Diastolic BP	.29[a]	–.03	.12	.06	.13	.55[b]
Body mass index	–.04	–.28[a]	–.21	.05	.08	–.004
Cognitive variables						
Knowledge	.33[a]	.07	.01	.02	.01	.25[a]
Self-efficacy	–.01	–.03	–.03	.25[a]	.00	–.05

[a] $p < .05$.
[b] $p < .01$.

Table III. Correlations in One-Year Changes Between Randomly Constituted Nonrelated "Family" Pairs Who Had Participated in Health Behavior Change Program

Observed changes	Spouses	Father–younger child	Father–older child	Mother–younger child	Mother–older child	Siblings
Targeted behavior						
3-day fat scores	.12	–.20	.28	–.04	.04	–.22
3-day salt scores	.14	.10	–.14	.13	.18	–.05
24-hour total fat	–.01	.14	.32	.24	.06	.02
24-hour total sodium (mgs)	–.10	–.19	.00	.19	.15	–.21
Food frequency index	.14	–.32[a]	.08	.15	.02	.11
Kilocalories expended during exercise	.09	.00	.24	.16	–.15	.02
Physiologic indicators						
Systolic BP	.03	–.01	.28[a]	.03	–.12	.10
Diastolic BP	–.09	.31[a]	–.19	.07	–.25	.08
Body mass index	.02	.25	.13	–.15	–.29[a]	–.17
Cognitive variables						
Knowledge	–.12	.05	.11	.00	.06	–.12
Self-efficacy	.16	.08	.10	–.07	–.05	–.08

[a] $p < .05$.

for diet and exercise was statistically significant. Three of the correlations for physiologic indicators and none of the cognitive variable correlations was statistically significant.

DISCUSSION

These data suggest that the aggregation of behavior change in families who had participated in a 1-year health promotion intervention program occurred, but the level of aggregation was moderate. We found more evidence for aggregation of change among targeted behaviors than among physiologic indicators or cognitive variables.

This pattern of aggregation would be expected because the program focused on behavior change, and physiologic change might be considered an indirect consequence of the behavioral change. The changes for cognitive variables are less clearly aggregated across family members. However, spouses and siblings did aggregate on knowledge change. Changes in siblings and spouse pairs were more likely to be significantly correlated than were parents and children across most of the measures. We also found differences in aggregation patterns as a function of dietary measure employed.

Examination of the total number of correlations that were statistically significant suggests that 21 of 66 (32%) of the correlations were nonchance. By chance, we would expect only three (5%) to be significant. In our randomly constituted "families" we found four significant correlations. These results indicate that the observed aggregation of change in families is a reliable phenomenon and cannot be explained by chance.

Of the correlations for behavior change targeted in this study 14 of 36 (39%) were significant whereas 4 of 18 (22%) of the physiologic indicators and 3 of 12 (25%) of the cognitive changes were statistically significant. It is possible that longer periods between assessments are necessary for subjects to make large enough changes to be reflected in aggregation of blood pressure and body mass index. However, the relatively weak concordance in cognitive changes cannot be explained in this manner. It is interesting that knowledge changes were significantly correlated for spouse and sibling pairs only, and in each of these cases the same form of the questionnaires was being compared. For parent–child pairs, separate adult and children forms were being compared. Thus the lack of association in knowledge for the parent–child pairs may have been due to different metrics. It is also possible that these forms ascertain somewhat different knowledge domains.

We found more evidence for concordance in change for sibling pairs (64% or 7/11 of sibling correlations were significant) and spouse pairs (45% or 5/11 of spouse correlations were significant) than in parent–child pairs

(20% or 9/44 of these correlations were significant). These findings suggest that family members are more likely to influence other family members of similar ages. Research on modeling (Rosenthal & Bandura, 1978) indicates that similar models are particularly influential, and age is a very salient variable. Although the mechanisms accounting for the robust spouse and sibling correlations are not known, the data suggest that intragenerational dynamics are more important than intergenerational dynamics within families in regards to health behavior change. This finding argues against targeting the "gatekeeper" or some other single family member, in hopes that change by this person will generalize to all other family members. These data also suggest that specific intervention strategies need to be developed to enhance intergenerational family influences.

We chose to include all of the outcome measures in these analyses, even those that did not change significantly after the intervention. The overall efficacy of the intervention program is examined elsewhere in detail (Nader et al., 1989). In general, in most age–ethnic subgroups, there were significant intervention effects in knowledge, blood pressure, and dietary salt and fat, but no differences in exercise. However, for purposes of the present study these findings are only of peripheral interest. Examination of the intervention data presented in Table I indicates substantial variability in change. Without this variability the present analysis would be pointless. For all measures, some subjects improve, some stay the same, while others get worse. The question addressed here is, are these changes similar within families?

We chose to use simple change scores in this analysis because they are readily interpreted. The problems with change scores are widely recognized in the literature. In particular, the error component of a change score is often large because it absorbs error from both the pretest and posttest. As a result, the reliability of a change score is expected to be lower than the reliability of either score on which it is based. The effect of this unreliability is to attenuate correlations among change scores, ultimately resulting in a conservative bias. In other words, the change score problem biases the analysis away from detecting significant relationships. Alternative methods, such as residualized change score analysis, resolve some of these problems but introduce other biases. Thus, we felt it was appropriate to use change scores because the well-known bias worked against our ability to detect aggregation. Given the conservative bias of the tests, we elected to use the standard .05 alpha level, despite the large number of correlations.

By using multiple dietary measures, we were able to compare the effects of assessment method utilized. The strongest concordance was found using the 3-day diet record, with weaker relationships found with the 24-hour diet recall and no relationship in change as measured by the food frequency questionnaires. These findings may be due to two factors. The first factor is reliability. The 3-day food record appears to provide a more reliable yet independent representation of an individual's diet when compared to the 24-hour diet recall. The major limitation of the 24-hour diet recall is that it supplies data for only one day, a day which may not be representative of usual food practices (Garn, Larkin, & Cole, 1978). Thus, this measure is more useful in comparing group means than for representing an individual's diet intake (Gersovitz, Madden, & Smicklas-Wright, 1978). This low reliability of 24-hour recall data is expected to suppress correlations. The second potential problem concerns the food frequency questionnaire. The data from this measure are expressed as a ratio of "healthy" to "unhealthy" foods. There was a restricted range in the change of this index that may have attenuated the correlations observed in this measure.

The present study clearly indicates that families who participate together in a health promotion program tend to make similar modifications in their health habits. These results are consistent with the Epstein et al. (1981, 1987) studies of family-based treatment for childhood obesity. The contrast between actual and randomly constituted families demonstrates that the observed level of aggregation was not due to chance. Although the intrafamily correlations are moderate in size, they provide support for the importance of family influences on health habit modification.

The findings of this study provide support for the strategy of targeting families rather than individuals in health behavior intervention programs. This intervention focused on involving all family members, increasing social support, and providing materials appropriate for each age group. The present analysis indicated that the intervention was only partially successful in stimulating intrafamily influences since stronger associations in change were seen within spouse and sibling pairs, when compared to cross-generation changes. It appears that, for fifth- and sixth-grade children, parent–child influences on changing diet and exercise behaviors are not strong, and it is important to involve both generations in health behavior change programs.

REFERENCES

Atkins, C. J., Patterson, T. L., Roppe, B. E., Kaplan, R. M., Sallis, J. F., & Nader, P. R. (1987). Recruitment issues, health habits and the decision to participate in a health promotion program. *American Journal of Preventive Medicine, 3,* 87-94.

Bandura, A. (1977). *Social learning theory.* Englewood Cliffs, NJ: Prentice Hall.

Baranowski, T., & Nader, P. R. (1985). Family health behavior. In D. C. Turk & R. D. Kerns (Eds.), *Health, illness, and families: A life-span perspective* (pp. 51-80). New York: Wiley.

Berenson, G. S. (1980). *Cardiovascular risk factors in children: The Bogalusa Heart Study.* New York: Oxford.

Birch, L. L., & Marlin, D. W. (1982). I don't like it, I never tried it: Effects of exposure on two year old children's food preferences. *Appetite: Journal for Intake Research, 3,* 353-360.
Blair, S. N. (1984). How to assess exercise habits and physical fitness. In J. D. Matarazzo, S. M. Weiss, J. A., Herd, N. Miller, & S. M. Weiss (Eds.), *Behavioral health* (pp. 424-447). New York: Wiley.
Block, G. (1982). A review of validations of dietary assessment methods. *American Journal of Epidemiology, 115,* 492-505.
Brownell, K. D., Kelman, J. H., & Stunkard, A. J. (1983). Treatment of obese children with and without their mothers: Changes in weight and blood pressure. *Pediatrics, 71,* 515-523.
Charney, E., Goodman, H. C., McBride, M., Lyon, B., & Pratt, R. (1976). Childhood antecedents of adult obesity. *New England Journal of Medicine, 259,* 6-9.
Curb, J. D., Labarthe, D. R., Cooper, S. P., Cutter, G. R., & Hawkins, C. M. (1983). Training and certification of blood pressure observers. *Hypertension, 5,* 610-614.
Degaudemaris, R. D., Folsom, A. R., Prineas, R. J., & Luepker, R. V. (1985). The randomzero versus the standard mercury sphygmomanometer. A systematic blood pressure difference. *American Journal of Epidemilogy, 121,* 282-290.
Dennis, B., Ernest, N., Hjortland, M., Tillotson, J. L., & Granibsch, V. (1980). NHLBI nutrition data system. *Journal of the American Dietetic Association, 77,* 641-647.
Eastwood, M. A., Brydon, W. G., Smith, D. M., & Smith, J. H. (1982). A study of diet, serum lipids, and fecal constituents in spouses. *American Journal of Clinical Nutrition, 36,* 290-293.
Epstein, L. H., Koeske, R., Wing, R. R., & Valoski, A. (1986). The effect of family variables on child weight change. *Health Psychology, 5,* 1-12.
Epstein, L. H., Nudelman, S., & Wing, R. R. (1987). Long-term effects of family-based treatment for obesity on nontreated family members. *Behavior Therapy, 2,* 147-152.
Epstein, L. H., Wing, R. R., Koeske, R., Andrasik, F., & Ossip, D. (1981). Child and parent weight loss in family-based behavior modification programs. *Journal of Consulting and Clinical Psychology, 49,* 674-685.
Farris, R. P., Frank, G. C., Webber, L. S., & Berenson, G. S. (1985). A nutrition curriculum for families with high blood pressure. *Journal of School Health, 55,* 110-112.
Feinleib, M., Garrison, R. J., & Havlik, R. J. (1980). Environmental and genetic factors affecting the distribution of blood pressure in children. In R. M. Lauer & R. B. Shekelle (Eds.), *Childhood prevention of atherosclerosis and hypertension* (pp. 271-279). New York: Raven.
Frank, G. C., Berenson, G. S., Schilling, P. E., & Moore, M. C. (1977). Adapting the 24-hour recall for epidemiologic studies of school children. *Journal of the American Dietetic Association, 71,* 26-31.
Garn, S. M., & Clark, D. C. (1976). Trends in fatness and the origins of obesity. *Pediatrics, 57,* 443-456.
Garn, S. M., Larkin, F. A., & Cole, P. E. (1978). The real problem with 1-day diet records. *American Journal of Clinical Nutrition, 31,* 1114.
Gersovitz, M., Madden, J. P., & Smicklas-Wright, H. (1978). Validity of the 24-hour dietary recall and 7-day record for group comparison. *Journal of the American Dietetic Association, 73,* 48-55.
Gottlieb, N. H., & Chen, M. S. (1985). Sociocultural correlates of childhood sporting activities: Their implications for heart health. *Social Sciences and Medicine, 5,* 533-539.
Harper, L. V., & Sanders, K. M. (1975). The effects of adults' eating on young children's acceptance of unfamiliar foods. *Journal of Experimental Child Psychology, 20,* 206-214.
Hollingshead, A. B. (1965). *Two-factor index of social position.* New Haven, CT: Yale University Press.
Israel, A. C., & Saccone, A. J. (1979). Follow-up of effects of choice of mediator and target of reinforcement on weight loss. *Behavior Therapy, 10,* 260-265.
Israel, A. C., Stolmaker, L., Sharp, J. P., Silverman, W. K., & Simon, L. G. (1984). An evaluation of two methods of parental involvement in treating obese children. *Behavior Therapy, 15,* 266-272.
Jacobson, M., Liebman, B. F., & Moyer, G. (1983). *Salt. The brand name guide to sodium content.* New York: Workman.

Karlin, S., Williams, P. T., Farquhar, J. W., Barrett-Connor, E., Hoover, I., Wall, P. W., Haskell, W. L., Bergelin, R. O., & Suarez, L. (1982). Association arrays for the study of familial height, weight, lipid, and lipoprotein similarity in three west coast populations. *American Journal of Epidemiology, 116,* 1001-1021.

Kirks, B. A., & Hughes, C. (1986). Long-term behavioral effects of parent involvement in nutrition education. *Journal of Nutrition Education, 18,* 203-206.

Klesges, R. C., Malott, J. M., Boschee, P. F., & Weber, J. M. (1986). The effects of parental influences on children's food intake, physical activity, and relative weight. *International Journal of Obesity, 5,* 335-346.

Morrison, J. A., Namboodiri, K., Green, P., Martin, J., & Glueck, C. J. (1983). Familial aggregation of lipids and lipoproteins and early identification of dyslipoproteinemia. *Journal of the American Medical Association, 250,* 1860-1868.

Nader, P. R., Baranowski, T., Vanderpool, N., Dworkin, R. J., & Dunn, K. (1983). The Family Health Project: Cardiovascular risk reduction education for children and parents. *Journal of Developmental and Behavioral Pediatrics, 4,* 3-10.

Nader, P. R., Sallis, J. F., Patterson, T. L., Abramson, I., Rupp, J. W., Senn, K. L., Atkins, C. J., Roppé, B. E., Morris, J. A., Wallace, J. P., & Vega, W. A. (1989). A family approach to cardiovascular risk reduction: Results from the Family Health Project. *Health Education Quarterly, 16,* 225-240.

Nader, P. R., Sallis, J. F., Rupp, J., Atkins, C., Patterson, T. L., & Abramson, I. (1986). The San Diego Family Health Project: Reaching families through the schools. *Journal of School Health, 56,* 227-231.

Parcel, G., & Baranowski, T. (1981). Social learning theory and health education. *Health Education, 12,* 14-18.

Patterson, T. L., Kaplan, R. M., Sallis, J. F., & Nader, P. R. (1987). Aggregation of blood pressure in Anglo American and Mexican-American Families. *Preventive Medicine, 16,* 616-625.

Patterson, T. L., Rupp, J. W., Sallis, J. F., Atkins, C. J., & Nader, P. R. (1988). Aggregation of dietary calories, fats, and sodium in Mexican-American and Anglo families. *American Journal of Preventive Medicine, 4,* 75-92.

Patterson, T. L., Sallis, J. F., Kaplan, R. M., & Nader, P. R. (in press). Influence of physical activity and diet on aggregation of body mass index in Mexican-American and Anglo families. *Journal of Obesity and Weight Regulation.*

Pennington, J. A. T., & Church, H. N. (1980). *Food values of portions commonly used* (13th ed.). Philadelphia: Lippincott.

Remmell, P. S., Gorder, D. D., Hall, Y., & Tillotson, J. L. (1980). Assessing dietary adherence in the Multiple Risk Factor Intervention Trial. *Journal of the American Dietetic Association, 76,* 357-360.

Rosenthal, T., & Bandura, A. (1978). Psychological Modeling: Theory and Practice. In S. L. Garfield & A. E. Bergin (Eds.) *Handbook of psychotherapy and behavior change* (2nd ed., pp. 621-658). New York: Wiley.

Sallis, J. F., Haskell, W. L., Wood, P. D., Fortmann, S. P., Rogers, T., Blair, S. N., & Paffenbarger, R. S. (1985). Physical activity assessment methodology in the Five-City Project. *American Journal of Epidemiology, 121,* 91-106.

Sallis, J. F., Haskell, W. L., Fortmann, S. P., Vranizan, K. M., Taylor, C. B., & Solomon, D. S. (1986). Predictors of adoption and maintenance of physical activity in a community sample. *Preventive Medicine, 15,* 331-341.

Sallis, J. F., & Nader, P. R. (1988). Family determinants of health behaviors. In D. S. Gochman (Ed.), *Health behavior: Emerging research perspectives* (pp. 107-124). New York: Plenum Press.

Sallis, J. F., Patterson, T. L., Buono, M. J., Atkins, C. J., & Nader, P. R. (1988). Aggregation of physical activity habits in Mexican-American and Anglo families. *Journal of Behavioral Medicine, 11,* 31-41.

Taylor, C. B., Coffey, T., & Berra, K., Iaffaldano, R., Casey, K., & Haskell, W. L. (1984). Seven-day activity and self-report compared to a direct measure of physical activity. *American Journal of Epidemilogy, 120,* 818-824.

Vega, W. A., Sallis, J. F., Patterson, T. L., Rupp, J., Atkins, C., & Nader, P. R. (1987). Assessing knowledge of cardiovascular health related diet and exercise behaviors in Anglos and Mexican-Americans. *Preventive Medicine, 16,* 696-709.

Wallace, J., McKenzie, T., & Nader, P. R. (1985). Observed vs. recalled exercise behavior: A validation of the Blair seven day exercise recall for boys 11 to 13 years old. *Research Quarterly for Exercise and Sport, 56,* 161-165.

14

Anxiety in Parents Seeking Pediatric Care[1]

Joseph W. Hatcher, Anthony J. Richtsmeier, and Sharen Westin
University of Health Sciences/The Chicago Medical School and Cook County Hospital

Interviewed parents of 103 children brought to a pediatric walk-in clinic, before and after seeing a physician. Previsit state anxiety was minimally related to parent perceptions of child's condition or the hospital. Anxiety, perception of child's discomfort, and perception of illness severity decreased while perceived understanding of child's illness increased postvisit. Parent perceptions of their child's condition and of the visit contributed little to the prediction of postvisit anxiety. Parent perceptions of their child's illness and the hospital were minimally related to their level of state anxiety when they brought their child to an acute care service. The visit with the physician decreased parent anxiety and improved parent perceptions of their child's condition, but these effects had little relationship to postvisit anxiety.

Many parents seeking pediatric care for children with acute illness appear distressed or anxious. Parent anxiety has been identified as a major non-symptom variable that appears to influence parent's decision to seek pediatric care (Bass & Cohen, 1982; Becker, Nathanson, Drachman, & Kirscht,

[1]This study was funded in part by the Hektoen Institute for Medical Research of Cook County Hospital. Portions of these data were presented at the 8th annual scientific sessions of the Society of Behavioral Medicine, Washington, DC. Anthony Richtsmeier is now at Department of Pediatrics, Rush-Presbyterian-St. Luke's Medical Center, Chicago, Illinois. Sharen Westin is now at Department of Psychiatry, Harbor General Hospital, Torrance, California. We gratefully acknowledge Frank Flossman for assistance in data collection, Robert Miller for assistance in completion of the study, and Betsey Benson for comments on a draft of this manuscript.

1977; Korsch, Gozzi, & Francis, 1968; Levy, 1980; Turk, Litt, Salovey, & Walker, 1985). Some authors have concluded that parents are anxious due to worries about their child's illness or physical condition (Bass & Cohen, 1982; Levy, 1980; Schmidt, 1980). This conclusion may not be warranted, as the relationship of parent perceptions of their child's medical condition to their level of anxiety at the time of the visit to the pediatrician has not been assessed.

Roghmann and Haggerty (1973) found that the probability of utilization of medical services was greater during periods of family stress, independent of the occurrence of illness. Mechanic (1964) found that mothers under stress reported more illness symptoms for their children and used pediatric services more frequently. These studies indicate that distressed parents are more likely to seek acute pediatric care, but their anxiety may be a function of more than their child's medical condition. These studies do not, however, provide information about the relationship of parents' perceptions of a specific illness episode to their anxiety level when seeking acute care.

The present study tests the hypothesis that parent concerns about their child's physical condition are the central element in the anxiety of parents seeking pediatric care for their acutely ill child. The study was designed to assess the relationship of parents' perceptions of their child's physical condition and medical care to their level of anxiety at the time of an acute care pediatric visit. Assessments were made both before and after the pediatric visit, to indicate the impact of the visit on parent anxiety and perceptions of the child's condition.

METHOD

Subjects

Each subject was the parent or guardian of a child brought to the pediatric walk-in acute care service of a large county hospital. A total of 103 parents participated in the study. All subjects were the primary caretakers of the child brought to the clinic (89 mothers, 10 fathers, and 4 other relatives). The hospital serves a predominately minority indigent population and the study population was approximately 80% black, 10% Hispanic, and 10% white.

Measures

State-Trait Anxiety Inventory–State Scale (STAI-S). The STAI-S (Spielberger, 1983) is a 20-question self-report inventory which assesses anxiety at a particular moment in time.

Previsit Parent Questionnaire. This is a 6-item investigator-designed questionnaire assessing parent perceptions of their understanding of what is wrong with their child, the amount of discomfort experienced by their child, and several parent beliefs about the hospital (e.g., "I have confidence in this hospital."). Parents indicated their response to each item using a five- or seven-point Likert-scale format. (A copy of the complete Previsit Parent Questionnaire is available from the first author.)

Postvisit Parent Questionnaire. This is a 16-item investigator-designed questionnaire assessing parent perceptions of their understanding of what is wrong with their child, the severity of their child's illness, the amount of discomfort experienced by their child, their understanding and agreement with treatment plans, their satisfaction with the pediatric visit, and their perceptions of several aspects of the pediatric visit (e.g., "I think that the doctor is medically competent."). Parents indicated their response to each item using a five- or seven-point Likert-scale format. (A copy of the complete Postvisit Parent Questionnaire is available from the first author.)

Procedure

A trained research assistant approached the parents after they had registered at the clinic main desk and their child had been seen by the triage nurse. Parents were asked to participate in a study of their perceptions of the present clinic visit. In obtaining informed consent, each parent was assured that participation would not affect their child's medical care in any way and that their responses would be kept confidential. All children whose parents participated in this study were identified by the triage nurse as not needing emergency medical attention. Approximately 40% of the children were diagnosed by the examining physician to have an abnormality of the upper respiratory tract. Another 40% comprised diagnoses relating to the ears, lower respiratory tract, gastrointestinal tract, skin, or viral syndromes. The remainder consisted of a variety of infectious, neurologic, musculoskeletal, and other medical problems. One child presented for help with a behavior problem and one adolescent presented to evaluate a suspected pregnancy. Only one child was admitted to the hospital.

All parents were interviewed twice. The first interview took place while the parent and child were waiting to see the physician. It comprised the Previsit Parent Questionnaire and the STAI-S. The second interview took place immediately after the visit with the physician and comprised the Postvisit Parent Questionnaire and the STAI-S. During both interviews all items were read to the parent and their responses were recorded by the research assistant. All interviews took place between 8:00 a.m. and 8:00 p.m. on weekdays during late winter.

RESULTS

Previsit Anxiety

The distribution of the previsit STAI-S scores of the study population approached normality. The scores ranged from 20 to 68 ($M = 38.7$, $SD = 10.8$). When converted to t scores based on the norms for the STAI-S (Spielberger, 1983, pp. 5-7), the scores ranged from 35 to 79 ($M = 53$). This indicates there was a wide range in the previsit anxiety scores with relatively equal numbers of anxious and nonanxious parents in this study. The mean of the study sample was not significantly different from the normative sample ($z = 0.67$), indicating that the sample of parents in this study were not more anxious than a group of "normal" adults.

A stepwise multiple regression analysis was performed to assess the relationship of previsit parent perceptions to previsit parent state anxiety levels. The results of this analysis indicate that two of the independent variables, satisfaction with past visits to the hospital (beta weight. = .27) and perceived severity of their child's illness (beta weight. = .27), were significantly related to previsit anxiety, $R^2 = .13$, $F(2, 99) = 8.54$, $p < .001$. The combination of these two variables accounted for 13% of the variance in previsit state anxiety levels, with 7% predicted by perceived severity of the child's illness ($p < .001$).

Effects of Visit With Physician

To assess the effects of the visit on parent anxiety the pre- and postvisit state anxiety scores were compared using a t test. This analysis indicated a significant decrease in parent state anxiety after the visit with the pediatrician, $t(102) = 3.88$, $p < .0001$. *T* tests were also performed to assess changes in parent perceptions of their child's condition which might be associated with changes in parent anxiety. These analyses indicated a significant decrease from pre- to postvisit in parent perception of severity of their child's illness, $t(102) = 5.06$, $p < .0001$, and parent perception of the amount of discomfort their child is experiencing, $t(102) = 2.57$, $p < .012$. In addition, there was a significant improvement in parent self-rated understanding of their child's illness from pre- to postvisit, $t(102) = 3.38$, $p < .001$.

Postvisit Anxiety

A stepwise multiple regression analysis was performed to assess the relationship of postvisit parent perceptions to postvisit state anxiety. To assess the impact of the parents' level of previsit anxiety, it was included in this analysis. This analysis indicated that three independent variables, previsit anxiety (beta weight = .49), overall satisfaction with the visit (beta weight = .23), and postvisit perception of child discomfort (beta weight = .16), were significantly related to postvisit anxiety, $R^2 = .38$, $F(3, 98) = 8.65$, $p < .001$. The combination of these three variables accounted for 38% of the variance in postvisit state anxiety scores. Thirty-one percent of the variance was predicted by previsit anxiety ($p < .001$), 5% of the variance was predicted by satisfaction with the visit ($p < .001$), and 2% of the variance was predicted by parent perceptions of the degree of their child's discomfort ($p < .001$).

DISCUSSION

The results of this study indicate that parent satisfaction with past visits to the hospital and perception of the severity of their child's illness are significantly related to the level of state anxiety present while they wait with their ill child to see the physician. The parents who were less satisfied with past visits and perceived their child as more seriously ill tended to be more anxious before seeing the physician. These perceptions, however, account for only a small portion (13%) of the total variance in previsit anxiety.

The visit with the physician did have a positive impact on parent anxiety. Pre- to postvisit improvements were also noted in parent perceptions of their child's discomfort, the severity of the child's symptoms, and self-rated understanding of the child's illness. These improved postvisit perceptions, however, had little relationship to postvisit anxiety. These results present an interesting picture. The pediatric visit reduces parent anxiety and improves parent perceptions, but both pre- and postvisit anxiety have little relationship to parental perceptions of their child's current medical condition.

Roghmann and Haggerty (1973) found that quickly accessible sources of medical contact, similar to the emergency room setting of the present study, are used more often at times of increased parent stress. This suggests that the group of parents in the present study could be a highly stressed population. The distribution of the previsit state anxiety scores was not indicative, however, of a highly stressed population.

Interviews of parents seeking pediatric care could be susceptible to response bias or social demand characteristics of the interview situation. The distribution of parent responses to each of the interview items inquiring about their child's medical condition approached normality, suggesting that the parents did not represent their children's condition to the interviewer in a biased manner. Thus, it appears that response bias and social demand characteristics do not limit the interpretation of the present results.

A broader approach in the assessment of parent anxiety, sampling more than one response channel, could prove useful. Future work should also examine the relationship of other parent perceptions, such as their perceived ability to care for an ill child and the presence of family stressors, to parent anxiety when seeking pediatric care.

The modest relationship of previsit parent beliefs about their child's condition to previsit anxiety fails to support the hypothesis that parent concerns about their child's medical condition are the central element in the anxiety of parents seeking pediatric care. The weak relationship of postvisit anxiety to postvisit perceptions strengthens this conclusion. State anxiety is seldom the product of a single stressor, but such a modest relationship is surprising. It appears that, for the more anxious parents, an ill child may be just one hassle out of many.

REFERENCES

Bass, L. W., & Cohen, R. L. (1982). Ostensible versus actual reasons for seeking pediatric attention: Another look at the parental ticket of admission. *Pediatrics, 70,* 870-874.

Becker, M. H., Nathanson, C. A., Drachman, R. H., & Kirscht, J. P. (1977). Mother's health beliefs and children's clinic visits: A prospective study. *Journal of Community Health, 3,* 125-135.

Korsch, B. M., Gozzi, E. K., & Francis, V. (1968). Gaps in doctor-patient communication: I. Doctor-patient interaction and patient satisfaction. *Pediatrics, 42,* 855-871.

Levy, J. C. (1980). Vulnerable children: Parent's perspectives and the use of medical care. *Pediatrics, 65,* 956-963.

Mechanic, D. (1964). The influence of mothers on their children's health attitudes and behavior. *Pediatrics, 33,* 444-453.

Roghmann, K. J., & Haggerty, R. J. (1973). Daily stress, illness, and use of health services in young families. *Pediatrics Research, 7,* 520-526.

Schmidt, B. D. (1980). Fever phobia: Misconceptions of parents about fever. *American Journal of Diseases of Children, 134,* 176-181.

Spielberger, C. D. (1983). *Manual for the state-trait anxiety inventory (Form Y).* Palo Alto, CA: Consulting Psychologists Press.

Turk, D. C., Litt, M. D., Salovey, P., & Walker, J. (1985). Seeking urgent pediatric treatment: Factors contributing to frequency, delay, and appropriateness. *Health Psychology, 4,* 43-60.

IV

A THEORETICAL PERSPECTIVE

15

Family Context in Pediatric Psychology: A Transactional Perspective

Barbara H. Fiese
Syracuse University

Arnold J. Sameroff
Brown University, Bradley Hospital

The degree to which the family is seen as a significant contributor to child health conditions impacts directly on the successful functioning of the pediatric psychologist. A transactional model of family functioning is proposed for pediatric psychology. Development is considered to be the result of a three-part process that starts with child behavior that triggers family interpretation that produces a parental response. Family interpretation is presented as part of a regulatory system that includes family paradigms, family stories, and family rituals. Corresponding to the proposed three-part regulation model, three forms of intervention are discussed: remediation, redefinition, and reeducation. Clinical decision making based on this model is outlined with examples given from different treatment approaches. Implications for the treatment of families in pediatric psychology are discussed.

Pediatric psychologists' treatment of children is often the treatment of families as well. Whether providing consultation to families under the stress of parenting a child with a chronic condition or providing direct services to children with psychosomatic complaints the family is often the most immediate and effective mediator of change and will be responsible for maintaining changes once the psychologist is no longer involved in treatment of the child. How pediatric psychologists think about families, what they consider the relation between the child's symptom and the family's functioning, and at what point the family is engaged in treatment directly influences the functioning of the pediatric psychologist. This paper is offered as a theoretical framework for understanding the family context in pediatric psychology. Hopefully, the model presented will enhance the pediatric psychologists treatment of children.

This emphasis is in line with the concern of health psychology with the role of family support in changing health behaviors (e.g., Baranowski & Nader, 1985) and the role of the family in maintaining illness symptoms (e.g., Jacob & Sielhammer, 1987). Pediatric psychology as a field has conceptualized the family from two broad perspectives: (a) the impact of childhood illnesses on the family and (b) the impact of the family on illness and disease symptoms. In the first instance a normally functioning family must adapt to stressful biological conditions in the child. How family members react to the birth of a handicapped infant (Affleck, McGrade, Allen, & McQueeney, 1985; Drotar, Baskiewicz, Irvin, Kennell, & Klaus, 1975; Roskies, 1972), how family members cope with children with terminal illness (Spinetta & Deasy-Spinetta, 1981; Spinetta, Swarner, & Sheposh, 1981), or how family members respond to the stress of a child with an acute medical condition (Cella, Perry, Poag, Amand & Goodwin, 1988; Melamed & Bush, 1985) are representative of this perspective. The family is considered by the pediatric psychologist to be capable of adequate functioning under normal conditions but may be in need of psychological intervention because of a special biological condition in the child.

The second perspective on family functioning prevalent in pediatric psychology is centered on the role the family plays in contributing to or maintaining a maladaptive biological condition in the child. The family has often been considered the breeding ground for somatic complaints. The classic example of Minuchin's psychosomatic families highlights this approach (Minuchin et al., 1975). According to Minuchin and colleagues, a child's physical symptom (e.g., "brittle" diabetes, psychosomatic asthma, or anorexia) is a response to conflict in families that can be described as enmeshed, overprotective, and rigid.

From a family systems perspective the child's symptom is a resolution of family attempts to avoid conflict and maintain peace in the family. The source of the symptom is moved from the individual taken alone to the family taken together. A family systems perspective emphasizes the role of family dynamics in symptom maintenance. Treatment is aimed at changing maladaptive family interaction patterns. A wide range of somatization disorders have been treated as family system problems (Routh & Ernst, 1984).

The distinction between the impact of the family on illness and the impact of illness on the family may be useful in cataloguing family factors in pediatric psychology; however, this distinction has provided little useful information for diagnosis or intervention. In distinguishing between conditions that may be considered primarily biological in origin or primarily psychological in origin the family is conceptualized as either reacting to or contributing to the child's symptomatology. Yet the disease process is rarely the result of a single factor nor do families function under single operating principles. If the family is considered only as a reactor to the child, there is little room to consider family process or organization as contributors to the child's condition.

It is surprising how sparse the pediatric literature is in regard to empirical evidence connecting family functioning and pediatric illness. There have been only a few attempts to specify organizational aspects of family functioning and its relation to pediatric illness. For example, communication patterns in families with recently diagnosed diabetics have been related to child adaptation (Hauser et al., 1986). This scarcity of research may be due in part to models that consider illness akin to a simple infectious disease process. Our view is that disease is rarely the result of a single cause but a complex interaction of several systems. The systemic properties of the disease process may be directly extended to understanding how the system of the family relates to the child's condition.

DISEASE AND CONTEXT

In its classic form, the medical model assumes that there is a single cause for a single disease (Engel, 1977). Infections, genetic abnormalities, or traumatic incidents are seen as direct causes of medical conditions. However, it is rare that there is a single cause in the majority of diseases. For example, exposure to the chicken pox virus should produce chicken pox. However, if the child has already had the chicken pox, he or she is immune and will show no consequences to the new exposure. Although the necessary virus may be present it is not sufficient for disease expression unless a context exists that can support the disease. Necessary and sufficient conditions for disease expression become even more complex when considering the psychological impact on biological conditions and, conversely, the impact of biological conditions on psychological processes.

Attempts at understanding the role of psychological processes and the course of disease has developed within the framework of identifying particular risk factors that may be associated with higher incidence of disease. The diathesis-stress model (Rosenthal, 1970) has been popular in explaining why certain individuals are more prone to certain health conditions. The vulnerability alone is not sufficient to explain a disorder without taking account of the stress in the environment. In adult health psychology, the linking of Type A behavior with heart attacks was seen as evidence that a personality type may cause a heart attack. However, recently it has been demonstrated that the personality type taken alone may not cause the heart attack. A host of contextual factors contribute to the recurrence of heart attacks. In fact, under some conditions Type A individuals may have a lower mortality rate if they survive the heart attack within the first 24 hours (Ragland & Brand, 1988).

Another single cause theory of disorder links stressful job conditions to coronary heart disease. However, when the job is perceived as stressful the prediction is enhanced (LaCroix & Haynes, 1987). Even in mice individual levels of physical risk, such as high cholesterol or high blood pressure, may not predict coronary heart disease as much as the controllability of the condition in which the animals are raised (Kaplan et al., 1983).

The current controversy over the critical components of Type A behavior pattern and the relation to heart disease may be resolved in part by incorporating contextual features such as occupational strain and psychophysiological reactivity along with crucial Type A behaviors (Krantz, Contrada, Hill, & Friedler, 1988). Although there is considerable controversy over the relation between Type A personality and chronic heart disease (Wright, 1988) there does seem to be agreement that the relationship is not a simple one and involves a complex interaction of individual risk factors, biological responsivity, and environmental context (Matthews & Haynes, 1986). A consistent conclusion of epidemiological and observational studies is that those factors considered risk factors for heart disease (e.g., smoking, obesity, Type A behavior pattern, psychophysiological stress) do not operate in isolation and, in fact, are very poor predictors of the occurrence of disease in the individual. In addition, focusing on single personality factors has proven relatively weak in attempts to predict adult behavior from child behavior patterns (Steinberger, 1986).

In pediatric psychology, the case of childhood asthma may be used to illustrate the complex system of personality and illness symptoms. Traditionally asthma has been considered a disease that is affected not only by emotional and personality factors but may also have a neurotic or emotional origin (Pearlman, 1984). If a simple relationship existed between emotional factors and asthmatic attacks then attacks should be preceded by an identifiable emotional arousal. In an extensive series of studies, Creer (1979, 1982) demonstrated that the emotional component of asthmatic attacks may be either a trigger for an attack or a response to the attack triggered by organic allergens such as pollen or dust. In addition, the intermittent nature of asthmatic attacks results in distinct coping styles of parents and children depending on the cyclicity of the child's attacks (Renne & Creer, 1985). Furthermore, the parents', and not the physicians', evaluation of the seriousness of the child's condition and probable triggers influences compliance to medical regimens and management of the disease (Deaton, 1985; Deaton & Olbrisch, 1987). If there is a strong emotional component to asthma then asthmatic children should be at a higher risk for emotional disturbances, yet there is very little evidence to support this contention (Creer, Harm, & Marion, 1988).

In order to resolve the paradox of whether the cause of illness is in environmental risk factors or individual behavior, a different theory of illness must be developed which takes into account the complex dynamics of disease processes. One such view that has been proposed is the transactional model outlined by Sameroff and Chandler (1975). We hope to demonstrate that this model can be directly applied to understanding illnesses seen in pediatric psychology, particularly as it relates to the family's role in child health problems.

TRANSACTIONAL MODEL

Placing the child's illness within the context of the family calls for a theory of context. The social ecology of Bronfenbrenner (1977) has been useful for describing the nested hierarchy of family and societal contexts (Belsky, 1980). From an ecological perspective, the family and child are part of a larger system including societal influences, socioeconomic factors, and current living conditions. Although an ecological perspective sensitizes us to the complexity of interaction between the child and the family system it has not been used to generate explicit assessment and intervention models for pediatric psychology. One proposal that adds a developmental dimension to the ecological perspective is the transactional model proposed by Sameroff and Chandler (1975).

The transactional model places the child in a dynamic system that is maintained by bidirectional influences between the child's and the family's behavior. One of the more important aspects of the transactional model was the emphasis placed on the effect of the child on the environment, as a complement to the more traditional unidirectional view that only saw the family's effect on the child. The experiences provided by the environment were not independent of the child. The child by his or her previous behavior may have been a strong determinant of current experiences. The child's environment includes not only the proximal environment of interaction between parent and child but also the more distal family and cultural environment in which the child is embedded. A diagram of the transactional model can be seen in Figure 1 (Sameroff, 1987a).

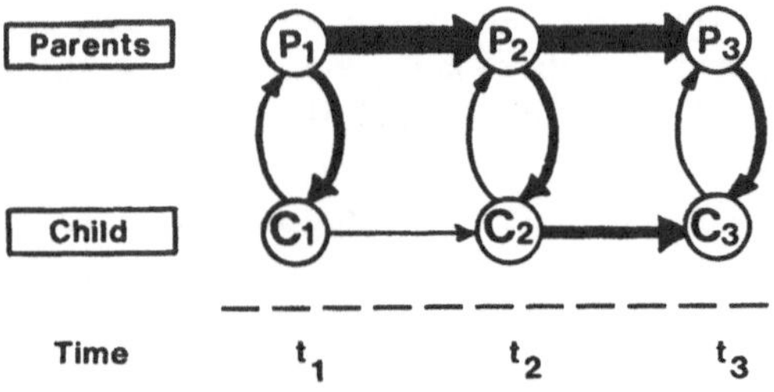

Fig. 1. Social regulatory model of development.

The child's outcome at a point in time (Cn) is neither a function of the initial state of the child (C1) nor the initial state of the environment (E1), but a complex function of the interplay of child and environment over time. A number of empirically validated examples of transactional processes in development have been described by Sameroff (1986, 1987b).

A transactional perspective has been recognized as central in understanding health-related issues in the family (Turk & Kerns, 1985). Patterson (1986) and his colleagues (Patterson & Bank, 1989) examined the origins of antisocial behavior in childhood using a transactional model. Pediatric psychologists are often called to consult on cases where the child's behavior is considered "out of hand" by parents and health professionals alike. Patterson argued that the lack of success in controlling the child's behavior may be due in part to a history of negative transactions between parent and child.

In the Patterson model, children normally engage in some proportion of noncompliance activities. If the parents are inept in disciplining their child, they create a context where the child is reinforced for learning a set of coercive behaviors. Parent ineptitude is characterized by a lack of monitoring, harsh discipline, lack of positive reinforcement, and lack of parental involvement with the child. The child develops noncompliant behaviors such as whining, teasing, yelling, and disapproval. These behaviors escalate parental negative coercive responses that promote further child noncompliance eventuating in high-amplitude aggressive behaviors, including physical attack. The high use of noncompliance with inept parents does not permit the child to learn a set of social strategies that are necessary with peers and in the school. When these aggressive noncompliant children enter the school setting they elicit poor peer acceptance that maintains poor self-esteem and poor academic performance. This constellation of antisocial behavior, poor peer relations, and poor school achievement has been demonstrated by Patterson to unfold in the developmental sequence of transactions described above (see Figure 2). The child's initial noncompliance does not lead directly to antisocial behavior, rather it is the inept parenting response that transactionally

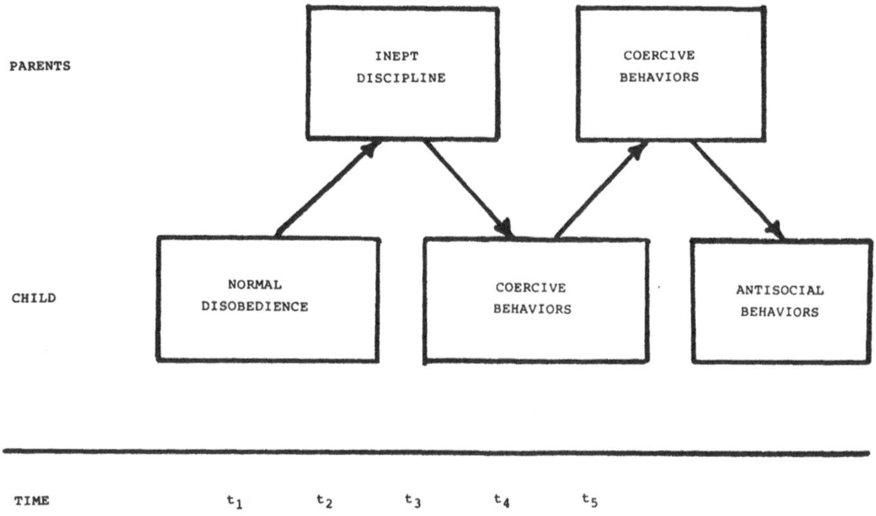

Fig. 2. Transactions leading to antisocial behavior. (Adapted from Patterson, 1986.)

converts age-appropriate expressions of autonomy into a coercive interactive style (Patterson & Bank, 1989).

Transactions have been hypothesized to produce adaptive responses in families with recently diagnosed diabetics (Hauser et al., 1986). Interactions were coded along dimensions of enabling and constraining behaviors while the family was engaged in a discussion about an issue on which they differed. The results of this cross-sectional study revealed significant differences between the families with a diabetic child and families with an acutely ill child. The families with a diabetic child engaged in more enabling interaction patterns, such as focusing, problem solving, and active understanding than the families with an acutely ill child. This pattern was particularly evident in mothers of diabetic children.

Hauser explained these group differences as a transaction between the child's illness and the parents' (particularly the mother's) reaction to the child's needs. From a transactional perspective, the diagnosis of diabetes influences the mother to become more involved with the child and perhaps express more focusing and problem-solving behaviors because she perceives the child as more vulnerable. The child, in turn, responds to this concern by higher levels of focusing, problem solving, and possibly a belief that compliance will alleviate some of the pain of a chronic illness. This pattern is in contrast to the lack of transactions in acutely ill families where there is not the perceived long-term vulnerability of the child. Acutely ill families are less likely to engage in enabling behaviors and less likely to engage in active understanding.

This difference may be due in part to less perceived threat to long-term functioning within the family. It is important to note that the patterns described by Hauser are patterns typical of diabetics under good diabetic control. In families where diabetic control is an issue it is possible that less enabling interaction patterns are evident (Fiese & Mead, 1988). Producing such changes is the goal of a redefinition strategy of transactional intervention described below.

A transactional perspective takes into account the influence of the child on the family and places an emphasis on the ways in which the family and child mutually create a context for disease expression. Thus far we have focused on how the family in general may transact with identifiable conditions in the child. We now turn to an examination of how the family context is organized and how specific components participate in transactional processes.

FAMILY CODE

From an ecological and transactional perspective, as children grow they are embedded in an increasing number of contexts that serve to regulate their development (Sameroff & Fiese, in press-a). It is important to recognize that individual behavior is always constrained by environmental structures, each with their own purposes. To the family is added the school and peer group within an overarching cultural and social system. Society regulates the family's behavior by statutes and normative rules. This cultural code may include regulations that insure optimal health for the general population. For example, every child is required to be immunized before attending public school and parents are not allowed to abuse their children. The family's compliance to these regulations is in part a compliance to the cultural code.

As society regulates family and child behavior through various levels of normative consensus in a cultural code, the family regulates the child's development through a variety of forms that make up the family code. The family code dictates the expected behavior of the child and family in a variety of situations. The family code is constructed in such a way that it incorporates the family's overall belief system or general view of the world, the family's definition of itself as distinct from other families, and finally the structure or organization of the family's daily routines. The family code may be considered a system of family definitions that are used as guidelines for the family's behavior. Following Reiss (1989) we have found three areas to be useful in constructing the family code: family paradigms, family stories, and family rituals (Sameroff & Fiese, in press-b). Family paradigms are global belief systems that define the social world for the family. Family stories include the transmission of values and define how one family is different than

FAMILY CODE

COMPONENT	DEFINING PRINCIPLE
Paradigm	How social world works.
Stories/Myths	How our family is different from other families in the social world.
Rituals	How our family works in the social world.

Fig. 3. Components of the family code.

other families. Finally, family rituals define how the family works and provide guidelines for the organization of the family's daily routines. A brief outline of the three components of the family code is presented in Figure 3. Each of these forms of regulation within the family vary along dimensions of articulation and accessibility to individual members of the family. We present a conceptual framework for understanding this family code as it pertains to pediatric psychology.

Family Paradigms

Family paradigms are the most general of the family regulations and the most difficult for family members to articulate. Family paradigms include a set of core assumptions, convictions, or beliefs that each family member holds about its environment (Reiss, 1981, 1989; Reiss, Oliveri, & Curd, 1983). Family paradigms dictate how the family sees "the relative safety and stability of the social world, the degree to which it is experienced as novel or precedented by past experiences, and the conviction that it treats the family as an integrated unit or as a group of unrelated individuals" (Reiss, 1989). The family paradigm regulates how individuals interact not only within the family but with members outside of the family.

The family paradigm is of interest to pediatric psychologists in at least two important areas: (a) how families understand their relation to health professionals in general, and (b) how families understand their child's medical condition. In the first instance, Reiss (1981; Reiss et al., 1983) identified a typology of family paradigms including environment-sensitive and distance-sensitive families. Environment-sensitive families are characterized by a tendency to organize cooperatively and to fully investigate subtleties in social information before coming to a family agreement. Distance-sensitive families, on the other hand, are described as isolated in a private world with little venturing out of the family context for problem solving.

What is particularly interesting is how these family paradigms may be related to how the family reacts to health professionals. In a study of degree of engagement in psychological treatment of adolescents, Reiss et al. (1983) found that environment-sensitive families with adolescents became more engaged in treatment than distance-sensitive families. In this regard, the importance of the family paradigm dictates, in part, how the family makes use of health professionals involved in their care.

A second aspect of the family paradigm important for pediatric psychologists is how the family paradigm may impact on the family's interaction with a child with a medical condition. There has been increasing interest in how parenting beliefs about children's development, in general (Sameroff & Feil, 1985; Sigel, 1985), and parents' beliefs about their own children's behavior, in specific (Dix, Ruble, Grusec, & Nixon, 1986), may influence parenting. In an extensive review of the literature, Goodnow (1988) outlined the multiple ways in which parenting beliefs may originate and may influence child behavior. Pertinent to the area of pediatric psychology is the family's belief about the cause of their child's medical condition. Affleck and Tennen (1988; Affleck et al., 1985) have described how parental beliefs about a child's disability influence parenting behaviors with the child. Mothers who blame others for their child's developmental disability are more likely to report caretaking difficulties and be less sensitive to their child than mothers who believe that they themselves are in part responsible for the child's condition. Affleck and colleagues described a complex set of results which may be explained by the parent's degree of willingness to attribute blame to themselves and associated coping patterns. It is also possible that a family paradigm that sees the world as threatening and blames others for family problems may be less likely to incorporate a disabled child and subsequently perceive the caretaking as more difficult.

Pediatric psychologists should consider how the family paradigm influences the family's view of the child's condition as well as how the family may react to health professionals.

Family Stories

A second form of family regulation is family stories. Family stories can be highly articulated and may be passed down from generation to generation. These stories may provide a context in which children learn family roles as well as family values. Although the act of storytelling can be differentiated in function from the content of stories (Reiss, 1989; Sameroff & Fiese, in press-b), it is the content that may be particularly important in pediatric psychology. Zeitlin, Kotkin, and Baker (1982) collected a large number of family stories and proposed that family stories may serve three broad functions: (a) to highlight conspicuous heroes or rogues in the family's history,

(b) to dramatize and conserve significant family transitions and stressful events, and (c) to enshrine and preserve certain family customs. Family stories may prove to be a rich source of family information for the pediatric psychologist. During the routine of clinical interviews, family members often offer a family story as a way of highlighting the ways in which the family responds to stressful conditions. For example, a story of loss may be told following a suicide attempt by a child; a story of survival may be told following the diagnosis of a chronic disease; or a story about the energy of an uncle may be told following a diagnosis of hyperactivity. Although family stories are spontaneously offered during routine clinical interviews and have been the subject of speculation and case studies (Byng-Hall, 1988; Carlson, 1981), they have not been the focus of controlled studies. A fruitful direction for future study may be to investigate how family stories provide family regulation. Such analyses may be particularly important in those illnesses where there is a strong generational component such as hereditary diseases (e.g., diabetes, asthma, or coronary heart disease) or high risk conditions that tend to recur across generations such as adolescent pregnancy.

Family stories may be based on the recounting of actual events as a means of transmitting values, assigning roles, and preserving family customs. Although a grain of truth is probably present in most family stories, they may become distorted, at which time family myths develop.

Myths. Family myths are beliefs that go unchallenged in spite of reality (Lewis & Beavers, 1976). For example a well-educated scientist may hold onto a family myth that his sister's tuberculosis was caused by "bad water" when she went away to college (Zeitlin et al., 1982). Myths may have a traumatic origin as well as strong affective component (Kramer, 1985). Family myths are not open for discussion nor are they readily recognized as distortions (Ferreira, 1963). Some family myths help to regulate role definitions. For example, a traditional family may consider females as unable to handle professional responsibilities of the work world despite the fact that they are able to organize a busy household. Family myths may serve a regulatory function through processes like role inflation. Subtle aspects of a particular role may become inflated and incorporated into the myth. For example, parents of a handicapped child may believe that the child is also cognitively handicapped despite examples of the child's intelligent behavior. A myth develops that casts the child in a "handicapped" role that encompasses behavior outside of physical limitation. In the same context, another family may create a myth that their mentally retarded child is unimpaired because of a bright-eyed look (Pollner & McDonald-Wilker, 1985; Roskies, 1972). Family myths are important in pediatric psychology because they may dictate a family's behavior in managing diseases. For example, the decision for independent management of the diabetic regimen is frequently based on the child's age rather than behavior (Ingersoll, Orr, Herrold, & Golden, 1986). A myth develops within the family that responsible management is in accordance with age and not the individual development of the child. Family myths may have detrimental effects in that they are rarely modified by the behavior of the targeted individuals.

Family Rituals

A third form of family regulation is family rituals. Family rituals are the most clearly self-aware of the family regulatory forms (Bossard & Boll, 1950). Rituals are practiced by the whole family and frequently documented. Rituals may regulate role definition in the context of family routines and activities (Wolin & Bennett, 1984). For example, at Thanksgiving the family member who sits at the head of the table and carves the turkey may be seen as the head of the clan. In order to participate in the ritual each family member must conform to the specific characteristics of the role.

Family rituals may provide a buffer against stressful situations in the family and protect family members from disruptive influences of other family members. Bennett, Wolin, Reiss, and Teitelbaum (1987) have demonstrated that families of alcoholics who are able to maintain distinctive family rituals at dinnertime are less likely to transmit alcoholism to the next generation. In a similar vein, families with diabetic children who maintain clear routines and regularly engage in social and recreational family activities have fewer behavioral problems than families that do not maintain regular routines (Wertlieb, Hauser, & Jacobson, 1986). In addition family organization may also be predictive of perceived competence in adolescent diabetics (Hauser, Jacobson, Wertlieb, Brink, & Wentworth, 1985).

REGULATIONS

The description of the family code presented above outlines different aspects of family life that may contribute to disturbances in pediatric populations. The particular aspect of a family that is disrupted may call for a different form of intervention. The forms of family practice are directed at regulating many aspects of the child's development. We have found it helpful to classify regulations into categories based on the duration of their consequences.

The longest time cycle is associated with macroregulations that are a part of a culture's and family's developmental agenda for the child. The developmental agenda is a series of points in time when the environment is restructured to provide different experiences to the child. Age of weaning, toilet-training, schooling, initiation rites, and marriage are coded differently in each culture, but provide the basis for socialization. Macroregulations set the guidelines for the family in terms of what is expected for children in general.

On a more repetitive and shorter time base are miniregulations that include the care-giving activities of the child's family. Such activities are feeding children when they are hungry, changing diapers when they are wet, keeping children warm, and maintaining discipline.

On the shortest time frame are microregulations that refer to the momentary interactions between child and care-giver that others have referred to as "behavioral synchrony" or "attunement" (Field, 1979; Stern, 1977) and are generally not consciously determined actions.

These three sources of regulation operate predominately at different levels of the developmental system. Within the cultural code, macroregulations are the modal form of regulations. Statutes, customs, mores, and fashions are passed down to caretaking members of society to aid in regulating the child's socialization and educational development. Macroregulations are known to most members of society and are rarely the source of disturbances in healthy families.

Miniregulations are the routines and caretaking practices the family develops in interaction with the cultural code. This form of regulation includes aspects of family stories, myths, and rituals that aid in daily care of the child. The relation between cultural macroregulations and the family miniregulations may be harmonious or disturbed. Disturbances may arise when the family's caretaking routines do not fit with the cultural code, as when the family is too severe in its punishment of the child or too lax in letting children become disturbers of the peace. Disturbances may also arise when the family code conflicts with the individual parent's regulatory code as when a parent may be too depressed or too busy earning a living to engage in appropriate child-rearing.

The individual behavior of the parent is constrained by microregulations that generally operate out of awareness of the individuals. The unique style that each individual brings to the family code aids in defining the individual characteristics of parents and children. Disturbances may arise when the individual characteristics of the parents or children do not fit with the family code or the family code cannot incorporate an unique aspect of the child.

MODES OF PEDIATRIC INTERVENTION

Based on the model proposed, we would like to outline how the family code and regulation model interact and how this model would facilitate intervention and treatment programs within a transactional framework. In a previous paper we described how the cultural, family, and individual codes interface with the macro-, mini-, and microregulations and suggested various forms of intervention in infancy and early childhood (Sameroff & Fiese, in press-a). Within the scope of this paper we would like to outline primarily interventions targeted for families with caretaking disruptions.

Each step in development is considered the result of a three-part process. The first part is the behavior of the child that triggers environmental response. This trigger could be as simple as a cry or as complex as a college grade report. The second part is the environmental interpretation of the child's behavior. In the case of the cry, the interpretation could be that the child is hungry or that the child is angry. In the case of college grades, the interpretation could be that the student is outstanding or flunking. The third part is the change in experience given the child after the interpretation is made. In the case of the cry, the response to one interpretation might be feeding, but the response to the other might be punishment. In the case of the college student, the response to both kinds of grades report might be to free the student from attending classes, but in one case the mechanism might be dismissal to the work force whereas in the other it might be admission to an honors program of independent study.

The intervention strategies suggested are targeted to one of the three parts described above for developmental tranactions. They are aimed at improving parent–child interaction by (a) changing the child's triggering behavior, (b) changing the parent's interpretation of the child's behavior, or (c) changing the parent's repertoire of responses to the child. For simplicity these forms of intervention have been labeled remediation, redefinition, and reeducation (Sameroff, 1987a). A schematic representation of the correspondence between the three intervention strategies and the three-part transactional model is presented in Figure 4.

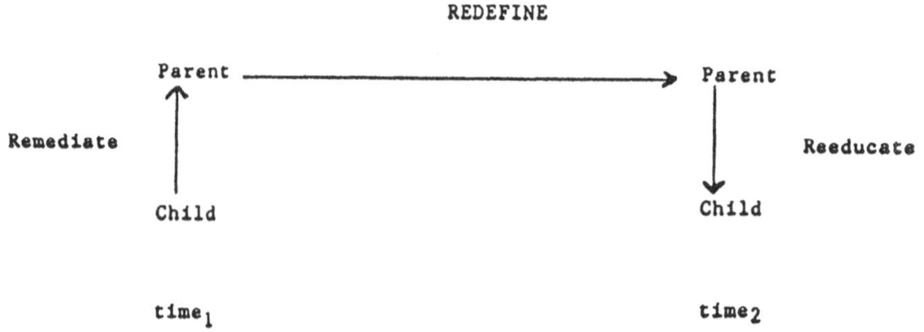

Fig. 4. Three R's of intervention in a transactional model.

Remediation

The strategy of remediation is the intervention aimed at changing the child. This strategy is based on the possibility that the child's condition can be altered and that routine caretaking may proceed once the child's condition has been changed. Frequently, this form of intervention involves repairing an impairment in the child's biological condition. Left alone, this condition would compromise the child's health and the family's ability to raise the child. The case of providing supplemental stimulation to premature infants is a case in point.

Feeding difficulties in premature infants present the pediatric psychologist with a particular challenge in dealing with parents. Initially, feedings are regulated through nasogastric tubes which may prevent the infant from developing normal sucking responses. In order for the family to better care for the child, a more normative feeding context must occur. Bernbaum, Peneira, Watkins, and Peckham (1983) have demonstrated that by pairing nonnutritive sucking during gavage feedings, premature infants gained weight more rapidly than infants who did not receive oral stimulation. The orally stimulated infants were discharged from the hospital sooner and were able to normalize their feeding patterns earlier and may have had fewer discrepant effects on their parents. Als et al., (1986) have demonstrated that individualized treatment of the premature infant is associated with higher degrees of social turn-taking, interactional synchrony, and overall quality of the interaction with their mothers during a free play session at 9 months of age. The remediation of the child as a neonate may have facilitated the parents' sensitivity in interacting with their child at a later age. In this regard, even though an intervention was targeted for the child it may have had positive effects on the family as a whole. An intervention administered by an oral-motor stimulation expert may actually be seen as part of the family treatment team.

There are other examples of altering the child's condition which may have an impact on the family functioning such as prescribing psychostimulants for hyperactive children which may have a positive impact on parenting interactions (Barkley, 1988).

Redefinition

Whereas remediation is indicated when the child's condition can be altered with subsequent effects on the parents, redefinition is indicated when the child's individual behavior cannot be altered and does not fit within the expectations of the family code. Occasionally the child is not incorporated into the family system due to some physical condition. For example, parents of handicapped children may engage in parenting activities based on their expectations rather than on the child's behavior (Maccoby & Martin, 1983; Minde, Brown, & Whitelaw, 1981). In this case, the family code includes only responses to normal developmental milestones regardless of the child's condition. Redefinition efforts are then directed towards expanding the family's code to include responses to a slower rate or different form of development.

Family rituals might have to be redefined in the case of children with chronic illness. A physically active family may have to redefine roles and routines to allow a child with cystic fibrosis to participate in family routines (Bronheim, 1978).

The need to redefine the child for the family occurs frequently when the child's condition does not fit readily into the family code. Redefinition may also be necessary when the parent's past parenting experiences impact on the child. For example, stories of health and illness in the parent's family may influence current caretaking practices. The family's beliefs about health-related behaviors may be passed down through the generations and have a significant impact on the child's overall health status (e.g., Epstein, Wing, Koeske, & Valoski, 1986). Family health beliefs also are related to compliance with medical regimens (Deaton & Olbrisch, 1987) and the degree to which parents will engage in preventive health measures (Becker et al., 1978).

Redefinition may require the alteration or elimination of family myths. In the case of diabetic adolescents, parents may base expectations of responsibility for independent management on age rather than on the child's behavior. The child may then interpret the parents' encouragement of independence as rejection and poor diabetic management results (Fiese & Mead, 1988). Overprotection or underprotection in diabetic families may result from myths surrounding the child's ability to manage their diabetes (Johnson, 1988; Parker, 1983).

The strategy of redefinition is indicated when parents do not admit the child into their caretaking system. Redefinition is a reasonable strategy when the parents know the cultural code and have adequate child-raising skills. However, in cases where the parents do not know the code or have inadequate skills, a third form of intervention is indicated: reeducation.

Reeducation

Reeducation is often the first line of intervention in families with children with illness. Educating families about diabetic regimens, asthmatic controls, breathing routines in cystic fibrosis, all involve learning a new set of routines and skills. Some degree of reeducation is necessary for any family with a child with a given condition. Educational programs have been demonstrated to be effective in early stages of disease acceptance and minimize family disruption (Johnson, 1988).

The effectiveness of educating parents in the treatment of obesity has been demonstrated in numerous studies (e.g., Epstein, 1985; Epstein, Wing, Koeske, Andrasik, & Ossip, 1981). Education efforts directed towards parents may have a positive effect on the child's weight loss particularly when it is paired with active problem solving as well as dietary information (Graves, Meyers, & Clark, 1988).

CLINICAL DECISION MAKING

The three transactional intervention strategies outlined above may be summarized in a decision tree aimed at aiding families of children with illnesses (see Figure 5). In most cases, the child is presented as having a problem. An initial question to ask is whether the child is treatable; that is, does the child have an identifiable condition that is subject to direct treatment so that the family is better able to care for the child. Examples of such treatment are providing supplemental stimulation to a premature infant for better feeding behavior, or prescribing medication for a hyperactive child. If the answer is yes, remediation is then indicated. Remediation is often in the purview of medical professionals such as pediatricians, occupational therapists, physical therapists, and nurses. Once the child's condition has been remediated there may be little continued disruption in the family.

If, however, the child's condition is not alterable a second set of questions must be asked. Is the problem that the parents do not realize that they have the requisite knowledge to care for their child? If the parents have the

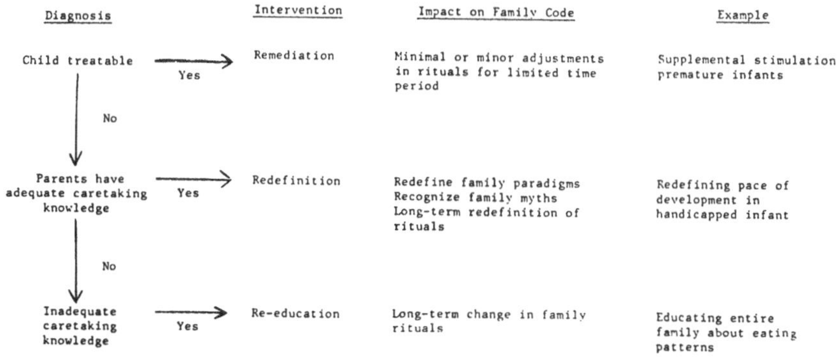

Fig. 5. Outline for clinical decision making.

requisite skills to care for a child whose condition cannot be directly altered, then a second form of intervention is indicated: redefinition. Redefinition is typically carried out in the context of the family by psychologists and other health professionals.

If special skills are needed to care for the ill child that are not in the parent's repertoire, reeducation would be the necessary intervention. Support groups of families with similar problems, educational seminars, or medical regimen training may be carried out by nurse practitioners, mental health professionals, or developmental specialists.

We have presented these forms of intervention as theoretically distinct from each other. It is possible in many cases that more than one of the approaches may be necessary. For example, as an adolescent mother is reeducated about caretaking behaviors it may be necessary at a later time to redefine her relationship with her child as she becomes a more competent parent. Even when an intervention is focused in one area, a transaction may also occur that calls for a change in intervention focus. Future research should be directed in this area.

HEALTHY FAMILIES

One of the requirements of the transactional model of intervention is to take a more dynamic approach to the family and rely less on single explanations of disease processes. From a transactional perspective neither the family nor the child is to "blame" for the child's condition. Rather, a current condition is the result of a series of transactions between the child's behavior and the family regulatory code during which parents and child tried to reach an adaptive state of interaction.

Given a systematic assessment procedure different members of the medical community can be called upon to provide services at the appropriate level for families in need. It is also helpful for families to see that parts of their family code may be functioning adequately, but specific aspects may need to be adjusted for particular conditions. By seeking strengths within the family, the burden of blame need no longer rest solely on individual family members. The area of pediatric psychology demands a complex view of families and health processes. We hope that the transactional model proposed here will aid in understanding how the family context contributes to health processes in pediatric populations.

REFERENCES

Affleck, G., McGrade, B. J., Allen, D. A., & McQueeney, M. (1985). Mothers' beliefs about behavioral causes for their developmentally disabled infant's condition: What do they signify? *Journal of Pediatric Psychology, 10,* 293-303.

Affleck, G., & Tennen, H. (1988). *Causal attributions for the birth of high risk infants: Implications for mothers' well-being, caregiving and future child bearing.* Presented at the Sixth International Conference on Infant Studies, Washington, DC.

Als, H., Lawhon, G., Brown, E., Gibes, R., Duffy, F. H., McAnulty, G., & Blickman, J. G. (1986). Individualized behavioral and environmental care for the very low birthweight preterm infant at high risk for Bronchopulmonary Dysplasia: Neonatal intensive care unit and developmental outcome. *Pediatrics, 78,* 1123-1132.

Baranowski, T., & Nader, P. R. (1985). Family involvement in health behavior change programs. In D. C. Turk & R. D. Kerns (Eds.), *Health, illness and families: A life-span perspective* (pp. 81-107). New York: Wiley.

Barkley, R. A. (1988). The effects of methylphenidate on the interactions of preschool ADHD children with their mothers. *Journal of the American Academy of Child and Adolescent Psychiatry, 27,* 336-341.

Becker, M. H., Radius, S. M., Rosenstock, I. M., Drachman, R. H., Schuberth, K. C., & Teets, K. (1978). Compliance with medical regimen for asthma: A test of the Health Belief Model. *Public Health Reports, 93,* 268-277.

Belsky, J. (1980). Child maltreatment: An ecological perspective. *American Psychologist, 35,* 430-435.

Bennett, L. A., Wolin, S. J., Reiss, D., & Teitelbaum, M. A (1987). Couples at risk for transmission of alcoholism: Protective influences. *Family Process, 26,* 111-129.

Bernbaum, J. C., Pereira, G. R., Watkins, J. B., & Peckham, G. J. (1983). Nonnutritive sucking during gavage feeding enhances growth and maturation in premature infants. *Pediatrics, 71,* 41-45.

Bossard, J., & Boll, E. (1950). *Ritual in family living.* Philadelphia: University of Pennsylvania Press.

Bronfenbrenner, U. (1977). Toward an experimental psychology of human development. *American Psychologists, 32,* 513-531.

Bronheim, S. P. (1978). Pulmonary disorders. In P. R. Magrab (Ed.), *Psychological management of pediatric problems: Vol. 1. Early life conditions and chronic diseases* (pp. 309-344). Baltimore: University Park Press.

Byng-Hall, J. (1988). Scripts and legends in families and family therapy. *Family Process, 27,* 167-179.

Carlson, R. (1981). Studies in script theory: Adult analogs of a childhood nuclear scene. *Journal of Personality and Social Psychology, 40,* 501-510.

Cella, D. F., Perry, S. W., Poag, M. E., Amand, R., & Goodwin, C. (1988). Depression and stress responses in parents of burned children. *Journal of Pediatric Psychology, 13,* 87-99.

Creer, T. L. (1979). *Asthma therapy: A behavioral health care system for respiratory disorders.* New York: Springer.

Creer, T. L. (1982). Asthma. *Journal of Consulting and Clinical Psychology, 50,* 912-921.

Creer, T. L., Harm, D. L., & Marion, R. J. (1988). Childhood asthma. In D. K. Routh (Ed.), *Handbook of pediatric psychology.* New York: Guilford.

Deaton, A. V. (1985). Adaptive noncompliance in pediatric asthma: the parent as expert. *Journal of Pediatric Psychology, 10,* 1-14.

Deaton, A. V., & Olbrisch, M. E. (1987). Adaptive noncompliance: Parents as experts and decision makers in the treatment of pediatric asthma patients. In M. Wolraich & D. K. Routh (Eds.), *Advances in developmental and behavioral pediatrics* (pp. 205-234). Greenwich, CT: JAI.

Dix, T. H., Ruble, D. N., Grusec, J. E., & Nixon, S. (1986). Social cognition in parents: Inferential and affective reactions to children of three age levels. *Child Development, 57,* 879-894.

Drotar, D., Baskiewicz, A., Irvin, N., Kennell, J., & Klaus, M. (1975). The adaptation of parents to the birth of an infant with a congenital malformation: A hypothetical model. *Pediatrics, 56,* 710-717.

Engel, G. L. (1977). The need for a new medical model: A challenge for biomedicine. *Science, 196,* 129-136.

Epstein, L. H. (1985). Family based treatment for preadolescent obesity. In M. Wolraich & D. K. Routh (Eds.), *Advances in developmental and behavioral pediatrics* (Vol. 6, pp. 1-39). Greenwich, CT: JAI.

Epstein, L. H., Wing, R. R., Koeske, R., Andrasik, F., & Ossip, D. (1981). Child and parent weight loss in family-based behavior modification programs. *Journal of Consulting and Clinical Psychology, 49,* 674-685.

Epstein, L. H., Wing, R. R., Koeske, R., & Valoski, A. (1986). Effect of parent weight on weight loss in obese children. *Journal of Consulting and Clinical Psychology, 54,* 400-401.

Ferreira, A. J. (1963). Family myth and homeostasis. *Archives General Psychiatry, 9,* 457-463.

Field, T. (1979). Interaction patterns of preterm and term infants. In T. M. Field, A. M. Sostek, & H. H. Schuman (Eds.), *Infants born at risk: Behavior and development* (pp. 333-356). New York: SP Medical and Scientific Books.

Fiese, B. H., & Mead, J. M. (1988). *Parental involvement and adolescent compliance in diabetic adolescents with recurrent diabetic ketoacidosis: A behavioral program.* Presented at Society for Behavioral Pediatrics, Washington, DC.

Goodnow, J. J. (1988). Parents' ideas, actions and feelings: Models and methods from developmental and social psychology. *Child Development, 59,* 286-320.

Graves, T., Meyers, A. W., & Clark, L. (1988). An evaluation of parental problem-solving training in the behavioral treatment of childhood obesity. *Journal of Consulting and Clinical Psychology, 56,* 246-250.

Hauser, S. T., Jacobson, A. M., Wertlieb, D., Brink, S., & Wentworth, S. (1985). The contribution of family environment to perceived competence and illness adjustment in diabetic and acutely ill adolescents. *Family Relations, 34,* 99-108.

Hauser, S. T., Jacobson, A. M., Wertlieb, D., Weiss-Perry, B., Follansbee, D., Weolfsdorf, J. I., Herskowitz, R. D., Houlihan, J., & Rajapark, D. C. (1986). Children with recently diagnosed diabetes: Interactions within their families. *Health Psychology, 5,* 273-296.

Ingersoll, G. M., Orr, D. P., Herrold, A. J., & Golden, M. P. (1986). Cognitive maturity and self-management among adolescents with insulin-dependent diabetes mellitus. *Journal of Pediatrics, 108,* 620-623.

Jacob, T., & Seilhamer, R. A. (1987). Alcoholism and family interaction. In T. Jacob (Ed.), *Family interaction and psychopathology: Theories, methods and findings* (pp. 535-580). New York: Plenum Press.

Johnson, S. B. (1988). Diabetes mellitus in childhood. In D. K. Routh (Ed.), *Handbook of pediatric psychology* (pp. 9-31). New York: Guilford.

Kaplan, J. R., Manuck, S. B., Clarkson, T. B., Lusso, F. M., Taub, D. B., & Miller, E. W. (1983). Social stress and atherosclerosis in normal mocholesterolemic monkeys. *Science, 220,* 733-735.

Kramer, J. (1985). *Family interfaces: Transgenerational patterns.* New York: Brunner/Mazel.

Krantz, D. S., Contrada, R. J., Hill, R. D., & Friedler, E. (1988). Environmental stress and biobehavioral antecedents of coronary heart disease. *Journal of Consulting and Clinical Psychology, 56,* 333-341.

LaCroix, A. Z., & Haynes, S. G. (1987). Gender differences in the stressfulness of workplace roles: A focus on health and health. In R. Barnett, G. Baruch, & L. Biener (Eds.), *Gender and stress* (pp. 96-121). New York: Free Press.

Lewis, J. M., & Beavers, W. K. (1976). *No single thread: Psychological health in family systems.* New York: Brunner/Mazel.

Maccoby, E. E., & Martin, J. A. (1983). Socialization in the context of the family: Parent-child interaction. In P. H. Mussen (Ed.), *Handbook of child psychology* (Vol. 4). E. M. Hetherington (Vol. Ed.), *Socialization, personality and social development* (pp. 1-101). New York: Wiley.

Matthew, K. A., & Haynes, S. G. (1986). Type A behavior pattern and coronary disease risk. *Journal of Epidemilogy, 123,* 923-960.

Melamed, B. G., & Bush, J. P. (1985). Family factors in children with acute illness. In D. C. Turk & R. D. Kerns (Eds.), *Health, illness, and families: A life-span perspective* (pp. 183-219). New York: Wiley.

Minde, K. M., Brown, J., & Whitelaw, A. (1981). *The effect of severe physical illness on the behavior of very small premature infants and their parents.* Presented at the meeting of the Society for Research in Child Development, Boston.

Minuchin, S., Baker, L., Rosman, B. L., Liebman, R., Milman, L., & Todd, T. C. (1975). A conceptual model of psychosomatic illness in children. *Archives of General Psychiatry, 32,* 1031-1038.

Parker, G. (1983). *Parental overprotection: A risk factor in psychosocial development.* New York: Grune & Stratton.

Patterson, G. R. (1986). Performance models for antisocial boys. *American Psychologist, 41,* 432-444.

Patterson, G. R., & Bank, B. (1989). Coercive families as determinants of antisocial behavior. M. Gunnar (Ed.), *Minnesota symposium in child development.* Englewood Cliffs, NJ: LEA.

Pearlman, D. S. (1984). Bronchial asthma: A perspective from childhood to adulthood. *American Journal Disease of Childhood, 138,* 459-466.

Pollner, M., & McDonald-Wilker, L. (1985). The social construction of unreality: A case study of a family's attribution of competence to a severely retarded child. *Family Process, 24,* 241-254.

Ragland, D. R., & Brand, R. J. (1988). Type A behavior and mortality from coronary heart disease. *New England Journal of Medicine, 318,* 65-69.

Reiss, D. (1981). *The family's construction of reality.* Cambridge, Mass.: Harvard University Press.

Reiss, D. (1989). The represented and practicing family: Contrasting visions of family continuity. In A. J. Sameroff & R. N. Emde (Eds.), *Relationship disorders in early development: A developmental approach.* New York: Basic Books.

Reiss, D., Oliveri, M. E., & Curd, K. (1981). Family paradigm and adolescent social behavior. In H. D. Grotevant & C. R. Cooper (Eds.), *Adolescent development in the family: New directions for child development* (Vol. 22, pp. 77-91). San Francisco: Jossey-Bass.

Renne, C. M., & Creer, T. L. (1976). Training children with asthma to use inhalation therapy equipment. *Journal of Applied Behavior Analysis, 9,* 1-11.

Rosenthal, J. (1970). *Genetic theory and abnormal behavior.* New York: McGraw Hill.

Roskies, E. (1972). *Abnormality and normality: The mothering of thalidomide children.* Ithaca, NY: Cornell University Press.

Routh, D. K., & Ernst, A. R. (1984). Somatization disorder in relatives of children with adolescents with functional abdominal pain. *Journal of Pediatric Psychology, 9,* 427-437.

Sameroff, A. J. (1986). Environmental context of child development. *Journal of Pediatrics, 109,* 192-200.

Sameroff, A. J. (1987a). Transactional risk factors and prevention. In J. A. Steinberg & M. M. Silverstein (Eds.). *Preventing mental disorders: A research perspective* (pp. 74-89). Rockville, MD: U.S. Department of Health and Human Services.

Sameroff, A. J. (1987b). The social context of development. In N. Eisenberg (Ed.), *Contemporary topics in developmental psychology* (pp. 273-291). New York. Wiley.

Sameroff, A. J., & Chandler, M. J. (975). Reproductive risk and the continuum of caretaking casualty. In F. D. Horowitz, M. Hetherington, S. Scarr-Salapatek, & G. Sigel (Eds.), *Review of child development research* (Vol. 4, pp. 187-244). Chicago: University of Chicago Press.

Sameroff, A. J., & Feil, L. A. (1985). Parental concepts of development. In I. Sigel (Ed.), *Parental belief systems: The psychological consequences for children* (pp. 83-106). Hillsdale, NJ: LEA.

Sameroff, A. J., & Fiese, B. H. (in press-a). Transactional regulation and early intervention. In S. J. Meisels & J. P. Shonkoff (Eds.), *Early intervention: A handbook of theory, practice and analysis.* New York: Cambridge University Press.

Sameroff, A. J., & Fiese, B. H. (in press-b). Conceptual issues in prevention. In D. Schafer, I. Philip, & N. Enzer (Eds.), *Prevention of psychiatric disorders in children and adolescents: A project of the American Academy of Child and Adolescent Psychiatry,* OSAP Prevention Monograph No. 2.

Sigel, I. E. (1985). A conceptual analysis of beliefs. In I. Sigel (Ed.), *Parental belief systems: the psychological consequences for children* (pp. 345-371). Hillsdale, NJ: LEA.

Spinetta, J. J., & Deasy-Spinetta, P. (1981). *Living with childhood cancer*. St. Louis: Mosby.

Spinetta, J. J., Swarner, J. A., & Sheposh, J. P. (1981). Effective parental coping following the death of a child from cancer. *Journal of Pediatric Psychology, 6,* 251-263.

Steinberger, L. (1986). Stability (and instability) of type A behavior from childhood to young adulthood. *Developmental Psychology, 22,* 393-402.

Stern, D. (1977). *The first relationship: Infant and mother*. Cambridge: Harvard University Press.

Turk, D. C., & Kerns, R. D. (1985). The family in health and illness. In D. C. Turk & R. D. Kerns (Eds.), *Health, illness and families: A life-span perspective* (pp. 1-22). New York: Wiley.

Wertlieb, D., Hauser, S. T., & Jacobson, A. M. (1986). Adaptation to diabetes: Behavior symptoms and family context. *Journal of Pediatric Psychology, 11,* 463-479.

Wolin, S. J., & Bennet (1984). Family rituals. *Family Process, 23,* 401-420.

Wright, L. (1988). The Type A behavior pattern and coronary artery disease: Quest for active ingredients and the elusive mechanism. *American Psychologist, 43,* 2-14.

Zeitlin, S. J., Kotkin, A. J., & Baker, H. C. (1982). *A celebration of American family folklore*. New York: Pantheon.

Author Index

C

D

G

H

T

Subject Index

A

B

C

D